Warric

MW00877802

Leading Her Son's Battle to Walk Again

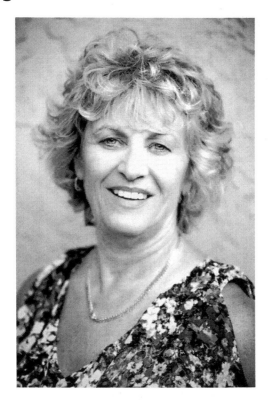

By Kay Ledson
Founder of Warrior Momz
Co-author – *Relentless: Walking Against All Odds*

Warrior Mom is the story of a mother's journey to give her son his life and independence back after he suffered a catastrophic spinal cord injury. Along the way, she had to fight to get her own life back, dealing with her grief and her own healing.

This is an epic journey of love, faith, determination, and healing.

Published by Readerplace, Inc.

Printed by CreateSpace

ISBN 978-1517437794

Cover Photo Credits

Front Cover: Alison Elizabeth Huntley – Del Mar, California
Back Cover: Nick Dale – Melbourne, Australia

Dedication

This book is dedicated to my son Josh Wood, my mother Dorothy May Ledson, aka "Dottie Dearest" (who travelled to another earth plane June 2010), my sisters Wendy Bennett, Susan Ledson and Ni Made Asri (Bali), and my furry grandkids, Montana and Thor.

My forever friends, who have travelled our journey, Marie Richardson (Perth, WA), Dominica O'Malley, (Salthill, Ireland); you have both given us so much love and unconditional support.

And to Sue, Brendan, and Grady Holland and their much loved son and Brother Bronte.

Finally, I dedicate this book to the families whose loved ones have suffered this unbelievably cruel, unrelenting, vicious spinal cord injury.

I have written this book to offer light and hope that anything is possible!

Authors note:

I never set out to write a book. I am not a professional writer. I am simply a Mum, who together with her son embarked on an incredible journey of healing after he suffered near fatal injuries from a snowboarding accident in 2000. It's a story of the setting of an impossible goal, never letting sight of it, and against all odds turning it into **I'M**possible.

It was not possible to write this book chronologically, so up front my apologies if you stop and think this is a little out of order. Also there are parts of the book where a little of the story is repeated to set a scene.

I have written my book for the families going through the stress of an injury or illness of a child or loved one. It's an honest, true account of our journey. If it helps one family, it has been worth the effort.

I make no recommendations in regard to healing therapies. All I am doing is telling my story while along the way letting you know what worked for Josh.

Table of Contents

List of Figures

Foreword

What can I say that isn't a cliché!

I have known Kay and Josh for nearly 20 years. While we live a long way apart geographically, today's technology keeps us in touch.

Kay was a social networker before the term existed. I remember being in awe of her ability to keep in touch with family, friends and colleagues alike.

She has always had support and time for anyone who needed her.

We were business colleagues first, and then friends, and now she is a sister by choice.

I remember her leaving my side in June 2000, to fly the late night flight home to Melbourne, after stopping over in Perth an extra day to check that I was okay. I was having treatment for breast cancer at the time. We joked that she was off to see what mischief Josh had got himself into this time. He was not unknown for having accidents, as his and her story attests.

The news the next day was devastating! My next clear memory was the next time I saw Kay in Melbourne, when I was well enough to travel and was visiting with Josh in the hospital. Kay and I hugged on arrival and she immediately apologized to me for not being more supportive and in contact while I finished my treatment.

Even in her darkest moments, she still thought of others before herself. Here I was feeling guilty because I hadn't been well enough to help her and Josh.

I have watched Josh's journey and have nothing but admiration for him. But he is his mother's son, so what he has achieved is not unexpected to a certain extent.

Kay is the person I would always have in my corner.

I walked the Kokoda track in Papua New Guinea in April 2013, and while the diggers were also in my mind, Josh's determination and ability to walk against all the odds was in my mind at the darkest hours, during the long days in the rain and the dark, when the very idea seemed ludicrous.

Having been at his wedding in the February and watching him WALK down the aisle was inspirational in a way you can't imagine.

I have faced business and personal challenges over the years but they all pale into insignificance when this story is read or spoken. I have had the privilege of hearing them both speak and it's gut wrenching and emotional, and every word is the truth.

Warrior Mom is a story of how a mother's love really does overcome amazing obstacles.

If you want to see a miracle, just tell Kay Ledson that it can't be done!!!

Resilience, attitude, and belief are words that Kay and Josh have brought to life for me and now for many others. In happy times and sad ones, she is a friend for life.

-    *Marie Richardson, Perth, Western Australia*

Kay "zoomed" into my life over a quarter century ago, I was a young Irish girl living and working in Australia. She joined the financial services organization I was working with, and from the outset was a "breath of fresh air". It didn't take long for me to work out that Kay was a "decent skin"- an expression we use in Ireland for someone we respect.

Her enthusiasm and work ethic was admirable.

With Kay there is no hidden agenda. For me, that's a measure of someone I can trust. Professionally we were successful together and personally we had some really fun times. Recalling them now still brings a smile to my face! We knew we could depend on each other, and maintaining integrity in our dealings with clients was a shared goal.

When I returned to Ireland, our friendship continued with regular contact and visits to each other.

I was a mother of two very young boys when Josh had his accident and so could understand Kay's despair and her determination to ensure Josh got the best care and treatment, and her willingness to do whatever was necessary to help him.

It changed her whole world and how she lived, worked and breathed. She has been an exemplary example of what "unconditional love" really

8

means.

Kay is one determined lady, driven and giving. She has run with whatever life has thrown her way, without complaint and always with positivity and enthusiasm.

We could all do with her positivity!

- *Dominica O'Malley, Salthill, Ireland*

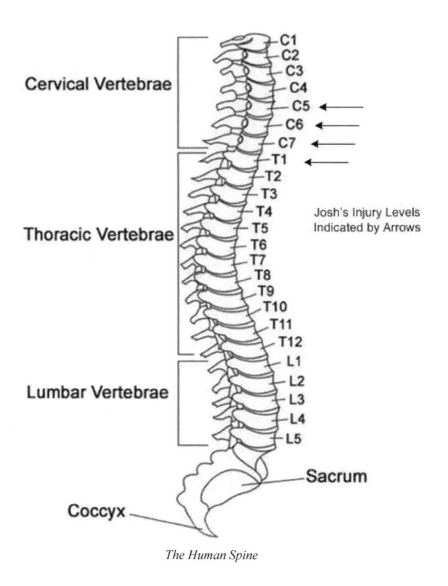

Cervical Vertebrae

Thoracic Vertebrae

Lumbar Vertebrae

Coccyx

C1
C2
C3
C4
C5 ←
C6 ←
C7 ←
T1 ←
T2
T3
T4
T5
T6
T7
T8
T9
T10
T11
T12
L1
L2
L3
L4
L5

Josh's Injury Levels
Indicated by Arrows

Sacrum

The Human Spine

PART 1 - The Darkness - Where NO Hope Is Given

Chapter 1. Setting the Scene
Ignorance is Bliss; We Never Thought It Would Happen to Us!

How often have we heard people say "Your life can change in a heartbeat" or "I never thought this would happen to me"?

In today's busy lifestyles, we rarely incorporate these thoughts into our daily lives in a positive way, taking the time to reflect upon our successes, and to enjoy and embrace our current life! Sadly, the "lifestyle" we create for ourselves forces us to focus on what we've done wrong, our failures, and missed opportunities. So often, we focus on what we need, buying something bigger and better. We rarely celebrate the precious things in our lives, our creations, what we have achieved - where our life is now!

Sadly, it often takes a "life changing event" to force us to really understand what is important in our lives, and to learn to differentiate what is simply the "clutter" and "stuff".

After reading my story, I hope you will take time each day to celebrate your lives, enjoy the moment, and learn the importance of celebrating the now!

As a parent there are probably three catastrophic events that can happen to your children:

- Death

- A life threatening illness, disease, sudden catastrophic accident

- Brain damage either through illness, act of violence or accident

Warrior Mom is my story of how a tragic event that occurred in my life when my only child, Josh (at 18 1/2 years), was involved in a near fatal accident leaving him living with the "life sentence" of "complete" quadriplegia.

My life and my son's life changed in a heartbeat. Our lives would never be the same again!

This is not a sad story. In fact it is one of empowerment, never giving up, and trying anything that made sense in pursuit of Josh's recovery goals. It is the story of my love for my son and the unrelenting trust we had in each other.

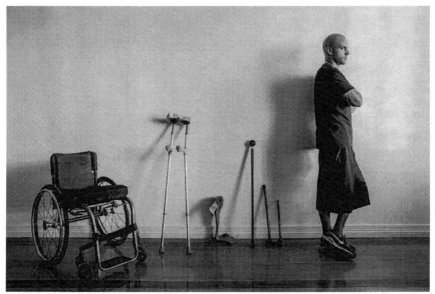

Josh: His Journey

With the recent release of my son's book: *Relentless: Walking against all Odds*, I decided it was time to share my story from the perspective of the parent, in the hope that I can offer support and help to others dealing and living with this cruel, sad injury. At all times, I have tried to be honest. I know some of you reading my story will find it confronting and upsetting, but I make no apologies!

Warrior Mom is the story of a mum and her son, who were catapulted into a crazy world that no one, and that no other life experience could prepare you for. A world of fear, hopelessness, frustration, and lack of understanding. A world that was beyond scary; the world of catastrophic spinal cord injury!

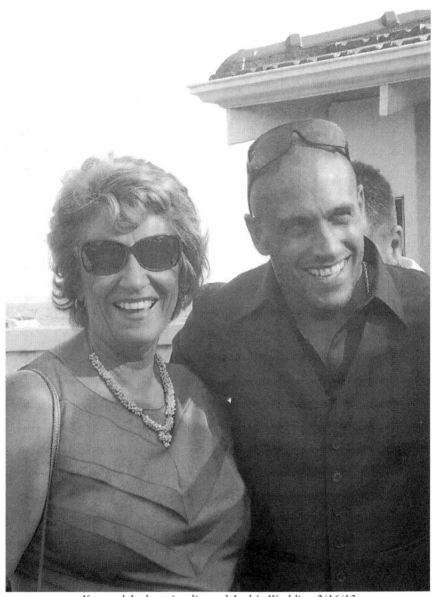

Kay and Josh at Amelia and Josh's Wedding 2/16/13

Sadly his medical team, who should have offered hope and encouragement, was totally the opposite, offering no hope, no encouragement, all the while preaching acceptance, while trying their best to save his life!

In an instant our lives changed, and although they were never the same, the experience brought us both so close, the trust we had in each other and the commitment we had to recovery, could really never be adequately explained, unless you were to endure a similar traumatic event.

From the moment Josh was airlifted by helicopter from the snowfields 200 kilometers north east of Melbourne, until he arrived at the Spinal Unit, we very quickly learned that the only thing his medical team was interested in was preparing Josh and all of us for his new life as a complete quadriplegic, "to never to get out of bed again" with less than 3% chance of any recovery.

His medical team didn't care that Josh was an athlete, that he'd worked through several serious injuries in the past, or that his mind was tougher than steel. Frankly, all they cared about was, "brainwashing" Josh and all who were close to him, into the acceptance of his "new" life.

We were all faced with a new destiny!

Oh my God, how we wished we could turn back time!

At 3.29 PM, on the 25th of June 2000, my son Josh, his father Garry, our family and close friends, and my life changed forever when Josh suffered near fatal injuries in a snow board jumping accident in the snow fields of the Australian Alps.

Josh attempted an aerial jump over a public asphalt road in the ski resort.

Josh was an experienced snowboarder, honing his jumping skills while on a student exchange in Switzerland.

As he mounted the jump he realized immediately that his approach was too fast. Instead of soaring off the jump, he hit it too fast, ending up flipping himself upside down. In those millionths of seconds, he tried to right himself in mid- flight. Landing on his back had to be avoided, so no matter what he had to land on his legs! He knew he would hit the road. He thought if all else fails he would manage a "commando" style roll, hopefully protecting his head.

As the asphalt neared, he relaxed his body to cushion the impact. He hit the road landing on the base of his neck, instantly breaking it, crushing his spinal cord. Luck was on his side; he remained conscious!

Here are Josh's words:

I approached the jump, everything was going well, and my speed was right. As I reached the bottom of the ramp something moved on my left line of vision on the road which momentarily distracted me. It was a split second, and I hit some soft snow that threw me off balance, causing me to be upside down in the air.

"I remember hitting the road. At that moment I realized I had broken my neck. I apparently bounced onto the snow but I do not remember this. I must have momentarily lost consciousness, but only for a few seconds. I remember Daniel and all my friends running up to me. I told them not to move me, because I knew my neck was broken.

"As I lay there, one of my friends ran to ski patrol, which was only about 30 seconds away. I understand Daniel called the ambulance straight after the accident. My neck began to convulse. I told Luke to lightly hold my helmet to stop my head moving around. At no time was I moved by any of my friends. They kept talking to me until ski patrol arrived, which would have been only a few minutes."

Chapter 2. "In the Beginning there was Life"

(February 1981)

I had been married for to Garry for 12 years, and for nearly eight of those years we had tried to have a child. We had been through every conceivable test. Our doctors could find nothing wrong, and there appeared to be no medical explanation.

IVF was relatively new, but we had been advised by our doctors that neither Garry nor I were committed enough to having children, so we were therefore "not good candidates" for it.

Obviously trying to fall pregnant for eight years wasn't commitment enough in our doctor's eyes. I had no idea what prompted them to make such decision on our behalf, and I guess it was simply doctors knowing best!

With what appeared to be our last chance gone, we decided to get on with our lives. I arranged to have my tubes tied after my 31st birthday in March 1981. Finally we had made the decision. We were both very sad, yet relieved!

We really needed a holiday; we made plans to go to Bali for three weeks, to celebrate my birthday.

Garry and I were runners. We had run with Royal Peninsula Hash House Harriers (RPHHH) for several years. Through the RPHHH Garry had run in and finished several Melbourne Marathons. With my pregnancy plans over, I decided 1981 would be my year. I committed to run the Melbourne Marathon in October. I was training hard, running and swimming laps several days a week.

As part of our training regime, and to allow me to build up my road miles, Garry and I decided to run a half marathon in mid-February.

It was on a Sunday, starting midday, which in hindsight was very late to start a half marathon, on a Melbourne summer day.

In those days, Garry and I were into partying. Never needing an excuse, with the run starting late the next day, we decided to throw a party. We partied late into the night, waking late morning, and going straight to the start of the run.

The entire run was on asphalt roads, through the back of Frankston, through farm land, down to Hastings. There was no respite from the heat. It was so hot!

The heat was unrelenting, scorching, burning hot, and the conditions were so tough that many of the elite runners pulled out, but I was determined to finish.

Garry was a much faster runner, so once he finished, he ran back to keep me motivated - keeping me moving through to the finish line.

Through pure grit and determination I finished; I was stoked, as several of our tougher, more seasoned runners had retired due to the appalling conditions.

A week later we left for Bali, looking forward to our much needed holiday.

In those days Bali was very much an undeveloped island paradise. There were only five or six hotels on the island; we stayed in a hotel in Kuta. Our plan for the next three weeks was simply to party, swim and sunbake.

A week into our three week trip I drank out of a dirty glass and within a few hours I was so ill! For several days I lived between our bed and the bathroom, hardly eating, barely drinking. I was in a bad way!

Bali was a relatively remote tourist destination with few doctors, and the local hospital was very basic. Fortunately, Garry met an Australian nurse, and he told her what my symptoms were. She gave him some pills to help settle me down.

Once on the medication, after a few days, I felt well enough to hit the beach.

I had lost so much weight!

The weather was fabulous. We thought we'd spend the rest of our time working on our suntans, body surfing in the "dumping surf", swimming, and enjoying daily massages.

But something wasn't right with me, my body ached all over, I felt nauseous. I felt really out of kilter.

On returning home I had lost 20 pounds, weighing only 112.

My doctor asked me if I could be pregnant. I said "no way"! And if I was, it would be a huge problem, as I quickly worked back to when I would have conceived my baby, and it was the night before I ran in the half marathon.

My pregnancy was confirmed the next day, and while we were both over the moon, quietly I was terrified because I had been taking the medication in Bali, I'd lost so much weight, and I had run the half marathon. This was hardly the best way to ensure the health of my baby.

I couldn't believe the irony of falling pregnant after all this time, with those first five weeks of my pregnancy being a total disaster, health wise, for my unborn baby. I made a decision that from that moment my pregnancy would be about me keeping fit, eating healthy food, no alcohol, and plenty of sleep. I had to make it up to my baby.

My Bali illness behind me, the rest of my pregnancy was uneventful, but I couldn't shake the nagging feeling from the events of my first five weeks; what if I had hurt my baby? Other than our families, we decided not to tell anyone about my pregnancy, until I was at least five months. In those first few months I only gained a little weight, so it was easy to hide my small "bump"!

I kept running with the hash, to maintain my fitness, until one night I got tangled in a barb wire fence, falling heavily, and that was the end of my running! Swimming seemed to be my safest option, and my only exercise in the end was doing laps in our local pool two or three days a week, which I managed keep up to the time I was hospitalized.

I progressed through to 36 weeks. I was healthy, I looked and felt terrific, I hadn't gained any excess weight, but unexpectedly the last weeks of my pregnancy saw me experience a series of health problems.

I was hospitalized three weeks before my due date for total bed rest. The doctors were concerned that my baby wasn't gaining weight, even with all the bed rest, so they made a decision to induce me.

Josh was born on Friday 13th November 1981, at around 2:30 - 3 pm. It was a very traumatic and stressful. No fun at all, forceps, birth! Josh was born into a state of drama and haste; he was two weeks early.

The placenta had died, but Josh had hung in there long enough to survive the birth. He was a long, skinny, very sick baby.

What was amazing, though, was that he had very dark piercing eyes. You knew he was an "old soul"! All the nurses said "this kid's been here before".

I had that instant connection with him. I truly believed he was indeed an "old soul", cleverly disguised in this tiny, sick baby's body.

The matron of the maternity wing commented to me, after seeing Josh for the first time, that she had a strong feeling that this was a special child. She told me she believed that Josh, (J. J. Wood she actually called him) would change people's lives in the future; he would grow to be a great man!

With all Josh's immediate health dramas, her predictions went totally out of my mind until many years later!

From the moment he was born, Josh had a fight on his hands, spending two weeks in the Special Care Nursery. He was so weak, he couldn't feed; the only way to nourish him was through a feeding tube fed directly down his throat.

For me, the Special Care Nursery was like a "Mum's boot camp", with a dedicated nursing staff available to assist me with every issue or problem. It was what I needed. It gave me time to gain confidence as a mother, something I was desperately lacking.

I was the one who always gave the children back to their parents when something went wrong. So now it was up to me; I felt totally hopeless!

I used to joke that I never played with dolls or anything girly, and yet here I was responsible for this tiny fragile life.

Finally we were released from Special Care, and with great excitement we took our son home.

I was convinced I was the most hopeless mother ever. I truly had no idea what to do, and how to look after this tiny child.

In spite of my hopelessness, Josh thrived. He was a smiling, active and happy baby. He never slept through the night for his first two years.

Although Josh appeared to be a happy, thriving baby, he was far from healthy. He suffered from continual ear infections, asthma, bronchitis, and eczema.

His first year was a succession of doctors and specialist visits.

Before he was a year old, he was on asthma medication, never ending antibiotics and antihistamines. I felt totally frustrated, freaked out by all the medication this tiny child was taking. Personally I hated taking any type of medicine, so from those early days I was constantly looking for alternative treatments for him.

When awake, Josh was always on the move. He loved music, his favorite pastime was laying in his bouncinette, looking out the windows of our family room, taking in the goings on outside.

As he grew older his "jumpy jack swing" mounted between doors was another favorite, his little legs constantly moving and bouncing. When he was awake he was never still!

Chapter 3. We Served a Very Unique Apprenticeship

For Josh's 1st birthday, my parents' present to him was a "mini" two wheeler BMX bike, with training wheels. Within a few hours, Josh was riding through the house, minus the training wheels. He could ride his bike before he could walk.

One night, I returned home from work to find Josh sitting in his building block's trailer. Next thing I watched in horror as he took off, literally flying down the pavement, using his feet as brakes, stopping just short of the road.

I wasn't happy, with either Josh or his dad, but my protests fell on deaf ears. Josh wasn't even two years old. I just shook my head. What hope did I have?

In everything he did, he loved speed, to go flat out, he was our tiny "stunt man", and his father did nothing to discourage him!

Being with his dad was what he loved best - we called him the "little man".

Garry had a 650 cc motor bike and Josh was often riding pillion, decked out with all his protective gear, well before he was three. The need for speed, even at this young age, was to become a major part of Josh's future.

Josh had his first serious accident when he was three years old. Helping dad cut down a tree, he was "safely" holding a rope which was attached to a safe part of the tree, when the branch lurched unexpectedly. Josh was airborne, landing heavily on his back. We rushed him to Emergency, where the doctor found his lower back was heavily bruised, but fortunately he was not badly injured.

This was to set up a pattern of injuries, which our mini action man would incur in his passion for speed and adventure.

Garry and I had been snow skiing for several years, and we were social members of a lodge on Mt Buller. We were anxious to return to the snow after we had Josh, and we wanted to introduce him to a sport we both loved.

It took us nearly two years before we had our first trip to Buller with Josh. Travelling to the snowfields with two couples and their children was the first snow experience for all the kids, so we weren't expecting too much skiing ourselves.

This trip with Josh set up his love of the snow. While other children cried or were cold, Josh reveled in the conditions. In fact he was out from morning to dusk. He started skiing, using a set of mini skis, given to him when he was born. He loved skiing! Initially we put him in the kids program, but it wasn't long before he was skiing with us. In fact he pushed us to go faster.

When Josh was seven, we decided on a "tree change". We bought farming land in the hills above Mansfield (Victoria), about 200 kilometers north east of Melbourne. We enjoyed the best of both worlds; snow in the winter and water sports on the various waterways nearby in the summer.

The move was a lifestyle decision. We planned to build a home, set it up as a "hobby farm", running some livestock, but enjoying a quality of life we didn't have in the city. The property was just over 100 acres. It comprised of some flat cleared paddocks, dropping down into treed valley.

I planned to re-establish my financial planning business in Mansfield, allowing me to work from home, in the office we had purposefully built off the garage, keeping it separate from our house.

As owner-builders it took us nearly two years to finally finish our home.

Our home sprawled across an escarpment, providing us with tremendous views of the snow covered mountains (in the winter), timbered valleys, and skyline.

We were very lucky. Being above the snow and fog line, we had the most beautiful existence, with every room in our sprawling home having the most stunning views of the surrounding countryside.

It was there Josh honed his motor bike skills. While his father and I built the house, Josh raced around on a purpose-built motor bike track we had constructed for him. There were always plenty of friends visiting with their children. It was truly a kid's paradise! They would be on the bikes for hours, sometimes switching to our four-wheeler for a change. The only rule was everyone had to ride the track, in the same direction. Even then there were accidents, banged heads, broken toes -- you get the picture.

Living in such wild open country, Josh developed into a competent horse rider; it was a joy to see him galloping across a paddock, horse and boy as one.

Over the years he owned two beautiful horses. The first was a Welsh pony "Snippet". Josh really learned to ride on him. Snippet was extremely well trained in eventing. All Josh had to do was hold on to the reins and balance, and the pony did the rest. Always highly competitive, Josh won many riding events, and with each competition he became more and more confident.

Turning 12, Josh needed a larger horse. Fortunately we found him a magnificent 16 hand chestnut named "Blue".

Boy and horse hit it off instantly. Blue had a beautiful nature. He was extremely well trained, quickly becoming devoted to Josh.

You would often find Blue lying in the house paddock, with Josh resting his head on his horse's huge body lying between his legs. Blue would follow Josh around like a dog, and more than once tried to come into the house with him.

Blue proved to be an excellent horse for Josh to further hone his riding skills; I loved seeing them galloping across the paddocks at break neck speeds. They had a fantastic trust of each other. As you can imagine, there were many bruises and falls around this passion, too.

Living on the farm, Josh was driving around the paddocks in an old car from age nine, quickly learning to back the car up to load the horse float. The tractor proved no challenge to Josh either; he used to have to sit on a cushion to drive it, and once he mastered it, the farm was really "Josh's slice of heaven."

The farm was sold after our marriage broke up, I thought about buying my ex out, as it broke Josh's heart when we sold it. Even though I loved the house and the property I was a city girl at heart, and extremely nervous about bush fires.

Our property was quite isolated, sitting atop an escarpment, above a treed valley, with one road in and out. On my own with Josh, they weren't odds I wanted to test, in case of a roaring firestorm occurring.

All these years later, Josh still misses "his little slice of heaven" and from time to time he makes a pilgrimage up to the property we called "Rocky Hollow".

Our property's proximity to the snow allowed Josh to develop his skiing skills; through his school, he was involved in snow program, which saw the students go to the snow weekdays as well as weekends.

By the age of 12, he discovered snowboarding, there was no stopping him, the skis and gear were discarded forever, quickly being replaced with snowboard gear and boards.

Snowboarding was just being introduced to Australia, so Josh and his mates became very early adopters of the sport. I loved my skiing, allowing me to be more involved in the snow side of Josh's life than his father, so for the first time since he was born we enjoyed a shared passion.

It wasn't long before Josh, his friends, Daniel, Chrisso, and other local boys were daring gravity, literally throwing themselves into snowboarding, the faster the higher the better.

Josh joined Team Buller. He was a competitive event snowboarder, who enjoyed competing at Mt. Buller, Falls Creek, Thredbo, and later Switzerland. Josh's favorite event was "board a cross", a fast, dangerous snowboard event incorporating break neck speed, obstacles, and random jumps - injuries were more common that not!

After our marriage break up, once Josh came to live with Wendy and me in Port Melbourne, he continued his snowboarding, representing Hobson's Bay High School (now Albert Park College) in the inter schools winter sports competition. Most weekends in the winter, he would travel on his own by bus up to the mountain, either staying with friends at the resort or in the township of Mansfield. I never really worried about him, as we knew so many people on the mountain. If he got into trouble I would have quickly heard about it.

When Josh was 15 ½ years old, he applied for and was accepted in a student exchange program which saw him travel to Switzerland, for four months.

Josh travelled from Melbourne, to Zurich (30 hours) managing transit stops in Singapore and Frankfurt on his own; he was truly able to travel independently at a young age.

He stayed with the Ernst and Regula Morger and their three sons, in a typical Swiss chalet, situated in a small picturesque village, Schänis, about 45 minutes, south east of Zurich. Josh truly felt he had found heaven.

The first week he arrived, Josh broke his elbow, messing around on a mountain bike. I was not happy with him! As always Josh was testing his body to the extreme!

For the four months he was in Switzerland, Josh was literally out of control, snowboarding, partying, and enjoying the good life.

I remember getting an email from Ernst. It went – "Josh is a good boy, he tells us where he is going, tells us what time he will be home, tells us who he is with, and we are very happy with him." From Wendy's and my perspective, he was out of control, doing whatever he liked.

I contacted the Exchange Organizers, voicing my concerns. They assured me not to worry. His Swiss family loved him, and importantly, they were enjoying their time with him.

Before Josh left Australia, I was advised to allow $250 per month for his expenses. Most months, though, he was racking up charges of over $1500 on the credit card I had given him. But he was having a fantastic time, enjoying the Swiss experience, so I just paid the bill every month.

Above all we knew he was okay, enjoying a wonderful experience with a fabulous loving family. It was during this time that Josh's passion for snowboarding, travel, and adventure was truly consolidated.

As part of the exchange, Josh was expected to attend the small village school every day. What usually happened was totally to the contrary – yes, Josh attended school as required. He would walk in the front door, say good morning to his teachers, and then head out the rear door, grabbing his snowboard gear, jumping on the fast train heading to the nearest snow fields at Flums.

Josh loved all things Swiss, especially the lifestyle it offered him, his host parents and their three sons.

The Morgers, for their part, were loving "parents" supporting Josh's passion for everything snow. Regula loved cooking and preparing Josh's favorite dishes, pizza, and chocolate mousse. For the first time in his life he was very spoiled.

Regula did everything for him; he wasn't expected to help around the house at all. Josh truly became their much loved 4th son.

While snowboarding at Flums, Josh became friends with a group of "purist" snow boarders. They were the best Josh had ever boarded with. Their passion was performing drifting aerial jumps on fresh powder snow, "off piste" away from the groomed runs.

Josh and the boys often hiked cross country to get to these areas. The conditions were always excellent. The snow you could only find in the stunning Swiss Alps.

Most of the time Josh was with them he was involved with building jumps; he was boarding and completing jumps at a level he had never experienced before.

While in Switzerland, Josh landed awkwardly on a rock while snowboarding, damaging his L5, and causing his first brush with a really serious back injury.

Initially, not being able to feel his legs, he dragged himself to an area where he could be treated. Very quickly, feeling began to return, so to save complications with language and reporting the injury, he decided to return to snowboarding and thought no more about it until he returned to Australia.

Returning to Australia, at the completion of his exchange program, Josh suffered chronic lower back problems. We turned to our trusted chiropractor Simon.

Josh's x rays showed a fracture to Josh's L5 - Simon commenced a two year treatment plan to repair Josh's damaged lower back.

Simon and Josh were relentless in his recovery regime. Visiting Simon twice a week for adjustments for nearly two years, and combining this with a structured gym program, Josh's back slowly improved.

In 1998, Josh and I travelled to Switzerland, enjoying a fantastic holiday with the Morgers. It was there, I realized that I had lost my son to this beautiful country, it was likely he would choose a life in the northern hemisphere, once he finished high school, pursuing his passion for a career in the snow.

After two years of grueling therapy, Josh walked out of Simon's practice, on the 23rd of June 2000, Simon's words echoing after him: "Josh, you have the back of an 18 year old. Well done -- your two years of hard work have paid off. Go for it."

Chapter 4. Josh's Rebirth: Celebrating a Second Birth Date

Saturday, the 24th June 2000, was a stormy day on the mountain. Snow, sleet, freezing cold -- the perfect day for Josh to spend at one of the resort's hotels, relaxing in the spa and pool with his friends.

It was my sister Wendy's birthday. Josh called her from the hotel, happy, loving life, wishing her a happy day. He excitedly told her that he thought he had a job, would have it confirmed Sunday night, and he was also hopeful he had somewhere to live on the mountain. He would also have an answer for that on Sunday night. (One of my rules for Josh was that if he was going to work on the mountain, he had to live on it. I didn't want him driving down the mountain road at night.)

After a month of Josh partying flat out, it was all coming together for him.

He called me that same day, asking me to lend him $4,000, the amount he needed to pay his share of the rent in advance. I was so relieved he had found somewhere to live on the mountain because the road down to Mansfield (the nearest town he could have lived in) was dangerous, especially at night. I was happy to lend him the money, knowing he would be safe and not needing to drive his car unless he was coming home for a few days.

Josh was in great form pursuing his dreams, creating his life. I was so excited for him!

Sunday, the 25th of June 2000

Josh

"As I had been living on the mountain for three weeks, snowboarding most days, so for a change I decided to build a jump. I asked some of my friends to help me.

"I decided to check out the old Village Run. I was familiar with this area of the mountain, as I had used this run for several years prior to it being changed when the road was asphalted.

"The combination of the long slope down, jumping over the road onto the lower slope over the road would provide a safe jump.

"I spent some time checking out the landing on the lower slope to make sure the snow was safe enough to land on. I then found the right place to build the ramp, which would give me the height and distance I needed to successfully make the jump. The ramp was located approximately 16 feet from road edge on the high side. Using this area of the slope, which was steeper, gave me a faster and smoother run down to the jump giving me more speed once off the ramp which would enable me to clear the road safely. I started building the ramp around lunchtime.

"To build the jump we smoothed out the run up and began to dig up snow from the area surrounding the run. We piled it to create the ramp height I needed (about five feet).

"Several friends came to help, and when they wanted to go for a run they left. There was always 3-4 of us working on the jump ramp and the run-up at any one time.

"As each section was completed I practiced the run down to the ramp several times. Every time we made an adjustment I tested it with a couple more runs down to the ramp.

"At approximately 3:00 PM the jump was verbally signed off.

"I completed several more checks of the run-down, the ramp, and the landing. I made several more practice runs down to the ramp to be sure. As an extra precaution, I arranged for the run-down to be salted. I also put speed wax on my snow board to ensure I had enough speed once on the ramp to gain the height and length I needed to make the jump safely.

"To gather greater speed, two of my friends assisted me to build up my initial speed with a sling slot action from the top of slope. We practiced this action over and over again. I then put on my body armor and helmet to get ready for the jump.

"We arranged for a couple of friends to watch the road to stop any traffic that was coming in front of the jumping area. I spent time reviewing the line I needed to take and the angle I would approach the jump. I then went to the top of the slope with Luke & Rooksie."

It was just after 3.30 PM. I was on the phone in my home office, chatting to a friend in the USA. The home phone rang, and given that it was only Josh's friends who rang the number I nearly didn't answer it - but, something said "get it."

I picked up the phone to hear Daniel's panicked voice on the other end, crying the words "Josh has had a terrible accident."

Daniel was one of Josh's closest friends.

He was sobbing, screaming, "Josh was really badly injured from a jump that had gone wrong."

For some reason I will never know, I didn't panic. I was extremely calm. I simply asked Daniel, "Was Josh conscious?" He answered "yes", and I asked "did Josh know where he was?" Daniel sobbed "yes". I answered Daniel "great, we have something to work with". I have no idea why I said it - certainly at that stage I had no idea the extent of Josh's injuries!

Having total confidence in Josh's ability to recover from all manner of injuries, I knew in my heart that he had no brain damage. He was conscious, and for now that was enough.

Geoff, Daniel's father, came onto the phone. He told me that Josh was "quite seriously injured, the medical team wasn't sure what they were going to do with him!"

I asked "should I come up?"

He said they were deciding what to do with Josh. There was a chance they could fly him to Melbourne.

Flying him back to Melbourne, in my mind, was the best option. I felt relieved, as I really didn't want to drive to Mansfield Hospital that night.

Much later Josh was to describe to me how he felt his body shutting down while he laid on the road. He said "everything was shutting down." He was about to say to Daniel "Look after Kze at the Ranch" (our property house name) but something stopped him.

At that moment, he was obviously given a decision to make: To live or die? Josh fought to stay alive. He made a decision to live!

If he had said that to Daniel, I know in my heart that Josh would have died!

It was many hours later I found out how close he was to not making it.

In the coming weeks, I would use that moment, the moment he decided to live, several times to remind Josh not to give up. When he had the chance to end his earth life, yet against all odds he had chosen to live.

Later I was told that Josh nearly died three times in those few hours after the accident, on the mountain, and within the medical center.

The fact the medical team where deciding what to do made me think Josh wasn't really badly injured. Maybe they were considering transferring him to Mansfield Hospital located at the base of the mountain.

In my mind, even though Daniel had been so upset, I felt quite calm. I was confident Josh would be okay.

I made a series of phone calls. I spoke to Josh's father, going over what I'd been told so far, I said as soon as I knew, I'd let him know which hospital he was being transferred to. I added, if Josh was transferred to Mansfield Hospital, he would have to drive me up there, as I was really tired, having flown home from Perth that morning on the "Redeye".

Wendy had been staying at our mother's in Frankston for the weekend. She was driving back to our home when I spoke to her.

Wendy

Wendy is my youngest sister, having no children of her own other than her precious furry kids, so Wendy was very close to Josh. Wendy had lived with Josh and me for several years in Port Melbourne.

I had recently sold my period home; Wendy and I were planning a property development in Port Melbourne with some friends. In the meantime we were renting a large home, and running a business from there together. Wendy was Josh's 2nd mum, as I travelled a lot with my work. When I was away Wendy was always there for Josh. We were a team; between us we managed to give a rounded family life to Josh, along with Wendy's miniature schnauzer - Madison.

Paula, (not her real name) was an extremely talented physic healer. Paula and I had been close friends for several years. People came from all over the world to see her. Paula had known Josh for several years, and it is fair to say they tolerated each other. They certainly weren't close.

34

I called her to let her know about Josh. I simply said, "Josh has had an accident on the mountain. I am hoping they will fly him home." She said, "I'll come straight around."

Living only a few minutes away, it didn't take Paula long to reach our home. She joined me in the kitchen. I asked her, "What can you see?" She answered, "I can't see anything." I said, "Is he still alive?" Paula replied, "I can't see anything." I remember saying to her "Don't you do this to me!"

Paula could always "see" when she wanted to. At that moment she wanted to but there was nothing. Again, I asked her, "Will Josh be all right?"

I could tell she was agitated; her mind was a blank. Paula went quiet as though she was in deep concentration, eventually saying "All the injuries Josh and I had dealt with over the years, all the alternative healing methods we had utilized instead of going the traditional medical route, had set us up for dealing with his accident - his injury." She said, "It was like we had served an apprenticeship."

Paula went on to say, "Whatever he has done was not in his destiny, this accident was not meant to happen and now his destiny would be changed forever." She still could not "see" anything in relation to Josh's immediate situation.

It's interesting that now in 2016, I don't believe Josh did change his destiny. I actually believe the accident *was* his destiny, giving him the ability to change people lives positively.

Earlier in 2000, Paula had done a physic reading for Josh. She had predicted that his close friend Daniel would have a serious accident while snowboarding, possibly dying. Josh and Daniel were together in her vision. I remember when Josh first left home to relocate to the mountain for the winter, when he told me he would watch over Daniel, making sure he would keep him safe!

I have learned over the years that often psychics are protected from seeing things when someone close to them is involved. Later when Paula and I had time to sit and speak about that crazy afternoon and evening, we came to the conclusion she had seen Josh, but she was "protected" from seeing him hurt. Daniel was with Josh when he had the accident. So it was a bit freaky!

In the past, when Josh had been injured, I always thought the worst, but for some reason this time I knew in my heart that Josh would be fine! I felt numb, but calm. Again, I had no idea what had happened, but having so much faith in Josh I felt that since he was conscious he would be okay.

Paula

Paula was a psychic healer. Her gift was precious and unique.

I had known her for several years, meeting her through a friend who encouraged me to have a reading with her.

Paula worked through spirit guides, birthdates, and numbers, using several packs of cards to confirm what she was "seeing" or the messages she was getting. She also used a collection of crystals throughout her readings or healings depending on what she was trying to achieve, or to gain a greater understanding of an issue.

My first reading with her was in the early 90's, and at the time I was married "not happily." I was struggling with my marriage that was in my view terminally damaged. We had simply grown in different directions. Really we had nothing in common other than Josh.

I felt scared. My greatest fear was that if I left Garry I would lose Josh. This first reading with Paula was very accurate. I was impressed, as she had never met me before, knew nothing about me at all, and yet she seemed to know everything.

From the first time we met we developed a friendship that would last several years.

Josh and Paula didn't really "get on" with each other. Often when she was at our home, she would casually mention in a conversation to be careful about something, or how long his current girlfriend would be around for; she always said, he would be a very successful actor.

Josh put up with her because she was my friend, but more often than not he would dismiss her and her thoughts!

It was fair to say they tolerated each other because they both loved me!

Little did we realize in those crazy early hours the crucial part Paula would play in Josh's recovery, how she would be the conduit in providing information to Simon, the other healers, and therapists, we brought into the hospital to work on Josh. She could "totally" tap into what was happening internally to Josh, especially in the first 12 months.

As the weeks progressed, it was Paula who was constantly seeking other alternative health practitioners to work with Josh. They always presented at the "right" time just when we were seeking more for Josh!

It was about 4:00 PM when I first tried calling the mountain's medical center. At that stage I don't think Josh had even been transferred to the facility, because the medics were still trying to stabilize him on the road.

Whoever I spoke to advised me, "They were not sure what they were doing with him yet." I was later to find out they were not confident he would survive any transfer, whether it was by air or road.

The medical team's reluctance to make a decision with what they were doing with Josh as far as the hospital transfer was concerned, only made me think Josh was not too badly injured.

I advised them that Josh had ambulance insurance, so if it was possible I would appreciate Josh being transferred by helicopter to Melbourne. The medical team must have thought I was crazy, but as I said, I had no idea really what was going on with Josh!

I rang the medical center every 15 minutes. Finally at around 5:45 PM I was informed that Josh was to be flown by helicopter to a Melbourne Hospital. I momentarily thought "That's the spinal injury hospital." Then I thought, "Oh well, he has probably hurt his back!" Truthfully at that moment, I was relieved that he was being transferred to Melbourne.

Josh had suffered so many accidents in his 18 1/2 years that I knew he had an amazing capacity for recovery, so I honestly always believed he would be fine.

By this stage Wendy was home. I rang Garry and we arranged to meet at the hospital. Neither Wendy nor I had any idea how to get to the hospital, which was located 20 minutes north-east of the City of Melbourne.

It was a typical busy winter's Sunday evening, taking us nearly 40 minutes to finally reach the hospital, having to weave our way through the busy city traffic and football crowds; using the reliable Melways (road maps); we didn't have GPS in those days. Thank goodness Wendy was an excellent navigator!

Chapter 5. Ground Zero! Hey! What the Hell Just Happened?

As we pulled up at the hospital, we heard the helicopter flying overhead, slowly coming in to land. It had flown directly over us and was landing on a helipad, near the hospital.

We made our way to the emergency room reception; on advising the nurse who we were, she immediately ushered us into a private room inside the emergency area, away from the Admissions foyer.

They say innocence is bliss? All I could think was how glad I was not to have to wait outside in the public waiting area. (I still hadn't figured out that Josh was critically injured.)

Garry and his partner Chris arrived about the same time as we did.

A male nurse entered the waiting room and explained to us that on Josh's arrival he would be taken into the ER. He would be checked by several specialists who had been called in. As soon as he was stabilized, Garry and I would be able to see him. He assured us not to freak out when we saw the number of doctors working on Josh; it was all very routine!

Just then another nurse arrived; Josh had been brought into the ER reception, and she said we could briefly see him.

There he was, conscious, but heavily medicated. He smiled at me, and I noticed he was breathing on his own. He was hooked up with wires and tubes to several monitors. I could see his chest moving up and down; you could actually see his ribs moving, his diaphragm pulsing, and his heart beat was very strong.

Seeing his heart beating against his skin! It didn't even register then!

(It was many hours later, after we knew Josh's prognosis that we realized you are not meant to see a heart beating against skin.)

Josh looked very strong, which confirmed my belief that he wasn't badly hurt. In my mind, all this attention he was receiving was really just a precaution. The only evidence of any injury was his lower arms and elbows were badly scraped from where he had hit the road.

The impact with the road was so powerful that even though Josh had a hoody and jacket on, his arms were both badly cut and scratched.

He mumbled something to me about keeping the three girls he was seeing apart. I thought, "Well, he can't be too badly hurt."

Garry, hearing Josh telling me about the girls, commented, "He obviously isn't that badly hurt if he was worrying about girls."

Garry commented to one of the attendants wheeling Josh's gurney, "He's a bit of a drama queen, loves all the attention." In hindsight, they must have thought us both mad! We returned to the waiting room, and as nurses came in from time to time we asked how Josh was. They said that he was stable, but they wouldn't know anything for several hours.

With all that was going on around us, I felt really calm, still having "blind faith" Josh would be fine!

Around 9:45 PM Garry and I were taken to see Josh in the ER. Josh was conscious, although heavily drugged. There were about six doctors and nurses working on various parts of Josh's body. Yet again, Josh seemed in good spirits, his vitals seemed to be functioning strongly, and we could see how strong his heart beat was from one of the monitors.

One of the doctors said "We are not sure what we are dealing with, as far as the extent of Josh's injuries are concerned, so, to gain better understanding, we are taking him for a series of X-rays, MRI's, and CT scans."

Seeing Josh breathing unaided and his heart beating so strongly, we both thought the medical team were being very thorough.

We returned to the waiting room, confident that Josh was in good hands and we would soon hear that he is okay!

Josh's step brother Andrew and his partner arrived. Andrew and Josh were very close, and he was totally devastated!

The room was becoming crowded. We were sitting talking quietly bringing Andrew up to date with what we knew so far, when the "messages" started hitting my mind! The messages I believe, were from the Universe, (not text messages -- have to clarify that these days.)

The messages were clear, definite and urgent!

"Massage his hands, fingertips, feet, and the tips of his toes. There are people around that will help you. I had to have faith; NEVER GIVE UP!"

It was almost like my brain was being hammered, hammered with these urgent messages, over and over again.

I later described it as someone standing next to me, yelling at me, repeating the same four messages, as if they were trying to embed them into my brain.

I told Wendy about the messages. Obviously at the time, neither of us realized the meaning of them, and what they were preparing us for. Still, they came, always the same, over and over again! At the time, I truly thought I was going mad!

It was about 2:00 AM when we were called to meet with the doctors. Finally, after all this time, we would know what was going on with Josh! Wendy came with us.

Walking through the darkened hospital corridors, my immediate thought was that they were going to tell us that they were keeping him in overnight and we could take him home tomorrow!

We were introduced to a doctor. I can only remember that his first name was Michael. We were advised that Michael was the duty orthopedic surgeon in the ER that evening.

It's strange what comes into your mind, in those early confusing moments. Michael wore a light grey casual cardigan, and he was black. (I don't mean this in a racial way. It's just what I remembered.) I was thinking "You are looking after my son and you are wearing a grey cardigan." He didn't seem appropriately dressed, yet here he was delivering us the devastating news about our son's future.

Michael calmly told us that Josh was critically injured. (These weren't the words I was expecting to hear.)

He went on to say that Josh had broken his neck, severely crushing his spinal cord. He mentioned C5, C6, C7, T1 complete, he repeated to make sure it sunk in, Josh was a high level quadriplegic...complete!

He was complete? "What the hell does this mean?" We very quickly found out!

Josh was totally paralyzed from the injury on down! Basically, in a heartbeat, he had gone from being a totally active "full on" teenager to

41

being, according to his doctors, a head and a brain!

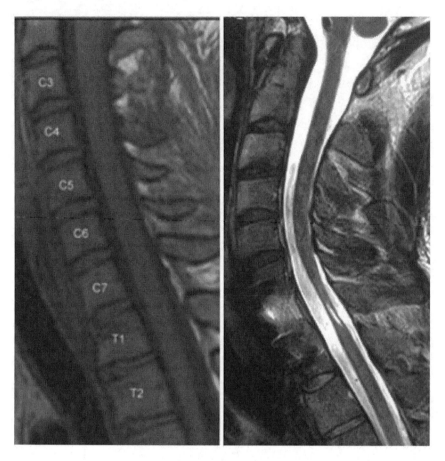

Josh's MRI (left, normal, right, Josh)

Michael advised us that, in his opinion, there was a less than 3% chance Josh would make any further recovery, so great was the cord damage. It was almost completely crushed... he was also concerned he may not live!

At that moment my heart broke in two, it snapped, and then went hard like concrete; in an instant, it felt like it weighed a ton, the pain was unbelievable!

I pushed the palm of my right hand into my chest to try and relieve the pain. Even though the pain in my heart was acute, mentally I felt rational, I didn't cry! Obviously I was in shock, at that stage I was too scared to cry, fearing I would never stop! I felt like I was in a trance, trying to take everything in. My brain was racing at what seemed a million miles an hour, all this, with this huge heavy aching lump in my chest.

Pulling myself together, I asked Michael "What does this mean?"

Michael was talking like Josh didn't exist anymore. He was saying Josh was now an 18 1/2 year old complete quadriplegic; he was categorizing him, pigeon holing him, in my mind, he wasn't dealing with an individual any longer, he was dealing with a statistic.

My grief turned to fury! How dare he make these assumptions about Josh's future? How could he make assumptions about Josh so quickly? It had been less than nine hours since Josh was admitted to the ER, yet Michael had written off any hope of recovery.

Again Michael repeated "He has badly crushed his spinal cord. He'll never walk again, but there is a chance he may have limited use of one of his arms. It is too early to tell, but it is likely he will never get out of bed so great is the injury."

In those early hours of the first night, Michael had already, in his mind, sealed Josh's fate. In his opinion, he repeated to us, Josh had less than 3% chance of any recovery, and he wasn't going to budge from that!

Michael appeared unemotional, like it was all very routine to him!

Yet again, as if to drill it into our broken hearts even more, Michael repeated his prognosis - Josh was completely paralyzed from his neck down.

My mind was racing, my emotions were going crazy, and the pain in my heart was epic!

I said, "You couldn't be right, Michael, as I had seen Josh move his arm earlier, you must be wrong" I rationalized - he must be a paraplegic!

Michael repeated, "Josh may have small arm movement, but we were not to expect too much." I tried telling Michael that Josh was an elite athlete, his mind was as tough as nails, he had worked through serious injuries before, he had fantastic tolerance for pain, and given time he would walk!

Michael said "a strong mind has nothing to do with this injury." I was struggling with Michael's total negativity!

While Michael was talking, in my mind I could see Josh standing there in his black suit, black shirt, and silver tie, leaning on the wall laughing at me saying "Kze, I'll be fine!"

Michael then said the words that I will carry to my grave, "Ms Wood (my married name), the sooner you accept your son's condition the better off he will be. Accept that he will never walk again. He may not even get out of bed."

I was crazy with grief, I retorted, "My son is tough, he will walk, he will never accept that he couldn't walk again, I would not accept it either."

After all these years I remember this moment like it was happening now!

I said to Michael, "You don't know my son and you don't know me. My son will walk again!"

Michael calmly turned to me and said "That's the problem, mothers like you, the sooner you accept your son will never walk again the better off you'll both be."… Another comment I will take to my grave!

At that moment, I could have ripped Michael's heart out. I fought to remain calm, and I simply answered, "My son will never accept your diagnosis and neither will I."

At that Michael said "I feel sorry for your son."

I remember at one stage saying "They grow babies in test tubes, and they'll be able to fix my son one day. We have to have faith!"

Although I was numb with shock, my mind was racing and the adrenaline was pumping through my body. At that moment I felt like I was two people: a devastated, heartbroken mother and a lioness gearing herself for the battle of her son's life!

More than anything, I wanted to wake up and find this was all a dream.

I felt sick. I kept on wanting the dream to stop. For heaven's sake let me wake up and find that I am dreaming!

This wasn't meant to happen to my boy, he was special, protected, so vibrant, living his dreams…how could he cope with such an injury?

All through this time, the one thing I was totally positive about was that

44

Josh was going to get better! Josh would walk. I never for one moment doubted it!

Wendy said to one of the nurses in the room, "This must be a dream," and the nurse unemotionally answered "This is reality. You have to accept it. You are not dreaming!"

We didn't realize it at the time, but from this first doctor's meeting, we were now part of the process of "acceptance"... this is as good as it gets!

We quickly learned to not rock the boat! Importantly though, we did not listen to and believe everything the doctors told us! No matter what the doctors said, no one would ever take away our faith in Josh recovering getting his life back.

Over the period of time Josh was in the hospital and later during rehabilitation, I watched the way the medical teams, doctors and most nurses took the injured person and their family's and friend's hope away! You know it only takes a few words to change one's future positively or negatively! I found this attitude horrific, cruel, and totally unacceptable!

As unbelievable as it sounds, the doctors don't know, especially in those early stages. In truth nobody knows! It is between the injured and God!

I understand the doctors have to be honest in assessing their patients' likely prognosis, give all the bad news to them, but should end it by saying, as bad as it is, we truly don't know!

Doctors can't be sued for being honest. They can't be sued for saying "they don't know."

It's really up to the injured person, and their family, to do whatever they can to achieve a level of acceptance and hopefully improvement. The medicos and nurses need to change the way they talk to parents and loved ones, too!

Their messages to us were all about acceptance. This is as good as it gets. Don't try and get the injured loved one to believe they can walk. They can't, so just accept it!

We understand they can't give anyone false hope, but it is immoral to take away all hope. It's inhuman and extremely cruel!

Everything Josh and I have written and commented on over all these years is not about giving people false hope, it's about giving them the will to live, to dream, to try and improve their condition – it's about giving them some control, importantly allowing them to maintain their self-esteem and not feeling that their lives are over.

It is extremely important during those early days to do everything possible to keep the injured person confident, calm, and focused.

It's been over 14 years since we met Michael. Strangely, after that first night we never saw him again, but I have a goal: firstly to locate him and secondly to make an appointment with him. Josh and I will enter his office, and I'll simply remind him of his words to me. I will say, "Michael, you are a doctor, you are not God. How dare you take away a patient's hope?"

That said, Josh and I will leave his office! Josh has said he is not interested in doing this, but if I ever get the chance I will, not for us, but all the others that have hope dragged away from them through this cruel injury.

Michael went on to inform us that Josh's surgery would be scheduled for some time in the next few days, and with luck it will be the only surgery he would require. The surgery would rebuild the damaged vertebrae, fusing the bones.

The surgeon will take a piece of bone from Josh's hip and fuse the C6 and C7 vertebrae, removing the shattered vertebrae from his spinal cord.

I thought my brain would explode with the mixture of unrelenting grief coursing through my heart and mind, my fury with the medical team's total negativity, combined with frustration, fear and the unbelievable amount of information I was trying to process.

There was too much information. I felt my head swimming. I was trying to take the whole scene in, and my brain was totally scrambled.

What I did know was that my son was critically injured, and the medical profession had made a decision about him, giving him a new title: teenage quadriplegic, C5, C6, C7, T1 complete. They didn't care about him or his dreams. To them, he was just another of what we were later to learn was called the "silent epidemic" of young Australians suffering this horrific injury.

The medical team had made their decision, and they didn't even know Josh. (Some weeks later, Josh was reassessed to C5, C6, C7, T1 complete, then incomplete.)

While, we were meeting with Michael, Josh had been moved to the ICU. Michael said we could see him briefly.

Garry was a mess; he was crying. I was numb. I felt angry, frustrated, sick, frightened, and my broken heart felt like a rock in my chest. It was so heavy, so sad, and I was in so much pain! I was so frightened. I knew if Josh saw us upset or even worried, he would get scared and then God knows what would happen. We had to remain positive and upbeat, no matter how hard it was.

I pleaded with Garry to stop crying, to try and calm himself. I said we had to be positive and not appear worried. We didn't want to scare Josh, because his life depended on us being positive.

Garry looked at me and said "You are a f@#*ing cold bitch". I retorted "In the 29 years we were together that statement proved to me that you never ever knew me"!

I then yelled at him "My heart is broken, but my son will never see me cry." To this day I have never cried for Josh's injury. I always thought if I started crying, I would never stop.

Wendy screamed at us to stop our arguing. We have to go and see Josh!

What Garry didn't understand, as we were preparing to see Josh, was that I was fighting with every emotion. I had to overcome the terror that was enveloping me. Frankly I was too scared not to be strong!

The messages I received in the waiting room were now starting to make sense. A voice inside my brain, kept telling me to have faith.

Almost instantly, I received another powerful, urgent message telling me that it will take 2 1/2 years for Josh to throw away his wheel chair.

The message was also saying that we must start to massage him as soon as possible. Truthfully, at that moment, nothing was making any sense to me. I was totally exhausted, physically and emotionally! But the messages kept coming into my brain over and over again! Was I imagining them, or was this just what I wanted to hear?

Again, I kept seeing Josh, clearly in my mind, standing propped up against a door jam, laughing at me, calling to me "Kze," telling me not to worry.

47

We finally saw Josh. He was very heavily sedated and really didn't know what was happening. We were glad we had made the decision not to say anything to him at that stage, as the medical team didn't know if he was going to live. But at that moment he was stable, drifting into sleep. He looked so vulnerable.

It's crazy that in all those years, even with all the injuries he had suffered, I had never thought Josh looked or was vulnerable since those first few weeks of his life. Now we are 18 years later and I am feeling the same emotions!

Seeing him, we were satisfied that we were right to decide to wait until after the operation to break the news to Josh about the crushing of his spinal cord and what the doctors' prognosis for him was. We just kept saying to Josh, "You really have to stay strong. You're having surgery, probably Monday or Tuesday. It will be long and be tough on you. You need to stay focused and positive. The doctors are going to rebuild your shattered vertebrae."

Josh was aware his neck was broken. He knew his vertebrae had been shattered, and he wasn't hearing anything from us he hadn't already known. At that stage he thought the paralysis was a result from the broken neck and the fractured vertebrae. I knew Josh. I knew he would think once the bones were fused he would be okay, and he would go back on the snow. As sad as all this was, for the time being it was important not to tell him the truth, really not to discuss it at all, just be confident and positive! The rest of the time we were in the hospital that night was a blur.

We begged Michael and the team not to tell Josh his cord was crushed until after his operation, and then not to tell him anything unless either Garry or I were present.

In our conversation with Michael, I had learned something that had significantly added to our fear. Josh was over 18 years of age, and the medical team did not legally have to take any direction from us. In fact they didn't have to tell us anything. Legally Josh was an adult, and legally they did not have to involve us at all.

At that early stage there was a chance that Josh would not survive the next few days; I knew he would not survive the operation if he knew the extent of his injury so we wanted everyone to be calm and confident. I threatened the doctors that under no circumstances was Josh to be told of the extent of his injury!

In the past, Josh and I had worked through some very serious injuries, particularly over the last few years. I knew if Josh thought we were scared, if he saw us crying, he would be scared, and from where he was, he couldn't move, the last thing he needed was to be frightened!

I had all these crazy thoughts tumbling around my brain, the doctor's lack of compassion and faith devastated me. I could not believe how negative they were, basically leaving us with NO ROOM FOR HOPE!

This was to set up a pattern between Josh and me with his medical team that sadly, all these years later, still exists – these early experiences with his medical team cost us the ability to ever trust them!

I rationalized, "Doctors! What do they know? They don't know Josh and they don't know me. I knew we would prove them wrong!" We had to prove them wrong; there was simply no other alternative!

It's crazy you have to feel like this. Even at that early stage, I quickly realized that it would be up to me to protect my son, and to keep him focused. At all times I needed to be totally positive in Josh's ability to recover.

This belief in Josh wouldn't be too hard for me as I was always so confident in Josh's ability to recover that I never really entertained the thought that he wouldn't. I knew he would walk and I knew it would take us 2 1/2 years before he no longer had to rely on his wheelchair. Wasn't that what the last message from the Universe said?

I had to have faith and never lose that belief no matter what!

Over the coming weeks I would be tested at every level to maintain my faith in Josh walking, but in truth, I absolutely believed he would. I never for one moment doubted this!

From that terrifying first night, all I remembered was that no one offered us any hope. His medical team to a one, were all categorical – "there was no hope"!

"The damage to his cord was so devastating, he would never walk again!"

Chapter 6. Thrown in the Deep End, Drowning in a Sea of Negativity

From the first night, I realized the doctors and nurses would make Josh medically stable, (mend him) but, that's all they would do. In their eyes "healing" him was not an option. All they were interested in was for us to accept Josh's new life, confined to a bed, or with luck be able to use a motorized wheel chair with mouth controls.

With this knowledge, I realized it would be up to us to find the answers to get Josh walking again, to give him back not only his independence, but his life.

Finally at about 3 AM, Wendy and I left the hospital to drive home. Wendy wanted to drive, but I needed to be doing something. I was totally devastated, and I insisted on driving!

Poor Wendy, she was dealing with her own emotions. She loved Josh and we had all gone through this harrowing, horrific, traumatic night.

In my present state, I was, frankly, oblivious to everyone else's feelings except Josh! My only thoughts and concerns were for Josh and what he was dealing with and how he would survive this horrible injury. It would take every ounce of strength and determination he had!

In May, after Josh had left home, I had bought my dream car. It was a navy blue MX5 Mazda Miata convertible; a typical car for an "empty nester." From the moment I first drove it, I always had the roof down, and tonight would be no exception!

So here we were. It was after 3 AM on a freezing Melbourne winter's morning with the car's heater on full throttle driving home! Poor Wendy was so cold, but she never complained! I was driving, but I had no idea where I was going. Fortunately, Wendy calmly told me to turn here, stop here, go left there. I do not know how we got home. Wendy was fantastic, and never once criticized my driving, and was amazingly calm. Yet like me, she was stunned; her heart was broken too!

I felt totally manic. Even in those early hours after the accident I knew in my heart and soul the world as we knew it had gone forever. We faced a whole new future, which as I drove home, was full of fear, lack of hope, and lack of any light!

Later the next week we were warned by one of the nurses hearing us that we needed to be careful driving when tired. Many loved ones were involved in car accidents driving home late at night after tragic events had occurred to family members. Driving while stressed, tired and not concentrating on the road often formed a dangerous combination of circumstances, leading to accidents! I can only think that during the whole crazy time when I drove home in the dead of night or early morning I was totally "protected", and I always expected to arrive home safely!

In those few short hours as we drove home, I had set a pattern in my mind, heart and emotions that would ultimately block out everything, except doing whatever I had to do to save my son and help him get his life back.

I would be oblivious to everyone else's emotions. I couldn't be my usual self, trying to make it easy, being the strong one for every one that simply could not be my role anymore. If I was to save Josh, I had to be totally focused on him, on him alone; there was no alternative.

I no longer had the strength to be there for anyone else but Josh, and above all else, I had to keep myself focused. I could not, would not, be distracted from this.

(This pattern still persists as I write this story even today.)

I often say Josh's accident taught me many things - two traits I didn't have at the time, but quickly adopted for my own survival: patience and the art of detachment.

For my own sanity I had to master these two skills, and master them quickly!

We finally reached our home in Port Melbourne at around 3:30 AM. I felt the adrenaline coursing through my entire body, and my mind was in overload.

I knew I had to get some sleep, but I was wide awake and not tired at all!

My brain ached, and my heart ached. I felt totally isolated from everyone and everything except Josh.

What on earth was I going to do to help Josh? With no medical training, all I had was my love and trust in his ability and strength of mind to somehow tackle this horrendous injury and gain recovery.

52

Recently, I had begun to meditate. Paula's daughter Jolie had trained me in TM meditation. I found it really worked and helped me in the past when I was stressed - tonight I would test it!

I was so overwhelmed with grief and information overload, I knew I had to download information out of my brain. Hopefully, meditation would help me!

As I climbed onto my bed, I felt enveloped in total despair. At this early stage I had no control on what was happening to Josh. I was so angry and frustrated with the negativity of his medical team, and, worst of all, I was sad, scared and devastated for him.

I felt, as a parent, I was letting him down. I couldn't believe the doctors. They were so negative, and yet they were supposed to help him. If they can't heal him who can? As yet I didn't have any answers. As a "can do" person I always found a way, but this, this was more than even I could cope with!

Sitting cross-legged on my bed in frustration I yelled "if there's a God I need the names. Who will be the ones to help me (as in the first message I had received earlier in the night)? I need those names now!"

Within an instant four names were propelled into my brain! Simon (Josh's chiropractor), Paula, Dana, and John.

Dana and John were an American couple I had connected with when I had attended the Anthony Robbins Life Mastery course in 1999. We had met at Honolulu airport while waiting in the line to board the plane to Kona, Hawaii. At the time we briefly chatted -- polite conversation. I ran into them several times over the next 10 days. We developed a friendship based on our shared experiences with Life Mastery. Since returning to Australia, I had kept in touch with Dana. I knew I could count on them both!

Feeling energized and slightly positive from my message, I rang Dana and John immediately.

As calmly as I could, I went through what had happened to Josh, including the attitude of his medical team. I remember saying how devastated I was with their total negativity and lack of any compassion.

Dana immediately offered to fly to Australia to help out with my business and supporting Josh in any way. I was amazed Dana would think of dropping everything to come to Australia, but I had already thought about confirming the Australian doctor's prognosis by getting a second opinion from an orthopedic surgeon in the USA. I persuaded Dana to be my eyes in the USA.

I asked her to locate the best orthopedic specialist in the USA. My feeling was with the much larger population there, the doctors would have greater experience with spinal cord injury than their Australian counterparts. I needed to somehow get hold of Josh's MRI's and x-rays, and get them over to Dana and John as soon as possible.

I desperately wanted another opinion from a spinal cord injury specialist away from Australia. I wanted someone that didn't know Josh, someone who hadn't actually sighted Josh, a specialist who was experienced enough to review his MRI's objectively. I had always loved the "can do" attitude Americans have, so it was crucial for me to have someone I could trust (Dana) asking the right questions in the USA.

Talking to Dana had calmed me down a little. I felt that I had a new "Team Josh member," someone I could trust, someone who would be positive, someone who would be on our side.

I meditated for about 15 minutes, trying to quiet my racing mind. I was exhausted, yet the adrenalin kept coursing through my body. I finally slept, waking about an hour later, fully alert.

It was around 5:30 AM. So much had happened, but little did I realize how much our lives were about to change. In fact my life up to that moment was over. I had a totally new life.

My mission was to give Josh his life back; to get him back the independence he treasured so much. I wanted him back to where he was before his accident!

In those few minutes after waking, I set my goals for Josh's recovery. I would do whatever it took, whatever it cost to:

- Keep him fit and focused,

- Make him confident in believing that anything was possible,

- Maintain his self-esteem, and never let that be challenged,

- Give him his independence back,

54

- and I would never cry for what had happened to him!

Strangely I felt better; I had the beginnings of game plan. I was positive it would become clearer as we understood more about the injury.

I also made an important decision, one that I would ask Josh to support - We would never research the Internet about spinal cord injury; I didn't want anything getting in our way of his recovery!

Monday, the 26th of June, was going to be the first day of the busiest week of my business year, when all my hard work in the past months paid off for me allowing me to earn significant bonuses. Seeing the investments flow into my clients businesses -- well, that was no longer important! That money would never be earned. My only priority was doing whatever it took to keep Josh alive. Nothing else mattered.

My business, of which I was the sole owner, was raising capital for startup agricultural projects. This year I had three clients. All were expecting me to generate significant capital for their businesses, and they were relying on me, yet my son was hovering between life and death. I had no choice but to walk away from my business. I had to be there for Josh!

Next I decided to see Simon, our chiropractor. In 20 minutes I managed to shower, dress, and drive to Simon's practice. Everything was fast forwarded into a sense of immediacy. Simon's practice was about five minutes from our home.

I arrived there just before 6 AM. Walking into the practice, I remember my emotions where at the breaking point. Simon was walking down the stairs and I blurted out "Josh has had a terrible accident."

I rambled through what had happened. Poor Simon. He didn't know what to say; he was also in shock. It had only been Friday that Simon had finally discharged Josh after two years of unrelenting therapy to repair Josh's L5 in his lower back. Now we were facing the future with an injury that even being positive, would in all probability, cause Josh to need treatment for the rest of his life.

I said, "What does it mean, Simon? They say his spinal cord is crushed."

Simon said before he could comment he had to see Josh's MRI's. It was imperative that I get access to them! Simon needed to see for himself what the damage was. He didn't want to commit to offering me too much at that stage.

He did say, "Josh was used to working through injuries. He was in great shape physically and he would be extremely open to recovery."

We talked for a while. Naturally he agreed to help us. He was so positive, saying that Josh was strong enough, his mind was so tough, and he had the experience, if he wanted it hard enough, to achieve anything.

He added that this would be his greatest battle, but Simon reiterated that "Josh was tough, he was positive Josh was up to it!"

As I left Simon called to me saying, "Kay, we need to see the MRI's."

The night of the accident, I had pleaded with Josh's doctors to allow Simon to be involved with Josh's treatment. I argued that Josh had been treated by Simon for so many years. They trusted each other; what was more important, we both had total faith in Simon. The doctors said it would not be possible, chiropractors were not allowed to practice at the hospital.

I couldn't believe that the medical team was so narrow-minded that they wouldn't let Simon be involved in contributing to Josh's recovery.

I argued that Simon knew Josh's body better than anyone; he had our total trust.

I understand the doctors being nervous about bringing anyone into the hospital they didn't know, but I was prepared to sign a waiver, but they weren't open to Simon being involved at any level.

Quickly, I realized it was pointless arguing with them, so I decided on a strategy that I would adopt for the entire time Josh would be in hospital and rehabilitation. I would lie!

Simon became Josh's snowboard coach!

I was later to introduce the rest of my team: Paula as my sister in law from the country, Isobel, my sister, Jackie, my aunt, whoever I thought of, to be part of our team, became an instant relative, coach, or friend.

On my way to the hospital, I called our family doctor, Graeme Baro. Graeme had been Josh's personal doctor for several years, since Josh had moved from Mansfield to Melbourne to live with me. Through all Josh's accidents, I found that Graeme had been open to our alternative healing practices, although he personally only practiced the "medical" approach.

I quickly brought him up to date with what had happened, including the doctor's early prognosis. At that moment there was little he could do, as Josh's medical treatment, for the time being, was out of his hands. But he agreed to keep me updated on Josh's medical reports that would be sent to him from Josh's specialist team. We trusted each other; Graeme became one of my most respected confidants, an important member of Josh's team.

Coincidentally, Graeme had gone through medical school with many of the hospital's specialists, so he either knew them personally or by reputation.

He assured me the medical team there was the very best. We were to later find out that the very best at mending could be total failures at healing.

My mission that first crazy week, along with everything else I had to do, was to get copies of Josh's MRI Scans to Simon, Dana and John.

Little did I realize what a mammoth task that would be!

We had found out the night of Josh's accident that neither his father nor I were legally allowed to act for him. We weren't able to determine his treatment and, for that matter, the doctors really didn't have to discuss anything related to Josh with us. You have no idea how totally stressed and inadequate this made me feel. I had worked in financial services all my life. I knew about medical power of attorneys, but never ever thought to get one on Josh.

I had one on my mother, but Josh was young, and in all honesty, it never crossed my mind.

"I never thought anything would happen to us!" Oh my God, how many times have I heard parents say that over these past years?

I rang my financial planner at 9 AM on Monday morning. He undertook to arrange for the medical power of attorney to be prepared "urgently."

I instructed him to increase my life insurance, actually to double it, and sell all of my investments. I was going to need the cash.

We weren't sure how we would get Josh to sign the document, as he was totally paralyzed, but all I could do in that moment was to stay focused on getting the document. I would worry about the signature later.

On my way into the hospital, I had arranged for Josh's snowboard gear to be brought into the ICU. Josh needed to know from Day One - he would get his life back.

Arriving at the hospital, I requested copies of Josh's MRI's, and they wouldn't release them to me. Legally, I had no right to access them; Josh had to approve this. Their argument was that the scans belonged to Josh, not me. But Josh wasn't in any position to do anything with them. I was terrified if I pushed Josh too much he would realize there was more wrong with him than a broken neck, so I had to tread very carefully.

Sometime during day the medical power of attorney was delivered to us at the hospital. I recall that someone held Josh's hand to make a mark, so the document was signed and it was all witnessed legally. Finally I had my document.

Whether they liked it or not, the medical team had to deal with me!

I can't even begin to tell you how terrified, stressed, tired, angry, and frustrated I was...but I don't give up easily. All I cared about at that stage was that Josh was going to be okay, that much I knew, so that is what I focused on. Then the energy flowed and I was rejuvenated.

I quickly realized that Josh wasn't in any position to fight for himself, so fragile was his condition, so I had to be the one to fight for him. I had to be his advocate!

Something early I insisted on with Josh's medical team: I did not want Josh referred to as being disabled; he was injured. In my mind, disabled was permanent, but injuries can be worked on, either healed or improved. Very quickly I realized the power of the medical team's "labelling" in bringing negativity into our new world.

In those days we learned fast, so often we were "flying blind." We learned very quickly to make our rules, and not be frightened to ask questions of his medical team or to challenge something we didn't understand.

These days, as I mentor so many families, the first thing I stress is that you must be your child's or loved one's advocate. Do not trust that the medical team will always have the best interests of your loved one as a goal. If you don't totally understand something, ask the question, educate yourself, and make the decision. Get them to explain why they are doing something or what those drugs were for. Don't be scared to ask; don't be too scared to challenge something you don't think is right!

It still took a few days for me to have the time to tackle the copying of the MRI's...finally the hospital's administration staff would have to co-operate.

I needed three copies of everything; a set each for Simon, Dana and John, and one for us. One of the doctors queried why I felt the need to send the MRI's to the USA, and I said I wanted a second opinion. He went off on a tangent saying I was wasting my time. Our Australian doctors were as experienced as any in the U.S.

I argued that with the Australian population being less than California's, doctors in the US would deal with significantly more spinal cord injuries. I would not be swayed. I reiterated I wanted a second opinion! The doctor was not happy.

Mission - get the MRI's! Armed with the medical power of attorney, I returned to the department for my copies. Even then they didn't make it easy. First I had to pay for the copies, (in cash, several hundred dollars) and then I had to do the copies myself. Seriously, this was beyond belief. I had no idea how to carefully copy these precious potentially "lifesaving" documents and now here I was having to do this without any assistance from the "experts."

I was fast realizing there was little I could expect from this hospital!

My Early Reality Check - Observations of the hospital we found ourselves in!

You have to understand that prior to Josh's accident our total experience with Australian hospitals was the quick visit for a cast to be fitted for a broken bone, a cut that required stitching, or a few day's stay in a local community hospital. Now, in what seemed a heartbeat, we were dealing with an ER, ICU, and Critical Spinal Unit. This experience was so far beyond anything we had experienced in the past that it was frightening and confusing. This doesn't take into account the medical language that was being blasted at us, the jargon!

Australia is a modern, wealthy country, and we expect our hospitals to be "state of the art." So when you are thrust into the Public Hospital system, your expectations are for our health facilities to be the best!

The hospital Josh was admitted to in the year 2000 was far from modern; it was in fact pre-World War II. Fortunately it has now been fully renovated, but in those days it was not much better than a 3rd world facility. You have no idea how shocked we all were! Our experience with the ER and the waiting room was what you would expect from any hospital. It was when Josh was transferred to the ICU that I was devastated. My initial observations regarding the hospital's ICU and the acute spinal wards were that it reminded me of a 3rd world hospital; something akin to the Sanglah Hospital in Bali.

As already mentioned, Josh was transferred to ICU in the early morning after his accident, having been stabilized in the ER. The ICU and spinal unit were located in a converted radio station attached to the main hospital building by an underground tunnel. It was a rabbit warren of narrow corridors, old stairs, and elevators. The building was well past its "used by" date!

In the ICU, Josh had "one on one" care by a nursing team 24/7 with an additional team in the background should something go wrong. The ICU unit was so old that it really needed a good painting, and a significant upgrade. I couldn't help but wonder how my son was going to progress in surroundings that gave you little confidence.

The ICU nursing team was fantastic, extremely professional, very caring, and we couldn't have asked for any more. But the ward itself was so old and depressing that it created more fear. I was thinking that Josh needs all the help he can get, but this hospital looks like it could fall down, it was so depressing and frightening. Given the dilapidated state of the ICU, it was still very sterile, hygienic and clean, but the paint was peeling on the ceiling, the curtains needed repairing, and everything looked old and worn out!

I guess those of you reading this would rightly think, "What was I doing worrying about the paint in the ward," but with Josh so critically injured, frankly I had no confidence in the physical facility. It just made me more and more frightened. I will stress though, the professionalism of the medical team was never a question in our minds. We were totally in awe of their kindness, care and attention toward Josh!

In the ICU, Josh was unable to eat. He was being fed through a tube that was placed down his throat; I found this extremely confrontational, as now I had to deal with the possibility that Josh could, according to his doctors, be bed ridden for the rest of his life. Here they were feeding him in the same manner as he was fed when he was a baby struggling in the Special Care Nursery.

According to the medical team, I faced the real risk of having an 18 year old, strong, healthy, fit son, who was now not much better, functionally, than a new born baby.

These times seriously challenged my confidence in Josh's ability to recover! I had to quickly pull myself together. I had no choice. I had to delete these thoughts from my mind instantly. I had to believe he would be all right!

I couldn't allow myself the luxury of sadness. I had to be confident in his ability to recover - no matter what!

At times like this I had to fight every emotion to stay positive; it was so hard!

Josh, thank goodness, was oblivious to his surroundings. Although he was conscious and able to have restricted visitors, he was so heavily drugged that I don't know how he got through those early days.

Because he hadn't been told the extent of his injuries, all his friends and our family were counselled by me before they visited him. They had to be positive and try to remain composed. I urged them to be as normal as possible, rather than standing around being sad. I asked them to massage his fingers and toes.

Late on the Sunday night Josh was admitted, Wendy and I had spoken to our brother, Gary, letting him know about Josh's accident. Collectively, we decided he would go to Mum's the next morning and let her know about what had happened to Josh along with the doctors' prognosis.

We asked him the impossible - to try and keep as calm as possible as Mum was such a worrier. She would be devastated; extremely scared for Josh.

Josh and Mum were very close. Mum had looked after Josh a lot as a toddler, and as we all lived close to each other, Josh spent a lot of time with her.

Gary arranged to bring our mother in early the next afternoon.

Chapter 7. Fighting the System, - Keeping Strong, Dealing with the "BS"

Monday morning, Day 1 - I needed to get word of Josh's accident out to his many friends. On my way to the hospital, I called Daniel and Geoff to update them on Josh's first night. When I finally reached them, they were already heading down the mountain in Josh's car, which they had packed up with his gear and clothes.

They were hoping to see Josh. I had asked them to bring his snowboard into the hospital, since I wanted it in ICU with Josh.

On their arrival I met them in the ICU reception. Taking them through to Josh, I grabbed his snowboard and placed it near Josh's bed where he could see it. The hospital staff said, "You can't bring a snowboard into ICU."

I answered, "I will do whatever I want to do. I will do whatever it takes to give Josh confidence he will get his life back. If he knows I am confident, he will be!"

THE SNOWBOARD STAYED! Josh needed to know without any doubt, that his life wasn't over. I would not allow it to be removed!

Over a few days, not only did the snowboard make it to ICU, but so did his snowboard boots and all his ripped and torn clothing from the accident. (Josh, after all these years, has kept the clothing he wore that day, resisting all my attempts to get rid of it. Every time I see them I feel physically sick.)

Much to the aggravation of the medical team, Josh's motorbike helmet and boots mysteriously made it to the ICU as well.

Many reading this section may think I pushed too much in bringing his gear into the ICU. I will never regret this. Very quickly I had figured out that this injury was as much "mentally challenging" as much as having to deal with the physical aspects of it. Josh needed to have confidence he would recover. He needed to be totally confident, and I knew beyond any doubt he would recover.

I wanted Josh to know categorically that I believed he would snowboard again and that I believed he would ride motor bikes again. So in those crucial early days he knew I was sure, and I was confident, and that really was all that mattered!

Much later, Josh said to me that he could smell the dirt on his motor bike boots when they were in ICU, and seeing his gear in the room with him, that he truly believed he would get his life back!

With all the negativity we dealt with every day, keeping Josh's mind believing that anything was possible was crucial!

We commenced massaging Josh's hands, fingers, feet and toes the first morning in ICU, Day 1. Josh hated the touching, but I said "Sorry, we have to do this; we need to keep the messages going to your brain."

Even though Josh couldn't feel anything, it was extremely annoying to him.

He understood why we were doing it, but he hated the fact his friends were having to massage him.

I firmly believe this immediate stimulation helped to set Josh up for his ongoing recovery, teaching him in those early days to commence the reconnection with his injured body.

Even though Josh didn't want his friends or family massaging him, everyone involved felt they were contributing to his recovery, and they were at least doing something positive! It took the focus off the sadness we were all feeling. It was positive focusing on his recovery.

It created a mindset of positivity, not despair!

We massaged him for hours every day, but the nursing team assured us that IT WOULD NOT HELP JOSH IN ANY WAY. We were wasting our time! We ignored them!

I come from the mindset "If you don't use it, you lose it." I was positive if we kept the messages "happening" from Josh's extremities, the spinal cord would remain stimulated, even though there was so little function.

I had already discussed the massaging with Simon earlier that morning, and he agreed stimulation was everything!

So began a process: when his visitors were sad we said "please just massage." Massaging made them feel like they were doing something positive for Josh.

Still his medical team said we were wasting our time.

Frankly, it wasn't my problem what they thought. I knew it would help Josh walk out of that aging facility. I was so positive!

My brother brought our mother into ICU the afternoon after the accident. It was truly a heartbreaking moment; the sadness in Mum's eyes was gut-wrenching. She was so brave, but in the end her tears flowed. They tumbled out of her eyes, and no matter what we said they wouldn't stop. At one stage everyone, including the medical team, had tears rolling down their cheeks,

Everyone except me. Honestly I was too scared to cry, fearing I wouldn't stop. Josh kept telling her, he was sorry he had caused her so much pain! Mum held him. She wasn't very tall, just 5 feet. It wasn't easy for her to reach him, so finally she sat on the edge of the bed holding his hand.

It was so hard. The medical team was so negative. They wanted us to accept what Josh's "new" life was going to be, and we seemed to be constantly at odds with them, trying to keep positive. It was a very challenging time!

Remember, at this early stage Josh did not know the extent of his injuries. We were constantly in fear that either one of the medical team or one of our visitors would accidently tell him. No matter what, I had to keep this information from him. I needed him to go into his surgery confident and full of hope!

We were lucky in those few days before his surgery. Although he knew his neck was broken, he was so drugged up with morphine and a concoction of other drugs, he fortunately didn't connect that the paralysis was a result of his broken neck.

Several of Josh's visitors were saying to me privately, "Take his gear out. You have to remove all his snowboard and motor bike gear." They said it made them sad to see it in ICU knowing what Josh's prognosis was.

I repeated, "I'm not getting rid of anything, because Josh is going to walk and get his life back." I never doubted it! You just have to believe. I don't know how. I know it doesn't seem possible, but he's going to walk. I know it; I know he will, we just have to have faith and never give up!

At times, it was hard to remain positive. Josh was so helpless! He couldn't eat, couldn't move, could barely communicate, the weight was falling off him before our eyes, but I knew he would walk. I guess it was too hard for me to think otherwise!

Chapter 8. New Beginnings, a New Destiny; There Is Another Way!

As I already mentioned, I had worked out very quickly that although the hospital's medical team would mend Josh, I knew that post-operation, from their view, their work had been completed and that from then on it would be about our acceptance of what they now believed were Josh's only options: living in a bed, or at best learning to manage a power chair with mouth controls.

Neither of these options was acceptable to me. I knew categorically that if I didn't have a plan for Josh to recover, I was certain he would die!

I have never been so terrified. My fear was beyond anything I have ever experienced, and yet I was outwardly in control!

Please don't get me wrong. As far as his doctors were concerned, I knew we had the best possible team operating on Josh that night. They were very talented and highly regarded, and they mended him with all their skill and precision – but that was where their commitment to Josh ended.

For the record, Josh never used a power chair. He realized very quickly that for him mentally to improve, he needed to set a goal to use a manual wheel chair once they got him out of bed.

Every day there always seemed to be another drama or surprise; something the doctors discovered through the myriad of scans, MRI's and X-rays was - Josh had only one kidney. It had shown up in his MRI's. His one kidney was "bell shaped" meaning it hadn't separated into two as he grew in my womb. The doctors felt something had happened early in the pregnancy; I thought it was ironic, after all these years to find this out. The issue probably could be traced back to my illness in Bali.

OMG, what else was going to happen? Every day there seemed to be something else.

There was nothing I could do to change the situation with his kidneys, so I quickly put this new development out of my mind and focused on the now, what I could do, what I could control. I needed to build Josh's recovery team. That had to be my focus, my primary goal, if I wanted to SAVE MY SON!

When asked what is my religion was, my answer was always the same. I believe there is a Universal God. Personally, I am not of one religion; I am an extremely spiritual person, believing in a higher spirit! If pressed I would elaborate, "I believe there is one God; personally, my spiritual belief is a blend of Christianity, Hinduism and Buddhism."

So I prayed in my convoluted way and asked for guidance, asking for those precious names of those who will help me save my son.

I already had the names of my initial team: Simon Floreani, Dana and John (our US team), Paula, my friend and physic healer...but who else would I need?

In truth I had no idea, but I remembered the messages from that crazy first night, in particular – "Never give up, there are people around that will help you" and then the 2nd – "Josh will be walking in 2 1/2 years and no longer using his chair" so I knew I had to believe, and have faith that the right people would come into our lives as we needed them.

Josh still had no idea of the extent of his cord damage. We just had to keep saying, we want to remove as much risk as possible, keep all the messages going through your cord, and that's why we are massaging your extremities.

Although it was only Wednesday, 3 1/2 days since our world had disintegrated, everything seemed as though we were in a time warp. Our old lives were so far in the past it was hard to imagine them. My new world was filled with fear, terror, and a new language, - convoluted medical terminology. The confusion and disbelief was overwhelming.

I was fighting every emotion to stay positive. It was critical for Josh that I always presented myself as confident and focused; truly, unless you have experienced something like this, there is no way you could imagine how you would manage this.

Josh needed to know that no matter what, I knew he would be okay!

There were so many visitors. They continued to wander into the waiting rooms, patiently waiting, some for several hours, for the chance of a few minutes visiting their broken mate. I made sure, as hard as it was, to always be upbeat and positive; for me there was no other option.

Our family and Josh's friends seemed to control all the available waiting room space in the ICU area.

While in the ICU Josh could only have two visitors at a time, so I made sure everyone had their turn. Every visitor, including my mother, had a pep talk from me before they saw him – "Josh will be all right; be positive, always be upbeat, massage his toes and fingers, and talk about the future as you would normally."

Although Josh was really struggling physically, seeing everyone made him happy; he even managed some jokes!

Although everyone was upbeat, as much as they could be, the one thing all his visitors could not hide from him was the sadness in their eyes. As injured as he was, Josh quickly picked up on this and much later, when we had the chance to talk about that crazy time "the first weeks," Josh told me how much it destroyed him that he had caused this sadness to his much loved family and friends. It made him more determined to recover; it was one of the driving forces for him.

We were looking forward to Wednesday night, when Josh's surgery was scheduled! Finally it was time. At last Josh was being prepped for his "lifesaving" surgery.

After my meltdown earlier in the day, when I let go with a barrage of questions to Josh's medical team on the qualifications and experience of all those involved in his life saving surgery -- were these doctors the best, the most experienced? It was the first time in those crazy days when I really felt totally out of control, with no idea how to deal with the fact that I was trusting a team of doctors who were largely unknown to me with my son's life. How could I have not asked these questions earlier?

I had a huge network of contacts in financial services, and many of them were financial planners who dealt with the medical profession as clients. I started calling them all, asking them for their contacts in the medical profession, and those that dealt with spinal cord injury.

For an entire morning I was totally manic trying to get those precious names, those professionals who could give me confidence, the reassurance that my son was in the best of hands.

Everyone I spoke to said the same thing: "We have the best doctors in Australia. They are very talented and experienced." I even phoned medicos from ER teams at other Melbourne hospitals, and again they all said that we had the best team to rebuild Josh's shattered vertebrae, and to remove the bone fragments from his precious spinal cord.

I know I was a nightmare. I was like this big lioness protecting my precious son. In my mind I was fighting for his life, his future, his potential to recover!

We stayed with Josh as long as we were allowed. Watching him being wheeled into surgery was gut-wrenching; I felt a mixture of unbelievable terror, yet a sense of relief because up until then Josh's neck had not been stabilized. Josh had started his journey to recovery. I needed to have faith!

It was going to be a long night, so Wendy and I decided to return home and try and get some sleep.

This was a decision I would regret for the rest of my life. I should have stayed!

It was such a confusing time, and I was totally exhausted. I had hardly eaten since the accident, and I was running on adrenaline; I still don't know to this day why I didn't stay at the hospital, being there, when he came through to recovery!

I had asked the duty nurse to advise me as soon as Josh was brought back to recovery. I wanted to be there when he woke up.

I also reiterated that under NO circumstances was Josh to be advised of his "complete injury," without either me or his father being present.

I was woken from what had been a fitful sleep early Thursday morning. It was the duty nurse telling me to get into the hospital urgently. I asked how Josh was, and she said "extremely upset." Why? She didn't answer, and my mind was racing. With urgency I asked her, "Josh has been told of his prognosis?" She answered me "Yes."

I remember screaming at the nurse "You are all bastards, my instructions were clear to you all." Now I have to figure out a way of dealing with Josh. Oh my God what would I say to him? I was beyond devastation!

All I could think was that Josh had been so callously delivered his devastating news and now he was lying in bed on his own. God only knows what he was going through.

How could I have let Josh down? I should have known better. I should never have left the hospital that night!

I was terrified, angry, and beyond scared. Josh had been told this horrific news when he was on his own; my worst nightmare.

At that stage I lost all trust in his medical team, and I can honestly say I never regained it!

I vowed this would never happen again. I would have to "camp" at the hospital if this was the only way I could protect Josh from the constant lack of concern for his mental wellbeing!

I threw clothes on over my pajamas, and sped through the freezing early morning Melbourne traffic to the hospital. I had the roof down on my car, heater cranked up, blasting the world with Andrea Bocelli, trying to figure out how I was going to convince Josh his life was beginning, not ending. I was so scared!

What would I say to Josh? How could I, using supreme confidence, convince him that he was going to recover, that he had to believe totally and absolutely that he would get his life back? In my heart and soul I had already understood this would be a long battle and from these early days, Josh had to know, that I believed he has the strength and courage to "get his life back."

In the end, I realized, I had to place my faith in the Universe that the right words would come to me!

Arriving at the hospital, I abandoned my car as close to the ward as possible.

I knew the "parking angels" would look after me, as in all the months of parking wherever there was a gap big enough for my small car I never received a warning or a ticket. Frankly at that moment I was beyond caring about anything other than what I would say to my son!

I approached the recovery ward with a sense of dread, feeling totally terrified; Josh was laying on the gurney. He had tears in his eyes, and he asked me to come close to him. Once again my aching heart cracked a little more! "Mum I can't live like this. You'll have to get me a gun, take me into a paddock, and somehow I'll figure out how to kill myself!"

I cannot describe my feelings; how I felt at that moment. Fear and horror aren't words strong enough. I knew what I said next was crucial; it had to be totally believable. It had to be the most important conversation I would ever have with my son!

With all we have gone through over all these years since, there would never be a conversation as critical to Josh's recovery as the one I had with

71

him that frightening early morning.

"Josh, I know I haven't been the perfect mother to you, but have I ever lied to you? Made you a promise I haven't kept? Well, you have to believe me, I know in my heart and soul you will walk again. You should have died on the road Sunday night, but you actually made a decision to live. I don't know when or how we will do it, but I will do whatever it takes to help you get your life back! I know absolutely you will walk again!

"You have to have faith and believe that I will not let you down, ever!"

Internally, I was a mess, but somehow the words flowed, amazingly, they made sense, even to me!

I kept saying "You had the choice to die on the road."

"I remember our conversation on the morning after the accident, when you felt your body shutting down, while you were lying on the road, you felt your life leaving you, you fought so hard to stay alive to live! Josh, you have to believe you will recover, together; we have worked through so many injuries in the past." I reiterated, "I seriously don't know what we'll do, but we have to have faith, and I will do whatever it takes."

Within a few hours, we became the Son and the Mum; nothing would stop our quest for Josh to regain his life! The rebirth of his new life, his new beginning; there would be no secrets, no hiding things. We had to be totally honest and trust each other.

The biggest asset we had going for us was our past experience with working through injuries. Importantly, our total trust in each other!

As Paula had said, "We have served a unique, successful apprenticeship in alternative recovery in the past!"

Josh promised to get a little bit better every day, and my commitment to him was to provide the money, and find the people who would help us in our quest for his recovery. Nothing would stop us; no stone would be left unturned in achieving his recovery goals.

This commitment between us was made on the 29th of June 2000, early in the morning.

I look back now, over 14 years later, and I am really blown away by how far Josh has progressed over all these years, looking at those impossible odds of less than 3% recovery to where he is today, and he is still

72

recovering. No one, even me, would ever have believed how far we would come!

Neither of us had any idea of the journey we had embarked on, that crazy Thursday morning!

Later that afternoon Josh was moved to the Acute Spinal Unit of the hospital. Like the ICU, it was so old that the curtains around each bed were mostly broken, hanging off hooks, but it was a new start.

Josh was in critical condition. His bed was the closest to the nurses' station, in case something went wrong. We were told that as he improved, he would be moved further down the ward. From memory there were eight beds, with every bed representing another family dealing with this horrific injury; another life instantly changed forever.

At the end of the ward, the sun streamed over the beds closest to the windows, and as sick as he was, Josh said to me "I want to move to one of the beds near the window." Remembering that he was the kid who always looked out the window, I was excited for him to have such a goal! A tiny goal, one of 100's that would be made, and each one represented another life milestone in his journey to recovery.

However, for the move to occur, Josh had to make significant improvement.

Sometimes in life, we overlook the little things, like the recovery power of the sun shining on your bed.

We introduced Simon to the medical team as Josh's snowboard coach.

At my insistence and after desperate pleading, Simon had come in the Sunday following the accident and spent nearly two hours trying to get a feel for what Josh's injury had done to his body. He was evaluating whether or what energy was still moving through Josh's broken system.

I remember Simon's wife Jennifer coming with him. She was heavily pregnant with their first child, due any time. Both Jennifer and Simon were totally committed to Josh's recovery; they were really the first "experts" to offer us hope!

Oh, "HOPE" was a word we hadn't heard in a week! How I loved that word!

It was only recently that Simon and I were reflecting on our journey.

When we first met, Simon had recently completed his degree, and his practice was only a few years old when he first started working on Josh and me. He was newly married, working with Jenny building their practice, and developing their wellness dream. Josh's journey was so much a part of Simon's belief in the human body to repair itself. I would love to see Josh and Simon write a book together one day.

I commenced a practice from Josh's first day in the acute unit to always close the curtains around his bed, closing them completely for "privacy," even if it was just a "normal" visitor. This was the beginning of creating a need for a "privacy plan" that would allow me the ability to bring in our healing team to perform their valuable work on Josh.

There wasn't a lot of room around his bed, as Josh's little area was plastered with pictures of him doing absolutely everything. They were stuck around the curtain frame, walls, and any other space in his tiny area. They were photos of some event or activity that would give Josh the ability to believe that gaining his life back was achievable. Importantly, he was starting to remember how he had done certain actions in the past. He was figuring out how his body had worked pre-injury.

Ironically there were no pictures of him walking, as he rarely walked, mostly living his life in the fast lane. Precious space was also taken up with his snowboard and motor bike gear. The nurses weren't happy, but even in that first week, I had developed an attitude that was totally focused on Josh's recovery and wellbeing, and frankly I was beyond caring what they thought.

As much as his old photos played such an important part of Josh's early stages of recovery, we took very few photos of Josh during all his recovery years. Josh refused to have pictures or videos taken of him; something we all now regret.

From the early days, I wanted to document his journey through pictures and videos, and yet I always respected his wishes.

My primary concern was keeping Josh fit, focused and healthy!

Lack of care nearly cost Josh his life in the hospital twice!

In those early days, we had no idea of the effect of a minor temperature change on Josh's wellbeing. We were "babes in the woods," totally innocent of the potential danger to Josh's state of health.

Even after all these years, we are still learning the effects of this injury on every aspect of his body and its function!

The nurses moved his bed slightly, leaving him near a draft. It was so light we didn't even notice it, but within a few hours, his weakened lungs (one of his lungs had collapsed since his accident) were struggling; in the end, within hours, Josh contracted phenomena.

His chest was already congested. Due to his injury, he couldn't voluntarily cough, so the nurses had to come in every few hours and basically "bear hug" him, while at the same time putting significant pressure on his diaphragm to clear the mucous from his lungs. Some of the nurses were very gentle, others were quite the opposite. It was painful for me to watch this, and many a time I had to speak to the nurses for being overzealous with their thumping of his chest. I was surprised he never suffered broken ribs from this challenging, confronting procedure.

This procedure occurred several times a day, and each time I felt totally inadequate, devastated this was happening, and with a little care it could have been prevented.

The second time was about a week later, when Josh was left forgotten in his bath for an hour.

(This incident was covered in *Relentless: Walking Against All Odds*, but I need to tell the story again albeit truncated, as the outcome would prove pivotal to Josh's alternative recovery.)

The nurse bathing him was interrupted, leaving Josh, and simply forgetting about him!

Unable to call out due to damage to his throat caused by his feeding tube, he panicked and once again felt his body closing down. It took everything he had to keep his body functioning and alive. Finally he was discovered by a nurse, when they found his hospital bed empty.

In my opinion this was beyond negligence, it was plain and simple a total lack of responsibility on the nurse's behalf, and at that time of the morning when there were always nursing staff everywhere, this was unforgivable.

Once found, Josh was quickly moved from the bath and wrapped in warmed blankets, combined with space blankets, to bring his temperature back up.

I had slipped home from the hospital around 6 AM, so I was oblivious to the drama at the hospital.

Since the accident, I had called Paula two or three times a day to update her on Josh's status.

Every morning since Josh's accident, Paula was meditating asking for guidance from her "guides" in how we could help Josh, but up until this morning, she hadn't been getting anything that would help. She was becoming very frustrated!

In my heart I knew when she was ready the messages would come to her.

It was around 8 AM, I had just reached our home, and the mobile rang. It was Paula.

"Something is wrong with Josh, something has happened. I was meditating and received a message to go to the hospital now!"

"Paula, I have just got home. Josh was okay when I left, they were about to give him a bath."

"I don't care, we need to go now, something has happened!"

"Okay, okay, I'll be right around to pick you up!"

We weaved our away through the city's morning peak traffic, trying to speed up but getting nowhere. Paula was extremely agitated. She was focusing on something, but wasn't sharing it with me. This would be the first time Paula had seen Josh since the accident, although Josh had asked several times when would she be coming in. I had just said "When she needs to!"

I guess the time was now!

I "dumped" the car in a space near the ward, and together we raced to the critical spinal unit.

When we finally reached Josh, he was extremely distressed. The area near his bed was chaotic, and the nurses were wrapping him in heated blankets and space blankets trying to warm him up! He looked like an Egyptian mummy with only his face uncovered. He was frightened and there were

76

tears in his eyes!

Even I, a nonmedical person, could see he was having a panic attack. Paula said "Leave this to me!"

I was beyond angry. "What have you done to my son? Who did this to him?"

As the story slowly emerged, all I could say "We are doing everything possible to keep my son alive and you guys seem to be doing everything possible to kill him!"

I was frightened, angry, and frustrated that something like this could happen!

I really lost all trust and confidence in what was happening to Josh when I or one of our family wasn't with him.

Meanwhile Paula, away from my ranting, was calmly speaking to Josh, telling him that she was clearing his crown chakra. She was quietly speaking to her "spiritual guides," asking questions, getting the answers, and working on Josh.

Her manner was quiet, thoughtful, and calming. She was speaking slowly and confidently to Josh, and he was totally engaged in what she was saying to him.

I noticed he had stopped shivering, and his body was calm. Paula quietly said "Mum and I are going to have a quick coffee. You sleep now. You'll be okay, and we will be back in 10 minutes."

This was a pivotal moment for all of us. Suddenly we knew there was another way and at that moment I knew as hard as the experience had been on Josh, Paula had shown us there was another way. I was totally confident an "alternative" approach to Josh's recovery would be the way we would progress.

For the first 10 days Josh was fed through a feeding tube. It was so confronting to me, especially the first time I saw it.

Thinking back to when Josh was born, he was so small and weak, for several days he was fed through a feeding tube.

Seeing my 18 1/2 year old being fed with a tube again after all these years shocked me and I momentarily thought "I have this vibrant son who is now struggling with a feeding tube, something he had when he was first born."

A defining moment - oh how I hated seeing that feeding tube! It was a constant reminder to me of those first few days of his life in the special care nursery, and it was also a reminder of Josh's new life if he didn't improve.

I had to learn to let it go and not dwell on what I couldn't control. I had to just keep myself focused!

Looking at the positive, his medical team advised us that within a few days he would be able to eat food normally again, although we would have to feed him. But it was a step, a positive step. We were finally, albeit slowly, progressing. I was so relieved.

Josh was losing weight at a scary rate; it seemed to be dropping it off his body in front of our eyes.

Getting some nourishing food into his nearly skeletal body would give him much needed nourishment.

But like everything up to then, we found there was going to be another shock!

I mentioned to the nurse, I was excited Josh would be eating normal food again. I asked her, "What's the food like!"

She answered that she wouldn't eat it. "The food wasn't fit for a dog."

The stupidity of the situation was that we had met with a hospital dietician earlier, who had asked us about his Josh's diet. She even made several recommendations. Remembering this, we wondered why she had even bothered talking to us!

Now we had another problem: the hospital food appeared to be inedible.

This was very concerning to me, since Josh, like me, was very sensitive to food textures. Neither of us could eat fatty or gristly meat. We always ate the best cuts of meat, and quality produce. I quickly realized that no matter what, I had to maintain and provide a healthful diet for him.

Years of living an inner city lifestyle we were in the habit of eating out a lot, so Josh was rightfully fussy about the quality of his food.

With the nurses agreeing the food was terrible, at least we had finally agreed on something!

Suddenly, we had a new and serious challenge! We couldn't believe the hospital would serve such disgusting food to patients who needed all the very best nourishment.

Our only alternative was to bring Josh "home cooked" lunches and dinners. We would cook all his favorite meals and bring them in every day.

We decided he could eat breakfast in the hospital; you can't really mess up toast and vegemite, or the hospital strength Sustagen he drank several times a day along with the seemingly gallons of cranberry juice to stop bladder infections.

Josh drank so much cranberry juice in hospital that he can't even look at it now, let alone drink it.

On the odd occasions when for some reason we couldn't bring his food in, I arranged accounts at several local restaurants. All Josh had to do was to get someone to call in his food order, and the restaurant would deliver his food to his bed.

Ironically there were menus from most of the local restaurants in the spinal unit... a very disappointing situation...a damning of the food the hospital served!

NOT GOOD ENOUGH!

Our favorite local restaurants stepped up to help Josh. As the word got out in our community about Josh's accident several restaurants we ate at regularly before Josh's accident offered to cook Josh his favorite meals. Whether it was fish and chips, Italian food (with extra freshly grated parmesan cheese), or Chinese, there was always someone calling asking us to come by their restaurant on our way to the hospital. On our arrival there would be freshly cooked very hot food, (they all knew his favorites), lovingly wrapped in foil to keep it as hot as possible.

It was the little things, those random acts of kindness, which made our crazy lives that little bit easier!

As soon as the feeding tube was removed, Josh craved McDonalds.

I am not a fan, but Josh was. I embraced his request, because for a few minutes, while we helped him eat the burgers, he felt he was getting some of his old life back.

He said eating Maccas helped him feel "normal," even though it was Wendy or me feeding it to him.

I found the closest McDonalds to the hospital. I went in and explained Josh's situation. The staff was great; they asked me to ring ahead with the order each time Josh felt like McDonalds, and they would have everything ready, wrapped in foil, when I arrived. Josh did not like cold food, so it was a challenge for me to keep his food hot.

I can't overstate the importance of letting the injured person get a taste of something normal even if it is McDonalds.

Early on we were starting to understand that it was the little things that were important; those small "normal" everyday activities like eating McDonalds for a few minutes were really therapeutic. In my opinion, anything that was positive from Josh's "old life" being reintroduced to his "new life" were small triumphs in Josh regaining his old life back.

Chapter 9. Oh, How I Hated the Nights; They Were Scary and Lonely.

During the time Josh was in ICU; there was no way I could stay overnight; there wasn't the room. Although leaving him was devastating for both of us, I was confident Josh was well cared for. He was on 24/7 "one on one care", being constantly monitored or checked. The ICU team was fantastic; nothing was too much for them. He was in the best place for his critical condition to be stabilized, slowly commencing his recovery.

Although I stayed until after midnight most nights, I felt confident he was being well looked after. He really needed sleep, and for that matter so did I.

The daily nonstop visitors were so important to Josh, helping to make the days pass quickly, that by night he was always exhausted. Even then though, he never wanted me to leave, so I waited until he was truly asleep before leaving him to return home.

Everything was so confusing; it was tough mentally, and emotionally. It was as if we had been transported to another world. Our old lives were so far removed that even at that early stage, life as we had known it was becoming more and more a distant memory. Our priorities totally changed. Our old much-loved lifestyle was no more – but it didn't matter.

Nothing felt familiar, or comforting; there was always so much happening and so much to take in!

My heart ached and my brain felt like it was so full it would burst!

I was still experiencing the nagging feeling of wanting to wake up from this nightmare, wishing over and over again we could turn back time!

To stay sane we had to quickly develop routines. We would gain a little confidence, but then in an instant, everything would change and we were back to ground zero again. I wouldn't wish this experience on my worst enemy!

Never leaving was the terror of watching your beloved son struggling to live, hearing him joking with his friends, yet seeing the terror in his eyes that never left them.

Josh stayed in ICU until he was stabilized after his surgery. He was moved to the Acute Spinal Unit, late Thursday afternoon, the 29th of June.

In the Acute ward, his bed was immediately next to the nurses' station, but he no longer had the "one on one" care he received in ICU.

Again I felt totally terrified that something would go wrong!

A pattern started to form. Each time Josh was moved, his temperature would spike and he would be struggling for a day or so. On top of his injury, this further made his life more miserable and extremely difficult.

I decided to stay with him at night, at least until he settled into this new environment, and his condition was more stable.

During the day there would be nurses buzzing around everywhere, yet at night there was only minimum staff on the ward, further adding to my anxiety.

At night his ward was totally different. If Josh needed something urgently I usually had to go find someone! He was so vulnerable, it was frightening.

Josh hated the nights, he hated being on his own. I was too scared to leave him, because I felt I was the only one who cared about him, who had his back, and the nurses always seemed to be so busy.

You also have to remember that we were less than a week from the accident, our lives had totally changed, and we were now part of this strange new world; a world no one can prepare you for!

On the occasions Josh slept, even at this stressful time, I realized the lack of night staff would work well for me in the coming weeks as I commenced smuggling in Josh's recovery team. But those first nights in the critical ward were a whole different story. I was embarking on a massive learning curve!

In the ICU, you are protected somewhat from the effects of the injury. I certainly had no idea about "The Turners"; what or who were they? I was advised by the duty night nurse, that the "turners" would come and turn Josh every two hours. I asked why and was told it would prevent him from getting pressure sores. Again I had no idea what she was talking about. What on earth was a pressure sore? There seemed to be a whole new language to learn; everything was new, so much to learn, so much to understand, and too much to take in!

Josh was in so much pain, he couldn't move to make himself comfortable. He was so miserable and frustrated. He was essentially trapped in his own body!

Josh was still on morphine, so not only was he extremely uncomfortable with the intense pain, he was getting all sorts of mixed messages from his mashed spinal cord to his brain.

I was terrified. I wasn't allowed to turn him, so I had to wait for these guys to come every two hours. There were times that Josh was so distressed he was in agony. One night he was in so much pain he was screaming at me to get the "turners." I had no choice. I went to find the them. I begged them to come now, to help Josh! As kind and caring as they were, they had a schedule. It was so frustrating.

The turners were great, explaining they couldn't break their routine. They would try and hurry to us. At that time, I felt totally useless, totally unable to help my son, totally out of my depth, struggling at every level, constantly feeling I was letting Josh down.

You know, you lose all pride. All I cared about was protecting Josh trying to make him comfortable, trying to keep him focused, trying to understand his and our new life; I didn't care what I looked like, what I wore, it was like you are in a bubble, nothing mattered but Josh and his survival!

It was a truly terrible time, and fortunately Josh doesn't remember much of those crazy early days.

The turners would finally arrive. They were always cheerful and encouraging. They gently moved Josh over, making him as comfortable as possible; Josh would settle for a little while, be calm, and then it would all start over again. I grew to love the turners; for small moments in time they made Josh comfortable and that was everything! They were really great guys, always cheerful and so positive.

As a parent it's a total nightmare!

During the two hour period while we had to wait for the next turning session, I tried to take his mind off things, but there was only so much I could do!

As a parent you are meant to have the answers and protect your children, but a spinal cord injury is like nothing you will experience. The worst was that yet again the medical team was totally negative, and every time we saw something promising they just said it's only temporary, it's an involuntary movement, and he is not controlling anything... blah, blah, blah.

This first night in the ward I decided I was staying the night, but the nurse told me I had to leave. But I wasn't going anywhere. Josh was so vulnerable there was no way I could leave. I asked if there was a rollaway bed I could bring in beside him.

"No there isn't; we don't allow anyone to stay overnight!" So NO for the bed and NO for staying!

I thought, "What is the worst they can do?" I prepared for a confrontation, and I wasn't going anywhere!

I didn't really care what the hospital's rules were. They would have to forcibly remove me!

The chair near his bed was small and uncomfortable. I couldn't sit on it all night, and I remembered the old sofa in the patient's waiting room.

I stayed with Josh until he settled yet again. Then I went down to the waiting room, somehow managing to drag the sofa into the ward, pulling it into the space on the left side of Josh's bed against the wall.

I searched for a pillow; something to cover the filth of the sofa.

I didn't care what it was. I just wanted to put something between me and the sofa. Oh how things ceased to be important at times like this, you almost adopt a "Caveman Survival Existence." I found their cache of clean sheets and pillows. There were no blankets, so I grabbed extra sheets. It was the middle of winter, after all.

Covering the sofa, I crawled onto it. Not sleeping; just the act of lying down was restful.

Josh would sleep fitfully, and then come awake, he was so agitated, uncomfortable and scared. Mostly we were on our own. Every so often a nurse would come in, but they never gave me any problems. I think by that stage they knew better than to challenge me!

The ward was so quiet. I lay next to Josh listening to his breathing, trying

84

to keep him calm when he was awake.

The quiet was punctuated by the turners arriving at Josh's bed every two hours.

While the days raced by, the nights dragged; the darkness was frightening, making everything strange and scary.

I kept my nightly vigil for the next few weeks, packing up my bed every morning, leaving around daybreak to go home, shower, try and eat, answer emails, phone messages then back to the hospital within 2-3 hours.

I have always been paranoid about fire, having been caught twice in wild fires as a child. Fire was something I feared, being trapped and not being able to escape it.

When Josh was three years old, we moved to a home near the beach, in Mt. Eliza (28 miles SE Melbourne). We all loved the house; it was nestled on a large treed site with an extensive native bush reserve behind it. As our first summer progressed, we developed a fire plan in case of wild fires that Josh could understand at that young age

We also developed a plan in case our home caught fire. Josh's bedroom was at the other end of the house from ours, so he was taught how to escape his room safely, and to not worry about us - to save himself. We taught him to get to the yard where he was safe, the place we would meet him.

I know it sounds stupid, but with Josh in hospital, I felt he was extremely vulnerable if there was a fire. Again, a stupid paranoia of mine, but he couldn't move, couldn't save himself and with everyone else potentially needing to be saved, it was another reason for me to stay in the ward at night.

I asked the nurses about what happens if there is a fire, and they just brushed me off, saying they had plans. You have to remember the hospital was very old (it's since been pulled down and rebuilt). In its past life it was a radio station, so it was more akin to a rabbit warren than a hospital. The only way I had peace of mind was to stay with him.

When Josh was transferred to the rehab center, I actually felt he was even more at risk. The facility was cavernous. It was serviced by a central staircase with two wings on either side of it. Obviously during a fire you can't use the elevators. There also were a lot less staff in the rehab center compared to the hospital. At night there was usually only five staff on for both wings.

On Josh's first day in rehab, I quizzed the nurses about security, and their fire plan.

I am sure no one had ever asked this question before. They assured me that staff would come from the main building and wheel the patients in their beds out of danger. At the time there were over 30 in rehab, and on my calculations this was a risk I wasn't prepared to take!

I am sure those reading this think what is wrong with this woman? Frankly I was so tired, had lost so much trust with Josh's medical team, I guess I wasn't prepared to leave anything to chance with making sure Josh was safe!

Josh was admitted to the rehab unit about seven weeks after his accident, and at that stage he couldn't transfer from his bed to his chair; it took time for him to master this skill. He could only slowly manage to roll over in his bed.

I felt he was so vulnerable! He could barely wheel his chair with his hands he was still so very weak.

Once again, Josh hated being alone at night. Usually the last of the visitors left around 8:30 PM, and I stayed after the last visitors. We always kept occupied, chatting, watching TV, and some nights, usually at least twice a week, I would bring either Paula or Isobel in for therapy.

The one positive aspect was that after about two weeks in rehab, Josh finally qualified for his own room. We had the room fitted out just as his room was at home. We brought in his television, stereo, bar fridge (stocked full of goodies), and his own linen and pillows. We tried to make it as comfortable and as much like home as possible.

All his sporting gear was brought in, if we could have done it, we would have brought his motorbike in!

Slowly Josh commenced gaining his independence back.

My goals always were to keep Josh fit and focused. I wanted more than anything for him to gain his independence. I didn't want him feeling lonely; his wellbeing was my main concern, so if it made him happy for me to stay, I would.

I stayed with him as long as I could every night, only leaving when he was ready to sleep. Usually it wasn't long until daybreak.

If the facility was in lock down by time I wanted to leave, I would have to hunt around for security to let me out.

I can say I was not popular with the staff and security due to my night time antics, but I was oblivious to what they thought. I just wanted to make sure Josh was okay.

For some reason once it was close to morning I felt he was safer.

I always enjoyed the crispness of the early morning, driving home with little or no traffic on the road. It was the one time I felt at peace. I enjoyed those precious minutes, alone in my car, roof down, stereo blaring.

Chapter 10.   Our World Became So Tiny

For many months after Josh's accident our world continued to shrink; it became almost minute - tiny!

Josh's and my worlds had been always so full. Prior to his accident we both enjoyed "bigger than Texas" lifestyles, and yet for those first six months, our world became so tiny, so confined.

Our days and nights consisted of hospital, rehab, visits from various therapists, home, maybe some work, but that was it! We learned to live in an isolated bubble/cocoon. Nothing was important, unless it directly affected Josh or his recovery. We appreciated the tiny goals Josh was achieving: scratching his nose for the first time, transferring from his bed to his chair, and rolling over in bed.

Small, tiny steps in his recovery, but every one was important!

I can honestly say, during this time, I totally changed the way I thought about my career; the measurement of success, what was truly important, and you know, I never went back to my old life, even when I had the chance to! Many friends, especially those in financial services, got tired of me refusing invitations and gave up, but some walked the journey with me and still do! I did continue working in financial services for several years, but something had changed in me. I lost the fire; in return I learned to live more in the now!

The days in the hospital and later rehab seemed to fly by. Slowly we forced ourselves into a routine and it worked, and made our "world" bearable.

If for some reason I had to do something away from the hospital, Wendy always tag teamed me! Sleep was a luxury for me; in truth there were never enough hours in the day. If I could grab two or three hours' sleep every 24 hours, I was good to go! Strangely, although I felt exhausted most of the time, I managed to survive on little sleep.

I went from a life of travelling all over Australia with my consultancy work, where I was away most weeks, four out of five nights, reading all the daily newspapers, including the financial journals, to basically living in this tiny cocoon, where nothing else existed. Ours was simply a tiny focused world called Josh's recovery.

I never thought about my old life; for that period of time it ceased to exist!

In some respects, especially in the early days, there were times that you felt you were living in a nightmare. Everything was immediate, new and frightening! The only way we could control anything was to keep it totally simple, trying to keep to our new routine!

We never complained, because we were so grateful that we still had Josh, but when I think back, it was such a crazy time.

I was never familiar with the north eastern area of inner Melbourne, even though I was born in South Melbourne. I was a "South of the Yarra" gal, and rarely ventured into the north! Oh how things changed! Everything changed in a heartbeat! The inner North became my new hood! Quickly, I learned where the coffee shops, restaurants, convenience stores, and gas stations were.

Always seeking coffee to keep me awake, I discovered coffee shops in areas I never knew existed. I even held the odd business meeting in between Josh's therapy sessions. I learned new roads, and amazingly found short cuts. It seemed that sometimes the car was on auto pilot, especially when I was going home alone in the early hours of the morning.

Most of the time Josh was in the hospital and rehab it was winter to early spring. The freezing nights, driving home in the wee small hours of the morning were the only time I felt centered and in control. It was my time for healing, regrouping my mind, reenergizing for the next day. I really enjoyed listening to Andrea Bocelli. I would play his CDs over and over again – "pumping out the opera!"

I loved the drive along Hoddle Street, toward home, turning off at Swan St, travelling past the Tennis Centre, crossing the Yarra - with the views of the City skyline always taking my breath away. It gave me a strangely calming effect.

There were few cars on the road at that time of the morning, and I selfishly grabbed every opportunity to be on my own, in my little world.

It was the little things, the normal things that randomly happened, that were making this dramatic change in our lives more bearable.

I was someone who never wore track pants or Ugg boots out of our home, yet there was many a night when I had to return to the hospital or rehab when I would throw track pants on over winter pajamas going into the hospital. Nothing was more important than being there for Josh. I truly didn't care how I looked or what I wore.

It was simply survival mode!

Mum moved in with Wendy and me to help us. I really think she needed to be with us as much as we needed her with us. Mum had to keep busy, to help her deal with her devastation.

All of our lives were dramatically altered. It was a time of teamwork, focusing on the common goal of getting Josh his life back.

We were taking all Josh's meals in, except breakfast. Mum would cook and clean - she kept busy.

I remember one morning she came into the house crying. She had been cleaning Josh's bungalow, and she found condom wrappers (before the accident Mum would have been angry). Now she was relieved that Josh had led a "normal" life prior to his accident, so there she was, celebrating opened condom wrappers!

Mum's day would be made when she came into the hospital, spending time with her precious grandson, massaging, massaging, and more massaging.

Every so often she would bring him a special treat; a small bowl of lemon cake icing - no cake, just icing. Josh loved it!

Mum's only respite was gambling on horse racing. Every Saturday, no matter what, Mum studied the racing form and placed her bets. We always teased her about her passion/hobby, but we all loved that she enjoyed horseracing so much. Really anything that was normal in those crazy days was welcoming!

Since the accident I had barely eaten. Every time I went to eat something, I felt sick. Mum started following me around the house putting food in front of me in the off chance I would eat something.

My heart ached all the time. Sometimes the pressure was so intense I would have to place my hand on my heart, pushing towards it with as much pressure as I could bear – it seemed to help.

And my brain continued to ache, feeling like it would explode from the information overload. It wasn't like a headache, it simply felt like it was going to burst. The pain was the pressure of overcapacity, too much information!

I had to do something! I made a decision to only focus on what I needed to. I simply deleted memories, experiences from my brain.

Me, who never forgot anything. I had a memory like an elephant, yet I deleted vast blocks of my life. (Still to this day those deleted memories never returned, causing much frustration to my family.)

I issued an instruction, a request to everyone, family, friends, and colleagues - from now on only give me the facts, no superfluous information. If you have something to tell me, or ask my advice about, just cut to the chase, just give me the bare facts!

The experience of managing everything after the accident taught me to detach! I learned to only deal with what I could solve, fix, or answer easily - anything else was too hard. I was not interested; find someone else!

I was no longer the "go to" person for my family. I had no interest in anything other than Josh's wellbeing.

I look back on those times now, and think what a nightmare I was. I totally detached myself from the day to day family and work issues. All I concentrated on was Josh, keeping him fit and focused.

I remember once Mum saying, "If Josh had died, I would have lost both of you." I agreed with her, saying "If he had died I would have disappeared, never to have returned, so great would have been my loss!"

Thank goodness I never researched spinal cord injury on the net.

As a parent, you have to remember that in those early days the web wasn't reliable at all, and there was no such thing as Google.

I believe the fact that neither Josh nor I bothered to research SCI helped us significantly in his recovery. There were never any barriers, or boundaries; in our belief he would recover.

The days always went fast. It was the nights that seemed to drag on and on...

I was quickly realizing that the medical profession didn't get the recovery possibilities of spinal cord injury!

Understanding this one fact allowed me to truly commit to the job ahead of us, moving forward, having faith that below-injury recovery was realistic, not a pipe dream!

I was learning to believe anything was possible!

I started to really appreciate the little things like getting my hair cut and colored. Just having those two hours sitting in the chair being pampered was so relaxing. I was careful to schedule appointments on days I knew Josh had plenty of visitors. Nevertheless, those times were so precious. Small beginnings in getting my life back to a sense of normal, even if only for a few hours.

Through this period I learned many things about what was important. Life, health, and a great attitude is everything!

Focus, belief and relentless optimism are what the priorities were to me in those crazy days.

I did learn an important lesson that greatly helped me. In those first crazy months, I was manic as far as Josh's recovery was concerned. Everything was about Josh and nothing else was important. I was barely eating, grabbing sleep when I could, and not caring what I looked like. Really, nothing mattered other than Josh. One day I mentally "hit a wall." I was exhausted, scared, worried about Josh's condition, and yet trying to be brave, positive, upbeat!

I experienced an epiphany – simply that I could never save Josh if I couldn't save myself. This was a huge realization to me! Simply put, I realized that I needed a time out! It was a time I called my period of "positive selfishness."

Every so often I announced to whoever was with me that I am having a few hours for me. I would have a massage, go for a walk along the beach, or have coffee with a friend.

Initially I found this very hard. I felt guilty, but I kept reminding myself simply to save Josh I had to save myself. I had to see that I had a chance of getting some things from my old life back, even if it was only for a few hours.

These days I mentor many mums and moms, and other loved ones. I take time to explain my philosophy on the importance of indulging in an hour or two of "Positive Selfishness." I emphasize how important it is for them to experience some "me time."

The reality is that no one, nothing, can prepare you for such a catastrophic injury to a child or loved one. In an instant your life is changed. You never get a chance to mourn **your** loss of freedom, losing the ability to be spontaneous; every aspect of your life changes!

You are thrust into a scary, frightening world, where you as a parent or loved one have little control initially.

You can keep going, pushing yourself, but in the end you can get caught up in this "new" world and begin to lose control.

I remember using the following analogy when I tried to explain the experience of those early days: "It was like being in quicksand. So often I felt myself wallowing in this sinking sludge, only to drag myself to the surface, only to lose my footing and fall back. Some days you had to fight with everything you had to free yourself from the quick sand of negativity, fear, and lack of control."

Chapter 11. Family, Friends, Strangers, Celebrations, Surprises, and Disappointments

I want to touch on the importance of support - family, friends, random acts of kindness, and the strangers who become lifelong friends, especially the mums/moms who are dealing with a child or loved one with a spinal cord injury.

I have thought long and hard about this chapter, and what I was going to write. I knew above all I needed to be honest; totally truthful.

I have taken a somewhat tough approach with some of my comments in this section. Where I have been critical, I agonized over including it, but the reality is, for me to write this book honestly, I have to discuss some extremely personal disappointments, as this is the nature of what can happen with an injury like this. Anyone reading this book needs to understand that along with the highs, there will disappointments, some real let-downs, once you are thrown into the crazy, frightening world of spinal cord injury.

It's now over 15 years since Josh's accident. As I look back over my life, I can honestly say I have met some truly amazing people, and had some wonderful and sadly, some tragic experiences on our journey.

In those dark days of 2000 there was little emotional "real experience" support for dealing with Josh's injury from the only experienced people; his medical team. We looked to them for help, but all they did was preach acceptance. According to them, Josh's life as we knew it was over.

Even in those early days we had realized his injury had destroyed Josh's goals, but it didn't mean he couldn't have a new even more rewarding life! Even when we didn't understand things, unless we were with someone in the medical team who was sympathetic, we got nothing from them.

I can truly say that I don't ever remember receiving one ounce of support for our view on alternative recovery, the power of energy, or our unrelenting massaging from one of Josh's medical team. All we ever got was "We were wasting our time."

Initially there were weekly meetings with Josh's medical team, but after a month they became less frequent. The night Josh was admitted we were promised counselling as a family - we are still waiting for that!

Looking back over the years, because of our determination in seeking alternative recovery options, initially it was an extremely frightening position for us, absolutely receiving NO support from the medical team. Yet once we realized that, and accepted that we were on our own, we got the power and strength that over the years has given us enormous knowledge and enabled us to help so many!

Our support really came from my family and our circle of friends, but in reality, no one had ever dealt with anything like this, so it was tough on everyone involved.

At times we felt so isolated, and as much as we tried to remain positive it was a battle!

Oh, how things have changed! These days Josh and I have a global network of friends and contacts. Through Facebook, we are part of a network of people who have been affected by spinal cord injury.

Our network is growing every day, and the friendships we have made along the way, especially with a small group of WARRIOR MOMZ, will last forever; we all share a unique, tragic experience.

For us these days, it's about paying forward. We have learned so much, but we are the first to admit that we can only ever advise families of what worked for Josh. We don't offer magic answers, we just simply tell his story.

In fact we always have told it as it is. As far as recovery is concerned, to achieve any level of recovery from this cruel injury requires dedication, commitment, extremely hard work, and a lot of time, energy and in many cases money! Those focusing on gaining as much back as possible need to train like an athlete, eat like an athlete, have the mindset of an athlete, and finally have unbelievable strength and courage to do whatever it takes!

For me, though, I can connect with a family newly affected by the injury and offer help and encouragement. There are no miracles. It's hard work, but I am so confident that below-injury recovery is possible that I can confidently give hope! I have seen so many gain-below injury recovery, which is everything! I cannot explain the bond I instantly have with mostly moms who have children with spinal cord injury. I am humbled at times that I am able to provide comfort for someone dealing with this horrific injury. It is the greatest feeling and makes all we have been through worth it!

It's interesting. I started writing this chapter early one morning and my computer crashed, losing all I had written. In all the previous chapters, the words have flowed easily. This chapter has had the most rewrites, and has caused me lots of joy and some great sadness.

Along our journey we experienced huge highs, joy, and lows to total devastation, but we survived. We are far wiser these days!

I can't overstate the importance of support during this critical period. There were certainly a group of visitors who really stepped up, and their support continues in some cases to this day.

Josh's accident opened up life opportunities, experiences we never dreamt of. I would like to spend a little time going through some of the highs and lows we experienced.

In acknowledging friends and family, there were so many people. I have just written about a few. I have not deliberately left anyone out.

Early days

The lack of support from Josh's medical team regarding the opportunity of any below-injury recovery possibility was both shocking and disappointing. I can honestly say that the only people who offered positive encouragement towards us were the hospital "cleaners" and the "turners". Those two groups of people were somewhat detached from the medical team, and they saw things that gave them hope. Patients who had been given a similar prognosis to Josh who were gaining improvement were treasured angels to us. They really used opportunities to tell you what they saw while they are doing their rounds of the wards. They were like a breath of fresh air to us; we looked forward to their visits.

Initially, we tried to let as many family members and friends as possible know about Josh's accident – what had happened to him; in those early days we really didn't know much more other than Josh's life was hanging in the balance.

It was important to keep Josh's spirits up and keep all of his friends and our family updated.

What we didn't realize was the far reaching effect of Josh's injury on not just our immediate family, but our wider family: his friends, my friends both in Australia and overseas, and people in our neighborhood who knew him or knew of him.

Josh attended Hobson's Bay High School in Port Melbourne, finishing and passing his VCE in 1999. He was a member of the Middle Park Life Saving Club, so he had a huge network of friends in our local community and they all seemed to hear about the accident at once. You have to remember that 15 years ago communications weren't as instant as they are now.

In 2000, mobile phones were not very effective with little or no network coverage throughout Melbourne.

Many nights I would return home for a few hours while Josh had visitors. The first thing I would do was to play the answering machine, picking up the messages that had been left. Most nights there would be 30-40 messages, many from people I didn't know, but they knew Josh.

One comment was left over and over again – "If anyone is going to recover it's Josh, he's such a wonderful young man, always positive. Please send our love to him."

I tried to call everyone back. I was so grateful for their support!

It inspired me to be more confident for Josh, and for a positive medical outcome! The messages, many from strangers, being so supportive proved to me that even they knew he was capable of improvement, yet no matter what we said, it made no difference to Josh's medical team!

In those early hours and days after the devastation on hearing the prognosis, the support of family, friends and strangers who sent messages of hope was an important process in our early recovery.

The morning after the accident, I rang Josh's close friend Lammo. (Josh had been staying at his family's ski lodge on the mountain when he had the accident.) I went through what had happened with Lammo, asking him if he could contact Josh's Port Melbourne friends and ask them to ring my mobile phone, or Wendy's, to get any updates on Josh's condition.

I promised to call him every morning to give him the latest on Josh's condition, so he could keep their circle updated.

I also asked Lammo to let a very close friend of both Josh's and mine, Bryony (Bry) know about the accident. Josh and Bry had a close friendship. They had gone out together for a year or so, and after they split up they had remained friends. I didn't want her hearing about Josh second hand.

Our home had always been a Mecca for the boys Josh hung out with; I had also asked Lammo to contact a group of girls that Josh had been really close to. They were his "chick" mates.

Oh, how handy Facebook would have been in those days; it would have been so much easier, but social media was non-existent!

There is never a perfect time for an accident to occur!

Josh's accident was the night before the commencement of my busiest week of the year!

Although I had two businesses, the one business that rewarded me the most financially was capital raising. The nature of this business was that I worked most of the year marketing, training, and promoting the investment and strategic nature of it, with the majority of financial investments being lodged and financed in the last seven days in June; the end of the tax year in Australia.

This aspect of my business was extremely hands on, very transactional.

For one crazy week, I would usually be working 15-20 hour days. I was involved in most transactions. Many deals needing finessing, to allow approval prior to the 30th June cut off.

Usually it was a week during which I would get little sleep, and by the end of it, I was always exhausted. Once all the deals were settled, I took a vacation for two to three weeks in July to recover.

It's early morning the 26th of June, and as a sole trader there was no one else to get those deals in but me. With everything else I was trying to get done that morning, no matter what, I had to call my clients and let them know what had happened. Our phones were diverted, alternative plans initiated. My clients, while disappointed, were supportive. They were briefed on where I thought the money would be invested, and I committed to call them later that morning with an update.

What I had already come to terms with was that all those dollars I would earn this week would probably never materialize!

In the year 2000, I had three main clients, and all were looking to me to provide them with crucial investment capital from external investors. Those clients needed the capital to continue, to grow, expand and develop their businesses.

With Josh's life hanging in the balance, the grief I was going through was unbelievable, and yet I knew somehow I had to earn as much income as possible in that week, as it could be months before I would possibly work again. Another nightmare!

It was critical, therefore, that I maintained contact with my investing clients and groups in that last week.

There was no way. I couldn't leave Josh for any lengthy period; I didn't know whether he would live or die!

Somehow, I had to get those "all important" deals in! I wasn't allowed to use my mobile in the ICU, and it was beyond a nightmare! Obviously my mobile was my only means of contact with the outside world.

My clients were very understanding. Somehow, I had to make everything happen.

The stress I was under cannot be described. Basically, if I didn't work I didn't get paid, and knowing what was in front of me, needing to spend the next several months with Josh as close to 24/7 as possible, it was crucial to get as many deals through as I could.

But miracles do happen!

Jenny

A close friend Jenny, hearing of Josh's accident, rang me early that stressful Monday morning, offering to help me. Although she didn't understand my business, she had a lot of experience with client relationship management, she had run her own business for many years, so with help from Wendy and me, she would be able to assist some of my clients. Jenny agreed to manage my office, follow up clients by phone, sending out faxes, etc. She was available to work for as long as I needed her. An angel!

Jenny became my unpaid assistant. She was brilliant, taking over for me with my clients.

100

I would call her each morning, after checking my emails, brief her on what needed to be done and she did it!

I arranged to call her through each day, and any problems she came across we would discuss. I would make a decision, and she would implement it!

Jenny basically kept my business running over that crucial period.

Not being "hands on" I didn't raise anywhere near my budgeted investments, but enough money filtered in over those crucial seven days to keep my clients happy and giving me some precious dollars to keep going!

Once things were less frantic, Jenny did all the research on the insurance policies Josh had. She arranged claim forms, completed them, and all I had to do was sign.

I will be forever grateful to Jenny and her support through that critical time.

Josh's Father

Josh's father and I had been together for nearly 30 years, and we had been married for 24 years by the time our marriage ended.

Josh was 12 when we separated. Even though his father had caused the breakdown, our marriage had been going through serious problems for about two years before it finally ended. Once separated, both his father and I were active in Josh's life. Josh and his dad had always been very close; best mates! Josh lived with him after our marriage ended for nearly 18 months; I was okay with this arrangement, as all I wanted was a happy child. My inner city lifestyle in those days held little joy for Josh.

At the time, it was important for Josh to stay in his current environment, with his friends and in a school he enjoyed. He was happy there, and most of all he wanted to maintain the snowboarding program through his high school in Mansfield. Through that period I paid maintenance and child support to his father.

All I cared about was that Josh was in a happy place mentally (the trauma of our marriage break up was still very raw to him), and he had been devastated. It was therefore crucial for him to stay in a place, surrounded by his friends and to continue snowboarding through the winter.

101

Eighteen months after our break up, Josh came to live with me in Port Melbourne. He saw his father most weekends and some holidays. They maintained their close relationship, which I totally supported. His father was always included in birthdays, Christmas, and all family events. Together we regularly discussed Josh's progress and any issues he may have had. It's fair to say until the night of the accident we worked together as a team of three, as far as Josh's welfare and wellbeing was concerned!

Sadly, one of my biggest disappointments, especially in the first six months, next to Josh's medical team's negativity, was his father.

We had just been told the devastating news. Coming from a life working in financial services, I realized very quickly that Josh's recovery was going to cost a lot of money.

His father made it very clear to me that he would not be in a position to help me financially, so from the first night, I knew I was on my own Thank God I had my family who, although not wealthy, I knew I could rely on if things got tough financially.

A few weeks later, Josh's father offered to help us, not directly, but through his motor bike club. They planned to hold a fund raiser to help pay for Josh's wheel chair. In the end the club raised between $5,000-$6,000, which nearly covered the cost of the chair. My mother helped out with the rest of the costs associated with his chair.

Josh's father has never contributed financially to Josh's recovery, or over the years, to Josh directly.

I was devastated by his lack of financial help. He had full time work, but I was self- employed. It was clear to everyone that if I didn't work there was no money!

Every investment I owned was sold.

I was lucky to have a strong credit rating, allowing me to access credit cards, which towards the end of the first 18 months saw me owing in excess of $60,000.

Seriously, I don't know to this day how we managed. Living with Wendy was a huge help. She was fantastic, and there was never anything that was too much for her. Whether it meant dropping everything to take Josh's lunch or dinner in to the hospital or race off to collect something he needed urgently. Wendy took over the 2nd parent role, so much so that

Josh often called her Mum by mistake.

His father's lack of support even went to meals!

I was in the hospital most of the time, and his father and his partner wanted to have time with Josh alone. I totally supported this, since a boy needs his dad! I asked one thing only; for them to bring Josh's dinner in one night a week. His father knew how fussy Josh was with food so I was very specific with what Josh would/could eat.

Josh had a high sensitivity to certain cuts of meat, so I specified the types of meals and meat to prepare for him.

Not having to worry about one meal a week gave Wendy and me the chance to have one night where we could relax for a few hours, without having to race to the hospital.

I always waited for his dad and his partner to leave before returning to the hospital.

This respite didn't last long. One night the phone rang and it was Josh's dad yelling at me saying how ungrateful Josh was. His partner had prepared a meal for Josh but he wouldn't eat it, he couldn't eat it.

Josh refused to eat the meal, and that's when the call came in to me!

After his father had finished berating me, Josh came on the phone. He was in tears and saying he was sorry. I was furious. His father finally came back on the phone, and I said to him "All I asked was one meal a week, and now I can't rely on you for that. Don't bother; we will bring his food in from now on!"

Thirty years of experiences, adventures, and happy times evaporated in a heartbeat!

As I hung up the phone, I realized that the moment was pivotal to me in finally finishing my relationship with him at any level. I was done, and I decided that I would never ask him for any help for Josh again.

Note: I want to reiterate that up until Josh's accident the relationship Josh enjoyed with his dad was positive; they were great friends and shared many passions especially around motorcycles and cars. To this day they are still close, especially since Josh has married and has continued to improve. My relationship can best be described as cordial. After all, he is the father of my son, and together we created an amazing man.

Outwardly I was coping, inwardly I was fighting with devastation, grief, and disbelief, but I knew I had to be strong for Josh and be always totally confident in his recovery!

Update of Paula's involvement:

The morning after the accident I had spoken to Paula. She, like everyone, was devastated, but she said something that became extremely important. "You must stay with Josh in the hospital for 4 -5 months. You must be there for him. You cannot trust that he will be all right, unless you are with him. If you can't be with him, Wendy must be there!" In shock I asked her how we would manage financially if I wasn't able to work for that long. Paula simply answered enough money would come in to pay what was needed, I needed to have faith. And not surprisingly every so often a check would arrive relating to work that I had done prior to the accident.

She went on to say that by giving Josh this time, you will give him a base for his recovery.

I asked her when she would come in to visit Josh, and she simply answered "When I am ready."

I knew her well enough to understand that she was gathering her energy for what was to become one of her greatest challenges, and in my opinion her greatest achievement.

Friends and Strangers

In those early days, I had many surprises, hearing from people I never expected to contact me, some I hadn't heard from in years, even old school friends. The fact that I never heard from a few of my closest friends, still makes me shake my head in amazement!

The delete button would become a well-used tool over the ensuing years. Once deleted they weren't just deleted from my phone, they were deleted from my life!

I never stressed or experienced any sadness, once someone was out of my life. There were the friends who had spent countless weekends with us enjoying our farm, their son (also an only child) riding motor bikes,

104

weekend after weekend, with Josh. I never heard from them.

These friends had been part of our lives for several years; they weren't casual acquaintances!

I get it that people don't know what to say, but for Heaven's sake say something!

I mention these few instances not to criticize these friends, but I understand that many reading my book will have similar experiences. So by documenting this, you will know you are not alone! This sort of thing happens to all of us!

On the other hand, the outpouring of support from strangers who knew Josh, the number of his friends who arrived at the hospital every day (some for months on end), patiently waiting their turn to visit with him.

The bevy of beautiful young women who were his friends certainly helped the male ICU and critical spinal unit teams get through the days and nights Josh was in their wards.

While there were many that went over and above to help us, there are a few I would like to specially acknowledge. One was:

"Daddy Lammo" (Lammo's dad) -

In those critical early days you would find him visiting Josh every day around lunchtime. He would encourage him, coach and mentor him, and give Josh the belief that anything was possible.

So frequent were his visits, most of the nursing staff though he was Josh's dad.

He came into the hospital day after day, until he was confident Josh was going to be all right. In those early crazy days, Daddy Lammo was an important male resource for Josh, as there were things going on with him that I am sure he didn't want to discuss with his mother.

Daddy Lammo ran his own business. He was a busy man, but no matter what, he always had time for his daily visit to Josh.

I asked him why he was so committed to Josh, and he explained that many years ago a close friend of his became a quadriplegic - sadly he passed away. I guess that was what drove him to support Josh; we were forever grateful!

The Weekend Parties

My goal from day one was to give Josh his life back, his independence.

Having an only child, our home was always filled with Josh's friends.

After his accident I knew we had to focus on Josh seeing he could get his life back. To see his life returning to some kind of normalcy, he had to get back into a situation where he could hang out with his friends, away from the hospital and rehab environment.

Once Josh was medically stable, he was allowed to come home on either Saturdays or Sundays for a few hours. The first time this happened, Wendy and I decided to have an open house, a BBQ, and invite anyone who wanted to see Josh back on his home territory.

We had a large rear courtyard, which amongst other things housed Josh's motorbike.

Many of his mates had asked me to sell the bike, but I refused. I kept saying you have to believe he will ride it again. My thoughts were that if I suggested anything like this to Josh he would think I was giving up on him, so the bike was left in its pride of place in the courtyard for all to see!

Even without social media the word spread like wildfire about Josh's homecoming for a few hours – there was going to be a party!

At the time, Josh was really struggling. He had lost so much weight he looked like a drug addict, but for a few hours he wanted to feel normal.

To be honest, nobody cared what he looked like. They were all so excited and relieved to see him in his own home, away from the hospital.

That first Saturday, we had about 60 come around to hang out with Josh. In those early days he could barely manage to be out and about for more than an hour, but as he got stronger, finally coming home for full weekends, everyone got to stay longer. At times it was like the old days.

The only difference was that Josh was not drinking alcohol. Paula had told him that his body needed to be free from anything other than nourishing food for up to two years, so no alcohol, no Coca Cola, just natural food and drinks. He still enjoyed an occasional McDonald's meal though, but no one cared!

I loved those days when the boys all came over. They were such an important part of Josh's rehab; just small steps in Josh getting his life back.

Seeing Josh's beaming face, loving being with his mates, made it all so worth it!

Bry

A truly loving, supportive, friend was Bry!

Bry and Josh had gone out together for a year or so when they were 16 and 17 years old. They had parted about 12 months before the accident. When Bry found out about Josh, she was in contact with me immediately.

Bry was in her final year of senior school, about to commence her finals, in the International Baccalaureate, so time off for her was a no-no - but was it?

Bry's parents, Susie and Allan, approached her school and gained permission for her to support Josh, initially while he was in the ICU, and later in the critical spinal unit.

Bry would be in the hospital with us most days, and when no one was visiting Josh, she would hold him, massage him, and encourage him to believe that anything was possible, for hours every day. In between spending her time with Josh, she would find a quiet corner, getting her all-important studying completed.

Bry was totally committed to do whatever she had to for Josh, to get him through this critical time. Bry would come into the hospital, when she had no classes, armed with her laptop, studying whenever time allowed.

In those crucial first weeks, she stayed with Josh and me until very late each night. Together we would go home; both of us devastated and so scared for Josh.

One night Josh was in agony. He couldn't get comfortable, and he was extremely frustrated. He was totally trapped in his own body, and he lashed out at us.

Bry quickly left the room; she was devastated! She kept saying what if we've lost the old Josh, what if we never get him back? I followed her out of the room, holding her, saying, "We have to believe he will be all right," explaining to her that he wasn't angry with us. His frustration was at a level we will never understand! In an instant, Bry pulled herself together, since she was determined not to let Josh down.

There were so many nights when we were both so tired, we would get lost driving home to her place, and somehow, I always managed to get her home safely.

Most nights, I returned to the hospital after dropping her home!

Bry's almost daily commitment to Josh lasted several weeks. Once he was in rehab, life was easier. You would find her bouncing in with her girlfriends making sure Josh was always in good spirits and having fun. They even managed a food fight one day in his rehab bedroom. I came in to see chocolate cake everywhere.

Times like this were so precious! I loved this, and we needed to have some fun after these months of sadness.

I will always be grateful to Bry's parents for allowing us to "borrow" her during this very critical time of Josh's recovery.

Bry, after all these years, is still in touch with me regularly. There is never a time when she doesn't ask how Josh is going.

These days, Bry and I enjoy a fabulous friendship. She is like the daughter I never had, and when we are together we always have so much fun!

Paul, aka Dutchy

Once Josh was transferred from the ER to ICU, there were many visitors, especially during the day.

One afternoon, Wendy was in the ICU waiting room, organizing his visitors, two at a time for no more than 10 minutes. I took the opportunity to sneak home for a few hours, to catch up with some emails.

Josh's friend Duchy's dad Bill had offered to take me back to the hospital in the evening to give me a break from driving.

There was not too much talking between us all as Dutchy, Bill, and I drove across the city back to the hospital.

Once we got to ICU, Bill and I stayed outside, letting Dutchy go in to see Josh on his own. I said I'd be in to see Josh in 10 minutes.

There was only one way in and out of the ICU wing so when I went in to Josh, he was sleeping and there was no Dutchy.

I thought he must be here somewhere in the ward, knowing he hadn't left.

Now Dutchy is a 6'6" Aussie Rules footballer. He and Josh had been friends since Josh had moved back to Melbourne to live with me about five years earlier. They were always together! In fact Dutchy had been snowboarding with Josh earlier in the week of the accident. They had been boarding hard and partying just as hard, both celebrating their freedom after graduating from High School. They were having so much fun!

So where was he?

I found a room all closed up, and there was Dutchy, his heart was breaking. He was sobbing for his mate!

It was devastating for me to see him so broken hearted! I sat down next to him, quietly saying Josh would be fine, he would recover, and we all had to believe that!

Dutchy was apologizing to me for being so upset. I assured him that I was fine, that we had to be totally confident Josh would recover, we had to have faith, and we had to believe in anything being possible!

After that first night, Dutchy would come into the hospital and without any prompting or hesitation start to massage Josh's feet and hands. Josh would always tell him to stop, but Dutchy would ignore him, and would keep on massaging, saying he wouldn't stop until Josh could walk out of there.

Once Josh was discharged and back in our home, there were many mornings that Dutchy would come by to take Josh to the gym. Some days he carried him to the car. He was determined that he would do as much as possible to help Josh recover. Dutchy and Josh are still mates to this day, both getting married within a month of each other in 2013. Dutchy never gave up on Josh; he always believed he would recover. Dutchy is such a special person to all our family, we will be forever grateful to him.

Daniel

Daniel and Josh had been friends since we moved to Mansfield in 1992. They attended the same school, discovered snowboarding, and had much in common.

They were always together, enjoying a friendship built on common interests. They were like brothers.

When Josh's father decided to move back to Melbourne from Mansfield, halfway through the school year, I arranged for Josh to board with Daniel, his brother Stephen, and their father Geoff.

I felt it was important for Josh to be able to complete his year at the high school.

Geoff was a single dad at the time, and I was conscious of Josh not putting pressure on Geoff with extra work, so I would drive up to Mansfield on weekends, to help him with cooking, cleaning, washing, trying to make it easier for them.

Through the snow season, I would be on the mountain with the boys most weekends, supporting them when they competed, being the cheerleader, gofer, and driver.

Their competitions were mostly at night. I would be up there on the mountain in the freezing cold, cheering them on, and afterwards driving them home off the mountain once their competitions were over. It was a busy, fun time, and we all became very close! Daniel was a talented snow boarder; at one stage he was ranked number two in Australia, representing Australia, and competing overseas.

Daniel was with Josh when he had the accident. Daniel was actually taking the photos of Josh doing the jump. Throwing the camera to the ground when Josh crashed, he was the first to reach Josh.

It was Daniel and another friend Luke (Dingo) who kept Josh alive while they waited for ski patrol. Daniel and Geoff came down from the mountain the day after the accident bringing all of Josh's gear back.

What Daniel went through that day I can't imagine, but I do know after it, he seemed to lose the passion for snowboarding. It was all very sad, and so many times Wendy said we need to help Daniel deal with Josh's accident, but I was always focused on Josh. I have many regrets about this now!

Daniel and Chris were with us the day Josh started snowboarding again.

Wow, what an afternoon that was. Watching the three of them back on the slopes boarding together was something I will remember forever.

I had received a lot of flak from many people by encouraging Josh to return to snowboarding. My answer was always defiantly the same: "He has worked so hard to recover that I would never stop him from doing anything he wanted. Why would he have committed so hard to his recovery, not to be able to do something he loved so much?"

I really believe Daniel and Chris were as excited as we were, seeing Josh glide off on his own, yet again proving that "doctors don't know the power of the mind to achieve recovery."

Daniel is an amazing man; he is always there for Josh, and he has totally supported him through his recovery, kept a watchful eye on him when Josh was in full party mode, and they are best friends forever.

Recently he was one of Josh's groomsmen! What a wonderful day that was, seeing them standing together!

Daniel is like my second son. We will always be so very close!

My mother and my sisters, Susan and Wendy

were sensational, always there when I needed a break, always there for Josh massaging, massaging, and then more massaging!

There was always a sadness in Mum's eyes after Josh's accident, something she carried to her grave.

Susan was so supportive, helping us whenever she had free time, with massaging, meals, love, and support.

Wendy has certainly been the extra "parent" to Josh, never stopping in her commitment to support and assist him, to recover.

111

There was never anything too much for her. Even though she worked for herself, Wendy would drop everything to bring a meal or something he needed in to Josh. When I was exhausted, Wendy, who was also exhausted, stepped in to help. When I had to do something taking me away from the hospital, Wendy would always be there assuming role of Josh's advocate.

Josh and Wendy love each other unconditionally, yet they argue, constantly "banging heads," but their support for each other is apparent to everyone.

I can honestly say it didn't matter whether it was day or night, Josh was surrounded by family and friends throughout his 4 1/2 months in the hospital and later in rehab. None of his friends deserted him; they were always there and all shared in the massaging.

Three years later when Josh celebrated his 21st birthday, he sent out over 300 invitations, expecting around 100 to attend. That night everyone who was invited came, it was truly a night of celebration for us all, everyone saying there was no way they would have missed his special night.

Dom

My friend, Dominica, "Dom" rang from Ireland nearly every day in the first months of Josh's recovery, and thereafter at least weekly.

Dom was a huge support to me personally. We had been friends a long time, originally meeting through working together.

She and her husband Pearse returned to Ireland in the 90's. We never lost contact with each other, and in fact our friendship grew stronger.

While they were living in Australia, Mum had them over for Christmas celebrations a few times, so they were well known to our family.

Josh and I had enjoyed a trip to Ireland in 1998, where he met her extended family, and becoming friends with one of Dom's nephews. They enjoyed a few nights out together. Josh really loved the Irish hospitality, and looks forward to the time he can return there.

After the accident, Dom's mother Dolly prayed and lit candles for Josh's recovery at her local church in the village of Tuam every day for several months, until she was confident he was recovering.

Marie

We had been friends for several years, sharing a passion for drinking great wines, too many memorable dinners and having fun. We were always up to some mischief together! I had been to dinner with her in Perth, the night before Josh's accident. Marie had been battling her own health issues and I had been supporting her through it. Her final words to me that night as I climbed into the taxi for the trip to the airport to fly back to Melbourne were:

"I wonder what Joshie will do to himself this weekend,", and my answer was "he's on the mountain -- he can't get himself into too much trouble."

Ugh -- famous last words!

Marie always felt bad, saying to me that she felt she had "mozzed" him that night, but as I said to her, "nobody had any idea this would happen, especially me. I always thought he was safe on the mountain."

Marie has been an amazing supportive friend to both Josh and me. She flew over from Perth for Josh and Amelia's wedding, saying to me "This was one wedding she wouldn't miss!" The day was such a celebration for us all!

Dana and John

True to their word, Dana and John took Josh's MRI's to an orthopedic surgeon in Los Angeles. He agreed with our medical team in Melbourne's prognosis. He believed on the basis of the MRI's that Josh would never get out of bed again.

Like us, this didn't deter them. They were a fantastic support.

Dana and John flew from the USA to join our family in Australia for Christmas 2000, spending about three weeks with us.

They were both totally committed to seeing Josh recover as much as was humanly possible, working with Josh every day on goal setting, physical activities, and keeping him focused. We all had a fun family Christmas together! For a change we decided on seafood for our Christmas dinner.

John and Mum took responsibility for peeling prawns and preparing the oysters, laughing and eating while they worked.

For that brief moment in time, for the first time in months, we were all happy. We were living the moment, enjoying normal Christmas celebrations.

Everyone was laughing and having fun. Quite a relief after all the months living with fear and sadness.

We decided to go to Noosa Heads in Queensland for a 10 day holiday together. Noosa is such a beautiful place, and we thought the change of scenery would do Josh good.

While in Noosa, John encouraged Josh back into swimming again, taking advantage of a calm lagoon on the outskirts of Noosa.

John set a challenge for Josh to swim to a yacht anchored in the lagoon, the challenge being to touch the rudder! Josh not only touched it once, but several times. This was when John started calling Josh "Rudder Boy."

We were all astonished! It wasn't five months earlier that we were given the prognosis of complete quadriplegia never to get out of bed yet here he was swimming. It wasn't his usual powerful stroke, yet he was able to move some distance without failing...not just once but several times.

Bit by bit Josh was getting his life back.

I loved seeing Josh back in the water. He was raised near the beach, and had his first swimming lessons when he was six months old. The water had been a huge part of Josh's life up until his accident, and seeing him back in the water was therapy for my broken heart.

Josh swimming again was just another positive step in rebuilding Josh's body. I was more and more confident we were on the right track with Josh's rehab.

While in Noosa, John and Dana set a series of new recovery goals with Josh. The payoff was, if he achieved them, they would pay for him to have sessions with a "Chi Master" Mark in California.

Achieving every goal they set for him, in May 2001 Josh was winging his way to Los Angeles.

Our Swiss Family

Josh's host family in Switzerland, Ernst, Regula and their three sons had planned a trip to Australia. They were to spend a week with me in Melbourne, a few days snowboarding with Josh on the mountain, after which they planned to travel by car up the East Coast of Australia to Cairns.

Josh had his accident about a week before they were due to arrive.

As you can imagine, our lives where in total chaos, certainly, in no position to play host to a family of five!

I called Ernst in Switzerland. Fortunately, he could speak a little English,

I explained what had happened to Josh, but I wasn't totally sure how much he understood. I basically told him that everything had to change. I was no longer free to spend time with them, and it would be difficult for them to stay with us.

As a temporary measure we would set Josh's bungalow up for them to sleep the first night they arrived.

We met them at Melbourne Airport early evening, after their long flight from Zurich. They wanted to go straight to the hospital; it was pretty horrific for them. Josh was so excited to see them, but the devastation showed in their faces!

I knew they loved him as their 4th son. It was a night that was truly bittersweet for us all!

For the first two weeks of their holiday, now totally changed, our good friend Jenny yet again stepped up, taking over from us, acting as their tour guide, and hosting them around Melbourne.

We were so grateful to her. Jenny made sure that they had a fantastic time, putting them up at her home, driving them everywhere, making sure they enjoyed our city. Yet their visit was tinged with sadness for us all!

There are so many to thank! You can never underestimate the power of support!

Those who tirelessly worked on Josh's recovery, Paula, Isobel, Simon,

115

Bing, Jackie, Ben Robinson (Josh's Personal Trainer for over four years); you are all amazing supporters, and most of you are still part of our journey all these years later.

Eating out!

A huge part of Josh's rehab, from my view, was for him to see he could get his old life back.

Once we were able to break him out of rehab, for a few hours or for the weekend, we would go to his favorite restaurants around Port Melbourne.

Arriving at a restaurant, he would transfer onto a normal chair, and his wheel chair would be discretely hidden away in the rear of the restaurant somewhere out of sight. This was important for Josh as he hated his wheel chair. That hatred spurred him on to walking; he always said he didn't want his life defined by a wheel chair.

For a few hours, out of his chair, Josh was able to feel normal.

A memorable restaurant experience was the first time we returned to Lynch's, in South Yarra.

Sadly, Lynch's is no longer there. It was a devastating day for Melbourne cuisine when Lynch's closed its doors.

For many years, when Josh and I had something to really celebrate, we always chose Lynch's. It was an exclusive, expensive restaurant. The food and wine list were phenomenal, and the service excellent.

Josh needed to get out of rehab for a few hours. We had so much to celebrate that we decided to have Friday lunch at Lynch's with Bry and a few of her girlfriends.

Josh and I arrived early. He was seated at the table, his wheel chair hidden somewhere out back, when the girls arrived. Josh had lost so much weight he looked really ill, but nothing was going to stop him from having fun today.

Josh and the girls were in fine form, lots of laughing and animated chatter! Slowly the restaurant filled with many of Melbourne's business community; Paul Lynch (the owner) was actually seated in a table behind us.

116

The more people arrived the noisier the restaurant became. It was always a big party when you ate at Lynch's; that was the charm of the place!

I guess many eating there wondered about the table full of vivacious young girls, a young man who appeared quite ill, and the old gal - me.

In those early days Josh, could go from great to "Mum I need to leave very soon." Quickly, we finished lunch, asking for his wheel chair.

As discretely as was possible, the chair was brought to the table. The whole restaurant section, hushed. As Josh wheeled his way out, Paul Lynch leaned over and said to me "It's such a shame; he's such a terrific young man."

I confidently answered, "Next time we are back, he will walk in, and he'll be fine."

True to my word, some months later we planned to dine at Lynch's to celebrate Josh walking. I phoned for a reservation, and I was told the restaurant was full that night. I immediately said "Remember the young man who came into the restaurant in his wheel chair? Well, he's walking and wants to come back to Lynch's to celebrate!" Immediately she said "We'll make room for Josh!"

Josh walked into Lynch's that night, and our table was the pride of the place in the center of the restaurant.

It's the little things that occurred on our journey, collectively helping to get Josh to where he is today. Yet again, everything we did was all about him seeing he could get his old life back!

Mum's Note

All though his hospitalization and later rehab, I never encouraged Josh to hang out with the others who were injured and sharing his ward or rehab, other than him being sociable.

The "no researching" the Internet was backed up with not bonding with the others going through the injury with him. Sounds tough and it was, but I didn't want Josh taking on other patient's frustrations and anger.

He needed to concentrate on himself!

I admit I was a nightmare, but I will never regret making and enforcing my rules.

Josh has achieved outstanding results against all odds, by never really understanding his injury!

My little "bans" didn't stop him getting into mischief with some of his fellow "inmates," challenging each other to electric wheel chair races around the rehab.

Our past attitude to support and help is the opposite of where we are now, where both Josh and I are constantly mentoring those enduring this cruel, unrelenting injury and their families ...and we love it!

Our past attitude with not hanging out with those with SCI while Josh was in the hospital and later in rehab is the opposite of where we are now, where both Josh and I are constantly mentoring those enduring this cruel, unrelenting injury and their families ...and we love it. We feel if we can help one family, our journey has been worth it. It's really why both of us chose to write our books. We are careful not to make recommendations, and rather just focus on telling our story and what worked for us.

Part 2 - The Glimmer - There is Another Way

Chapter 12.   Doctors: Great at Mending, Sadly NO Good at Healing!

Since we were thrown in to this crazy world, after all these years, I am still amazed at the lack of much of the medical profession embracing the evidence of the potential for "below-injury recovery." The majority of doctors across the world continue to ignore the successes of those, who against all odds, have shown below-injury recovery over their original medical prognosis.

It's now 2016, and there has been so much progress in research and knowledge of spinal cord injuries, and yet many doctors look at an injury and they continue to categorize recovery, or lack thereof, by statistics; i.e., Josh was an 18 1/2 year old male, C5 – T1 complete quadriplegic. He wasn't a name, he was a statistic, he was pigeon holed, "Less than 3% CHANCE OF ANY RECOVERY, life in bed, maybe if lucky a motorized wheel chair with mouth controls."

This opinion was made in the first nine hours of Josh's injury.

Thank God we didn't listen; his medical team, the experts, were totally wrong!

How many lives have been ruined by a negative early prognosis of recovery opportunities and options?

How many lives are lost? How many of those who are injured just give up?

Sadly, in 2016, this negativity is still prevalent in most of the medical communities throughout the world. The comments I receive on the Warrior Momz Facebook page echo our early experience with those first weeks of Josh's hospitalization. Frankly, I just don't get it!

Our recent feedback is telling us, even today, that when your loved one is admitted with a spinal cord injury to a hospital there are doctors still of the belief that where there is (in their opinion) no chance of recovery, they may choose not to repair some of the damage or fail to reattach a muscle.

They basically make the decision that this person won't walk or recover again!

A friend in the medical profession once told me how she instructed the surgeon operating on her son to operate on him as if he would walk again, don't assume he is never going to get function back in his legs. I questioned her, saying I thought all doctors would have a view to give the patient the best possible chance to recover. Her answer was not always.

Over the years I have heard of many such stories. Frankly, it makes my blood boil, with the research in stem cell, re wiring neuro pathways, and below injury rehabilitation programs breaking new ground every day, I believe the surgeons should share the view that science and research will provide recovery options, so every patient should have the best possible recovery chances set up in their surgeries.

We believe that Josh's right hip flexor muscle may not have been re-attached properly during his surgery.

To rebuild Josh's fractured C6 and C7 vertebrae, a surgeon removed bone from Josh's right hip. The bone was crushed and molded to reform the damaged vertebrae.

Josh knew something had happened to his right leg.

After waking up the morning after his surgery, Josh instinctively knew something had happened to his upper right leg during his surgery. He repeatedly said to me, "Mum listen to me, my right leg feels empty. They have done something to it."

At that stage Josh could not feel anything below the injury level of C5, but as strange as it was, Josh knew mentally that there was a detachment from his physical body to his right leg.

We requested film of the operation, but there was none available. Josh's Specialist Consultant assured us the operation was uneventful "text book" and had progressed to plan.

Exhausting every avenue, we felt there was nothing else we could do, yet Josh was adamant – his right leg "felt empty."

When Josh started his recovery it was determined there was a problem with his right hip flexor muscle. No matter how much rehab Josh did, his right hip flexor muscle was always a problem.

During his first visit to Project Walk in 2011, the recovery therapists focused on this area of his upper leg, resulting in a slow process of the hip flexor slowly showing some life, confirming the significant problem with this very vital muscle.

A Timorese Sharman, (2011-2012) not knowing anything about Josh or his injury, or for that matter that he had even had surgery on his right leg, stated the first time he met Josh that, "This man's right hip flexor muscle had not been reattached to his leg during a surgery."

This talented healer confirmed to us something we had long felt; he diagnosed the problem from watching Josh walk. He didn't need MRI's. He simply watched him walk and came to his conclusion from what he observed!

Not good enough, not acceptable!

As previously mentioned, the night Josh was first admitted to hospital, his doctors didn't care that he was an athlete, that he was used to training and setting goals, or that he had worked through many other injuries including an L5 fracture.

They didn't take into consideration that he had been under the care of a chiropractor for two years who had essentially repaired and rehabilitated his L5 injury with adjustments and massage, combined with an exercise program. Sure, it took two years, but Josh's back was healed without the need for surgery.

All the doctors cared about the night Josh was admitted was that we accept their prognosis for "Josh's benefit." Their final prognosis was made within nine hours of him being admitted. As one they all worked on the belief that we needed to accept that his life was now confined to a bed - we needed to help Josh accept this; we needed to keep Josh focused on his new "life."

All these years later, I know that if I had accepted their prognosis that fateful night Josh would be dead; my son could never have accepted the life they predicted for him.

Josh and I have stated on many occasions that we were grateful for the excellent work done by his medical team at "mending" him, but "healing" him was not on their agenda.

The one exception to this was our general medical practitioner, Dr. Graeme Baro.

Graeme had been our family doctor for several years. Graeme had known Josh since he was 12, and he had been privy to some of the alternative options we had used in the past for dealing with his various injuries.

I contacted Graeme the day after the accident, and he quickly became a fantastic resource to me. Josh's injury was beyond anything I could understand. I felt I was failing him on so many levels through my lack of knowledge. Graeme patiently talked me through so many of my fears, and as simply as possible explained the injury.

I was slowly building my recovery team and Graeme would become an integral member, a truly valuable resource for me.

As we knew the extent of Josh's injury, Graeme continued to explain in layman's terms what we should expect. He agreed with our view on the massaging of Josh's extremities, and he explained to me why it was important, basically echoing what Simon had said.

Graeme had studied medicine with some of Josh's specialist team, so he was aware of the various personalities we were dealing with. This was great, as he was proactive with some very helpful insights.

Graeme was extremely positive regarding the talents and expertise of Josh's surgeons. This made me feel a lot more confident with the planned surgery taking place late Wednesday evening.

Without hesitation Graeme gave me his mobile phone number saying to call him whenever I needed any help at all. Yeah! I finally I had a doctor I felt I could speak freely to and what was more important - he knew Josh!

Graeme was very aware of Josh's determination and his never-give-up attitude, so he was able to provide me with great comfort, helping me to slowly gain some confidence.

Because he was Josh's primary doctor, the specialist team was obligated to provide him with reports on his progress.

Graeme, like all the others in our team, has been on an amazing journey with us, which still continues to today.

Graeme believes Josh's story needs to be told and he is prepared to help us in any way possible.

Josh and I have been highly critical of the lack of positive support from his medical team after his operation, particularly not offering any encouragement to him at any level.

The medical team never changed their view that Josh would never recover any function or improvement below his injury - **against all their predictions, he did improve, and he walked!**

Their medical talent was never a question in our minds. We always believed we had the best team to rebuild his fractured vertebrae and remove the bone fragments from his cord.

We completely respected their knowledge and expertise. As professionals we believed they were amongst the best in Australia, but as we've previously mentioned, they were great at mending but not healing.

Today, when members of his medical team are asked about Josh, they now say Josh preaches "false hope" when he is asked by families to visit their injured loved ones in the hospital! They discourage families from speaking to Josh or inviting him into the hospital.

Please don't ask me to explain false hope versus no hope! (Which is what they still preach.)

Neither Josh nor I understand this, given that we know they didn't misdiagnose him!

Actually, it's very disappointing and closed-minded on their behalf!

Knowing that they did not misdiagnose Josh's injury, and seeing what he has achieved, I often wonder if they ever think about how far Josh has progressed, and wonder how he has done it?

There was however, a wonderful story involving one of his specialists that took some months to evolve.

(To protect the doctor involved, we are not using his real name - I will refer to him as Dr. Jeff.)

A quote from Dr. Jeff (after we finally met him some months after his surgery on Josh): "To think two strangers helped save each other's lives!"

Josh's specialist surgical team wanted to give Josh the very best chance to for recovery, we were advised the surgery would be very delicate especially the removal of the fragments from his cord. His surgery was delayed for a few days while equipment was brought in from the USA.

It was a stressful time for us all, because his neck, where the break was was unstable, and there were fragments of bone still in his spinal cord...and of course at that stage Josh didn't know the extent of his injury.

As I mentioned on several occasions earlier, I needed Josh to go into the operation focused, and confident that he would be healed and okay; anything less he would not have survived.

It was a nightmare keeping his condition from him for those three days, but we knew his life depended on it!

The surgery was finally scheduled for Wednesday 28th June 2000, three days after he had been admitted.

The surgery didn't commence until late in the evening. It was scheduled to go for several hours.

Although there were many in his team that night, there was one surgeon who would share a unique and special experience with Josh, taking several months to unfold.

Dr. Jeff was responsible for the delicate work around the break; he was probably our most critical surgical team member.

After the operation was concluded, Josh was sent to recovery.

The next morning Paula rang me saying whoever had operated on the cord area had set Josh up for recovery; his surgical skills were magnificent. She received this "message" during one of her daily meditations.

She reiterated this again some days later when she finally saw Josh.

To keep the family informed, Josh's medical team held weekly meetings with us to update Josh's condition and ongoing care. After what Paula had said, we were keen to meet Dr. Jeff. He didn't attend the first meeting or the second. I asked when we would see him. The doctors were very evasive, refusing to give me an answer!

By coincidence I ran into one of my colleagues in financial services who was asking about Josh and enquired who the orthopedic surgeon was. I said Dr. Jeff; he knew him well, through his football club, but then he said "Well, it's terrible what's happened to him."

124

He had heard that Dr. Jeff had been admitted to a hospital with an acute illness and wasn't expected to survive. From what I was able to find out, it would have been a day or two after he operated on Josh.

Josh and I were devastated. This man had done such intricate, specialized surgery in repairing Josh's vertebrae that night, potentially saving his life, and now he was fighting his own battle for life.

Josh asked me to write to him, thanking him for his amazing work, telling him of his goal to walk out of rehab before his 19th birthday on November 13th 2001. (Just over 4 1/2 months from being admitted.)

Josh asked me to encourage him to use his amazing talent to heal himself.

Months went on, we didn't hear anything, and we didn't know if he was alive or dead.

On the 11th November 2000, Josh was discharged from rehab. He walked out of hospital at about 2:30 PM, never to return as a patient. I took photos, and once again we wrote to Dr. Jeff. We included photos and Josh outlined his plans for the future. We both thanked him again, wishing him success with his own battle.

Still we didn't hear from him!

One morning the phone rang. It was Dr. Jeff's receptionist, asking Josh and me to visit his surgery office for a check-up. We were elated that Dr. Jeff had survived and was back at work!

Arriving at his Melbourne surgery, we were taken straight to his office. We walked in, Josh using his elbow crutches.

Dr. Jeff warmly greeted us, shaking Josh's hand. It was a special and unique moment.

Dr. Jeff went on to say how two strangers had saved each other's lives. He said "In my darkest hours I read your letters, and knowing in my mind it was impossible for you to walk, I was greatly encouraged when you did. I then thought anything was possible, and I focused on my own recovery."

Josh immediately said "So you're cured?" Dr. Jeff said "I'm in remission."

Josh looked at Dr. Jeff and said "If you don't see yourself cured you will never be."

Another powerful moment!

I was totally blown away with Josh's response. It offered me more insight into how he thought, and I realized this is exactly how Josh thought every day of his recovery – he always saw himself healed.

Some weeks later (time would have been March/ April 2001), Dr. Jeff contacted us and asked if we could come in to speak to the hospital's spinal team about Josh's ongoing recovery. It was to be held in the teaching area of the hospital.

The catch was that we had to be there at 7 AM.

Getting Josh anywhere, even today, at 7 AM, is always a challenge!

Somehow I managed to get Josh's wheel chair into the trunk of my Miatta; a major achievement!

Although Josh was walking at the time, he still relied on his wheel chair. He continued to use the chair for a further 2 1/2 years, before finally "retiring it" in favor of elbow crutches.

Josh had managed to transfer up, from the car seat into his chair, so to all those who told me to sell my car - I said "Nothing is impossible when the will is strong!"

Josh was suited up, in "business dress". This was an important day for him!

On our arrival, we were shown to a changing room, Josh was asked to strip down to his jocks. Neither Josh nor I were happy at this request and we challenged the medical team over it. Apparently the team wanted to examine him.

Josh was not happy, and what was worse, we didn't know any of the doctors involved. Finally Josh agreed, he quickly undressed changing into a theatre gown, and he climbed onto the gurney.

To lighten Josh's disappointment I joked with him "At least you had your Calvin Kleins on."

Josh was wheeled in to a mini auditorium, with seats circled around a presentation area. The female doctor who was examining Josh was apparently the head of the rehab unit Josh had been in. At least that was what we were told.

She knew nothing about Josh, didn't know any of his history with the hospital or rehab other than what she had read! She made no effort to ask Josh about what he had been doing to progress his recovery from a complete injury to walking.

There were about 50 people, nurses and doctors all grouped the team examining Josh.

The doctor commenced her examination...This is how it went:

Josh's legs were still prone to quite intense spasms and that day was no exception!

The doctor noted that Josh had high spasticity in both legs, saying "If he was currently walking it would be short lived." She went on and on and on, saying "He would be back in his chair in no time, and in her opinion, Josh would never walk in the long term."

I could see Josh getting very frustrated. He was devastated; rather than the team being positive, we were once again subjected to the same old negativity we experienced while in the hospital and rehab.

I was ready to explode. It was the same old S&^t, blah, blah, blah...

I was so angry, I looked at Dr. Jeff, who was across the room from us and mouthed what the F^$%* is happening here? I could not believe this was happening all over again, what was wrong with these people?

He stood and said, "In my opinion, Josh should never have walked because his cord was so badly crushed. Josh has done something no one with such an injury had ever achieved, in his experience, in Australia before. He walked!!!" He then made a statement that rocked us to our souls...

He said "We need to sit down with this young man and find out what he has done to walk. WE NEED TO LEARN FROM HIM!"

Josh and I looked at each other and smiled smiles of relief. Finally we were getting through to these people! Finally they would learn something that may change the way they speak to the newly injured and their loved ones!

Just maybe change their attitude to one of the possibilities of below-injury recovery. Be interested at least in working with Josh on a research study, which he was more than willing to participate in!

127

So we waited for them to ask us questions, none came!

This is an extract from a private letter "Dr. Jeff" sent to Josh. I have replicated word for word. Part of it I omitted so there was no way he can be identified:

Dear Joshua,

I finally have improved sufficiently to catch up with work related matters. During this process I came across your letter dated the 4/2/2001, which I was very pleased to receive. Thank you for the photograph that was taken when you were discharged from hospital. It was fantastic to see you walking again. Our lives have crossed in a most curious fashion in that you sustained a devastating injury to your neck which had a terrible impact on your life and 2 days after I performed surgery on you namely 29/6/2000 I presented to my local doctor .... No doubt you have improved further since you wrote me in Feb 2001, and I hope your life is coming back together again. I was very appreciative of your letter in 2001, when I was recovering from the effects of .... like you I felt as weak as a church mouse and even going for a short walk was difficult. When I read about your progress it lifted my spirits. I was thrilled because most of the spinal cord injured patients that break their necks don't do well and remain bed bound or stuck in wheelchair. It is fantastic when a spinal cord recovers as it has in your case and hope that you get back most of your body functions and that you can regain a full lifestyle again".

Chapter 13.   Things Need to Change!

There is something that has been challenging to me for many years. Recently it has caused me huge frustration and ENORMOUS sadness.

We were told Josh's prognosis nine hours after he was admitted. The one constant thing that devastated us more than anything was that his medical team GAVE US NO HOPE!

No matter how we asked questions: But what if? How can you be so confident there will be no recovery? It's only been a few hours. One of Josh's arms moved slightly, what caused that?

At all times, we were totally shut down, basically ORDERED to accept the medical team's prognosis. They were so always so adamant that there was no hope of any recovery!

About three days after Josh's accident I was peppering his Consultant Specialist with questions. In frustration he said "Look, Kay, we just don't know!"

I hugged him, telling him, "This was the best news we had in three days, why didn't you tell us this Sunday night?"

He never answered me...

Look, I don't want to get into doctor bashing, but this is potentially life threatening. Something has to change; somehow doctors must not shut out hope of even a small amount of recovery.

Maybe it's as simple as telling the person who is injured, their family and loved ones, all the really bad news. They do this already, but finish by saying, look we don't know, everyone is different! We can only go by our experience!

In my opinion this approach would be far more humane than by simply shutting out hope altogether!

December 2012, I was contacted (through Josh's website) by a woman whose husband had sustained a spinal cord injury. She asked me a lot of questions about what we had done. She also wanted to arrange for Josh and Simon to visit him in the hospital. It was the same hospital Josh had been admitted to over 12 years ago. Josh and Simon arranged a time for their visit. The gentleman was very ill, but certainly brightened up when he met Josh and Simon, listening intently to the type of recovery therapy Josh had done and the work Simon and Josh had done together.

The next day his wife was called to the doctor's office. The doctor chastised her for bringing Josh Wood into the hospital, stating that Josh preaches FALSE HOPE. She was devastated by this doctor's attitude and arrogance. (This doctor was Josh's specialist consultant, who knows they did not misdiagnose Josh.) He knows against all their predictions, Josh walked and continued to improve over 14 years later. Has this man no conscience?

How can he continue to ignore the fact that Josh and the others (at least four) who were patients at that same hospital he practices at, all diagnosed complete, and they have walked, and all have improved significantly from the initial prognosis!

We are not naive enough to say everyone will walk. Frankly that is between the person and God. What we are confident in saying is "If you do the work, have the right attitude, take care with your diet, keep focused, be prepared to work harder to achieve a goal than you ever have in your life, anything is possible!"

Certainly below-injury recovery is possible. We are experiencing this on a regular basis with people we are mentoring or become friends with, or read about on social media.

Neither Josh nor I have ever made false promises, given false hope to anyone, nor have we ever misled anyone of what is possible! All we have ever done is tell our story, as the others do, solely for one reason: to give the person who has suffered this devastating injury, and their families and loved ones, a belief that anything is possible. Maybe they get some hope from this; we always take care to point out that every spinal cord injury is different.

You cannot base your recovery on someone else!

It is important that you understand that neither Josh nor I have ever charged anyone for supporting them through this injury. Even though recently our funds have been decimated, we have flown to fund raisers at our own cost, and I have personally donated money to several fund raisers on behalf of people with spinal cord injury.

Josh has donated several copies of his book to help individuals gain an understanding of the road ahead if they focus on getting their lives back.

Sometimes it's not easy making time in our day, but we do. We have never shied away from helping someone who has asked for it.

I repeat, at no time do we offer false hope, we look at it as providing someone with a light, that with hard work, anything is possible.

We are experiencing first hand people having some form of recovery from this injury. Maybe they are not walking - this is not everyone's goal, maybe they are just gaining more independence, able to feed themselves, look after their personal needs, gaining a sliver of independence; any recovery over what was predicted by the medical "experts" is a bonus and should be celebrated!

As Josh says, "It's the loneliest injury anyone can suffer, as no one injury is the same!" And therefore NO recovery can be the same.

Like the injury, everyone going through this has different goals and motivations. Therefore, in our view, with the right motivation, therapists, and trainers anything is possible!

We do know - fitness, the right mental attitude, a training regime, and correct diet and supplement program is crucial to any form of below-injury recovery! You must adopt the mentality of an athlete; training, combined with all of the above is critical.

It is now 2016 and Josh is still walking, still improving, still beating the odds, and we are patiently waiting for one of Josh's original medical team members to ask Josh how he has done what he has done! How has he achieved the impossible?

This is not a witch hunt against the hospital. Far from it...but they need to understand that not just Josh walked, but there have been others.

My goal is that one day his doctors will be brave enough to have that talk with Josh and finally learn from him...and of course the others.

Here's what the doctors never told us:

There is so much I could write here if I thought about everything it would be a chapter in itself. I have tried to include what I believe were the main issues.

Every injury is different, yet it appears patients are diagnosed according to their injury level and given the devastating news. These days they are given an "ASIA" rating. Seriously, we never bothered with what Josh's

131

rating was, as it didn't concern us. In our view it was just another label.

Someone could break their neck or back, and if there is no or minimal damage to their cord, they could achieve a near full recovery.

The real danger with spinal cord injury is cord damage, and this varies significantly depending on impact, and what caused the injury. (Yet the doctors persist on the "one diagnosis fits all.")

Autonomic Dysreflexia

This is probably the most life threatening condition that strikes suddenly, sometimes with little warning, and needs to be urgently dealt with. I have included below a medical reference of the condition.

Autonomic dysreflexia is a potentially dangerous clinical syndrome that develops in individuals with spinal cord injury, resulting in acute, uncontrolled hypertension. All caregivers, practitioners, and therapists who interact with individuals with spinal cord injuries must be aware of this syndrome, recognize the symptoms, and understand the causes and treatment algorithm.

Briefly, autonomic dysreflexia develops in individuals with a neurologic level of spinal cord injury at or above the sixth thoracic vertebral level (T6). Autonomic dysreflexia causes an imbalanced reflex sympathetic discharge, leading to potentially life-threatening hypertension. It is considered a medical emergency and must be recognized immediately. If left untreated, autonomic dysreflexia can cause seizures, retinal hemorrhage, pulmonary edema, renal insufficiency, myocardial infarction, cerebral hemorrhage, and death. Complications associated with autonomic dysreflexia result directly from sustained, severe peripheral hypertension. - *Ryan O. Stephenson, DO, Assistant Professor, Department of Physical Medicine and Rehabilitation*

We were warned about this condition really early in Josh's admittance to the hospital, but with all the information we had to digest it was just another issue we had to deal with and to be honest, other than Wendy remembering those dire warnings, we never really thought about it until –

It was several years after his accident that Josh suffered his first autonomic dysreflexia. Initially we thought he had a migraine, but as he worsened his body started to close down. We raced to the hospital with him realizing what was happening to him.

Because we were going to a traditional ER (non-spinal cord injury ER) with little experience with the condition, we gave them our limited knowledge and finally Josh commenced the treatment he needed.

For us the frightening consequence of autonomic dysreflexia on Josh is he becomes a "complete quadriplegic." His body is in such a panic he loses the steely control he usually has of his brain.

Josh is pretty switched on to his body these days, but in 2012 Josh suffered a near fatal event. It rocked us to our souls; it occurred at a time when Josh's life was going well, he was getting married, everything was fantastic, then in a heartbeat we nearly lost him.

Swollen Spinal Cord

The damaged cord can be swollen for over one to two years. Paula could "see" Josh's cord and she maintained it was swollen for over three years. It was actually Paula who told us about the swollen cord, not a doctor. When we questioned one of his doctors about the cord swelling we were advised that we should not expect any major recovery after the 1st year. In his view any recovery after this period was extremely unlikely.

Standing Frames

We were never told about the importance of a standing frame, again something else we worked out for ourselves. We didn't even know about standing frames! Once home Josh used to wheel himself to a bench or table and attempt to stand. After a lot of practice he would stand holding onto something, for as long as he could. Josh's motivation was to teach his body to remember standing. He used visualization to reconnect his body with standing and the feeling of his legs standing on a surface. As he became more confident he would practice standing on different surfaces, concrete, grass, sand – visualizing the effect it had on his balance and movement. Josh felt this was an important part of him teaching his legs to walk again.

We have learned the importance of standing frames for your organs. While standing your organs hang normally, in a chair they are somewhat restricted.

Pressure Sores – THEY CAN KILL YOU!

I talked about the "turners" in an earlier chapter. No one ever really explained the danger of pressure sores to us. Fortunately for Josh, once he was in the rehab, he was active enough to roll over and in truth has never ever had a problem with them. But I have seen so many people that have nearly died from a pressure sore that hasn't been attended too urgently.

Unattended scratches or small skin tears in an area that could cause a pressure sore can very quickly turn into a life threatening situation. Great care is needed especially from care givers to be ever vigilant in minimizing the risk of a pressure sore occurring. If one is detected urgent medical advice needs to be sought.

Importance of Diet and Fitness to Maintain Bone Density

A professional recovery program should not be commenced without a bone density scan to avoid unnecessary bone breaks or fractures.

Finally, there is more and more proof these days that those suffering spinal cord injuries that maintain their fitness, eat a healthy diet, limit unnecessary medications, alcohol, and drugs, spent much less time in hospitals. This saves the community significant medical costs. We hope medical insurance companies start to understand the health benefits of therapy for spinal cord injury and begin to support families who want to attend one the many Recovery Centers being established around the USA. Out of pocket expenses for recovery are usually funded through the family, causing huge financial pressure on households. It's not easy to be constantly fund raising.

Personally I believe if medical insurance would cover below injury recovery programs it would, over a period of time, take a lot of stress away from hospitals.

Josh has been injured over 15 years. He has been in the hospital fewer than 10 times, and two visits were for infections in his elbow.

For us, hospitals represent stress, because we have to educate the admitting medical team on Josh's injury. They have to be extremely careful in his treatment.

Families attending a hospital with a loved one with SCI agree this is a huge, potentially life threatening problem. We made a decision never to return to Josh's hospital for any treatment, so traumatized were we from his stay there. This means we have to attend a hospital that is not as experienced with spinal cord injuries. Fortunately that hospital now has a file on Josh, but nevertheless in an emergency situation, it does add a significant level of stress.

Chapter 14.   The Power of Prayer, a Journey of Gratitude and Healing

My great passions for reading, travelling, spirituality, and conversation have extensively opened up many experiences to me over the years.

They have certainly given me a very broad, open perspective on health and alternative options for recovery, healing, and life.

I had read several books and had personal experiences of the spiritual healing aspects of American Indians through their Shamans, the Australian Aborigines, their spiritual doctors, and the Balians from Bali.

Over the years I had been open to the powers of the many different healers I had encountered and experienced, all being an important part of my personal journey towards alternative healing.

From a young age, Josh had been exposed to an alternative way of looking at healing, through his "crazy mum's weirdo ways" as he used to refer to it.

Importantly, he had been exposed to my beliefs, so from that aspect, looking at another way of healing his injury wasn't anything he was afraid of; in fact with nothing more positive on offer, he embraced it!

Even without the immediacy of social media, we managed to get word out of Josh's accident to our family, our friends in our community, our wider communities within various parts of Australia, USA, England, Ireland, and Switzerland.

In turn they joined with their various communities in support, through prayer and healing ceremonies for Josh. These ceremonies continued for several months.

Our family in Liverpool (UK) held several prayer gatherings in the Cathedral for Josh, his host family in Switzerland held many prayer services in their beautiful church in Schänis, there was an Indian Prayer Circle organized by our friends from Southern California, and prayers were offered at Salt Hill and Tuam Cathedrals (Ireland). My Irish "sista" Dominica's mother, Dolly, lit candles and prayed for Josh daily in Tuam Cathedral for several months.

Our local community of Port Melbourne, Josh's friends, and their families gave us, as a family, never ending support.

There were so many people, family, friends, and strangers involved in prayers for Josh's recovery, it was truly humbling to us, and it certainly helped us in coping, especially in the early stages in dealing with the trauma of his accident.

In May 2001, Josh went to California, in the care of our friends Dana and John. They had arranged for Josh to attend healing sessions with a chi master called Mark who was based in California. Dana and John had generously offered to pay all expenses for Josh while he was in their care. My responsibility was to fly Josh over there and back once his chi energy healing sessions were completed.

With all the travelling I had done with my business, I had earned enough frequent flyer miles to fly Josh first class return on United Airlines.

Josh called me from the plane before taking off, saying this was the only way he wanted to travel in the future. Hahahaha! I told him to enjoy himself and make the most of it because it would be the last time on my watch.

Josh flew out alone, on a direct flight from Melbourne to Los Angeles.

As Josh still ran the risk of thrombosis and blood clots from flying, he actually had to inject himself in his stomach to eliminate the potential of things going wrong during the long non-stop flight from Melbourne to Los Angeles.

Dana and John, understanding Josh would need a solid healing support team, flew Paula and Isabel over to the USA to support him. They stayed in the same hotel as Josh, making sure he looked after himself, ate properly, while both maintained their individual healing sessions with him.

Reflecting on this, all these years later, I shake my head asking myself, "What was I thinking?"

Josh wasn't even 12 months post injury, and here I was sending him 1/2 way across the world for alternative healing. I realize now that we really operated on blind faith - always moving in the direction of alternative therapy, always believing Josh would be greatly improved from his experience. Certainly Mark came to us with excellent credentials. He was a personal friend of Dana and John's so the decision to send Josh to the

USA seemed to make so much sense.

The plan was for Josh to stay in the USA for around 6 - 8 weeks. His trip would be a mixture of Chi Energy Therapy with Mark, ongoing massage and crystal healing sessions with Paula and Isabel, while enjoying some down time with John and Dana.

We were all exhausted after 12 months of stress, celebration, and riding the never ending emotional rollercoaster that comes with a spinal cord injury; we were grateful for the support we had experienced from our family and friends.

My mother and I decided to take the opportunity, with Josh being in the USA, to visit those who had prayed for and supported him in their various countries.

We made arrangements to travel to Europe and the USA to visit family and friends, to thank them personally for their support through prayers and communications, which had been so very important to us all, especially in those early scary months.

It was mum's first trip to Europe, and although she had travelled frequently over the years, it had been mainly to Asia and the USA, so this trip although tinged with sadness, was a dream come true for her.

Our first stop was Zurich, Switzerland. We were met by Ernst and Regula, Josh's host parents, and their boys. We planned to spend four days with them. Mum was very tired from the flight, but that didn't deter our friends, who whisked us out of the airport and took us to a stunning alpine restaurant for breakfast.

As a family they had been devastated by Josh's accident. He was their 4th son. Since they visited Josh in those early days a few weeks after his accident, we had been in touch with them regularly, keeping them updated through email of Josh's progress.

They showered us with love and attention, taking us to all Josh's favorite places. I had been to most of them before, but for Mum it was all new; she loved it. We were very spoiled - Regula took great delight in cooking and preparing for Mum and me Josh's favorites, pizza and chocolate mousse.

Ernst enjoyed sharing Swiss wine with us, always asking for my opinion. Mum and I felt so welcomed.

We stayed in a typical Swiss Chalet, owned by a family member. It was a huge room the size of an apartment. The furnishings were typical to the Swiss, so comfortable.

Josh and I had stayed in the same home when we had travelled there a few years earlier.

There was a small dairy on the property. Every morning Mum and I woke up to fresh milk, butter, and cream on our doorstep. We felt truly indulged, feeling special after months of living with fear and grief.

We visited the little church where the prayer services were held for Josh's recovery - it was very beautiful, extremely ornate, nestled in the beautiful village of Schänis.

After all these years, we keep in touch with our "Swiss family." They are still keen to keep up with what Josh is doing and how he continues to progress.

From Switzerland we travelled by TGV (fast train) to Paris, my one indulgence of our trip. There was no one to thank there; I just wanted to take Mum to a city I loved so much.

Travelling by train allowed Mum to enjoy the scenic views of the little villages, and the countryside between Switzerland and France. It was a journey I had enjoyed on many occasions, loving these tiny glimpses of country life within the most stunning scenery. Mum was in 7th heaven.

I was excited to show mum Paris, a city that was so special to me, holding so many precious memories.

Paris was where Josh and I had spent a fantastic week with Bry, during our Mum and son Europe trip in 1998. In 2000, around 2 million party goers and I had celebrated the birth of the new millennium in Paris, in front of the Eiffel Tower, just over 12 months earlier. Wow, what a night that was. I was so filled with excitement and promise as to where my life was going, how turning 50 (March 2000) was going to be my year; OMG so much had changed.

From the moment we arrived at the beautiful old style railway station, Mum was not impressed with Paris. She felt it was too busy, too dirty and no matter where I took her, initially she didn't embrace the city at any level. My mum, a very stubborn woman, refused to use the Metro, and didn't want to walk too far. Without the Metro and the ability to walk any distance, Paris is not the easiest city to get around.

For the week we were there, I seemed to be constantly begging the taxi drivers in my broken French to take us short distances.

We paid a fortune in tips!

Finally, after a few days, Mum got into the swing and ambiance of the city, enjoying our luncheon cruise down the Seine, visiting the Eiffel Tower, and especially the scenic elevator ride up to the top.

Finally, we enjoyed fun experiences and memorable times there. Overall, while it wasn't her favorite place, she did agree it was a stunning, beautiful city.

On our final night in Paris, I treated Mum to a night at the Sheraton Charles de Gaulle, making it easier to catch our early flight to Shannon, Ireland the next day.

Dominica (Dom), met us at the airport. On the way back to her home we stopped for lunch at Clarinbridge, near Galway. Dom planned this welcome lunch especially for Mum, as she knew of her love of oysters and all things seafood; she wanted to give her a taste the fabulous Irish oysters. It's fair to say Mum was yet again in 7th heaven.

Dom's family had met Josh while we were in Ireland in 1998. They were all so supportive and interested in his ongoing recovery.

Mum and I were staying with Dom, her husband Pearse, and their boys, Shay and Brian, in their period home in Salt Hill one block from Galway Bay.

Mum embraced everything Irish, forming a great friendship with Dolly, Dom's mum. They remained close friends for many years, a friendship that lasted until my mother's passing 2010.

Our goal to thank all those who had supported us was turning into a healing time for Mum and me.

Dom's family welcomed us, as one of theirs. We visited the cathedrals that prayers for Josh's recovery had been held in, and enjoyed being pampered by Dom's siblings and parents. We immersed ourselves in the wonderful Irish culture of family, drinking the Guinness, eating the seafood, along with a lot of laughter and friendship.

Dom decided to take us on a mini road trip. For two days we travelled the rambling Irish roads, visiting the stunningly beautiful Kylemore Abbey, and the Cliffs of Mohr. Unfortunately it rained all day, yet nothing could be taken from the wild rugged scenery.

We travelled through many tiny villages, staying one night in a B&B in the ancient seaside town of Clifden. Mum loved the wildness and beauty of Clifden, she especially enjoyed the old pub, where we went for dinner; she ended up chatting up several locals, being the center of attention.

(Later in 2011, after my mother had passed on (2010), my sisters and I travelled to Ireland to visit Dom and her family. We brought with us a precious package (a small amount of our mother's ashes) as my plan to bring my mum back to Ireland. I wanted Mum's ashes to be in places of great beauty, giving her amazing views. We chose a beautiful rock pool in the shallows of the wild Irish ocean off Clifden and in the shallows of the beautiful peaceful Galway Bay. Whenever I think of my mum, I know she is sailing the oceans of the world and I am at peace!)

Our last night in Galway was celebrated with a traditional Irish seafood dinner at the famous O'Connell's Pub, a meal my mother would reminisce over for many years.

The following morning we left for Dublin, spending two days with Dom's sister Imelda and her family. We were so spoiled, loving our time with them, loving the old streets of Dublin.

After a wonderful week of enjoying Ireland and all it offered, we flew to back to Heathrow, where I rented a car. Our plan was to drive to Liverpool, the city where my grandfather (paternal) was born. He grew up there, before he and his brothers migrated to Australia in the 1920's.

Our Liverpool family had strong ties to their church; we spent a week with them, touring and getting to know them. Mum had corresponded with them for many years, but meeting them was an amazing experience for us both. Once again she embraced the lifestyle offered by England. For me, being a lifelong Beatles fan, I enjoyed walking along the Mersey, discovering the areas my Grandfather had grown up in, and the parts of Liverpool made famous by the Fab 4.

We visited Liverpool Cathedral, where the prayer services were held for Josh. It was an impressive ancient building, a very large, historical structure.

All too soon it was time to leave our family. After Liverpool we enjoyed five days in London.

Mum discovered her "spiritual home" in London. We went to Buckingham Palace and managed to visit all the tourist sites. We walked and sailed the Thames. Mum found a second wind, enjoying exploring the city, feeling rejuvenated in the beautiful summer weather London provided for us.

There were places from World War II mum wanted to visit. She was like a kid in a candy shop. Our last night in London, we found an old pub that had survived the blitz, we enjoyed an early dinner, and Mum had fun chatting to the locals. It really was a fun time! I even managed to get her on the tube! Surprise, surprise she loved it!

With our Europe trip finally over, we left London and flew to San Francisco, where we planned to meet my cousin, Steve Ledson.

Steve owned the magnificent Ledson Winery and Vineyards in Sonoma, Northern California.

Steve and I had been discussing creating a joint venture wine project, utilizing my contacts in the Australian boutique wine industry. Our plan was to bring high end premium bulk wines from Australia for distribution through the Ledson Wines USA; something I found very exciting.

Both Mum and I had been to San Francisco before, so only having a day to look around we decided to spend it at Fisherman's Wharf, enjoying the seafood and characters of the area. Our plan was to stay overnight at the Sheraton Fisherman's Wharf, meeting Steve for dinner. We enjoyed a very special dinner with Steve at a restaurant on one of the private wharves there. Mum was in her element, tackling the fresh seafood with her usual gusto.

Steve stayed overnight, and the next morning drove Mum to the airport for her flight to Orange County, California. Mum was visiting her old friend Bernice, staying the week with her, thanking her family for their part in arranging the Indian Prayer Circle for Josh.

I was staying with Steve in his home in Sonoma, catching up with the US Ledsons, hearing the family history. In those early days, unbeknown to me, within a few months my life and Josh's would be taken in a whole new direction, although in those early days it wasn't apparent.

On our return to Australia, I have to confess, I was challenged a lot by the way my mother totally relied on me for everything on the trip. It made me realize she was getting old (73 years), which at the time I found confronting. I began to learn that our relationship was changing from mother and daughter, to me assuming responsibility for taking care of her - our roles were certainly reversing.

Mum and I would look back fondly on those six weeks we had together. The memories, the people, the friendships, and especially just before she passed we chatted about the trip very often. In a quiet time she said she realized how difficult she had been especially in Paris. Ha-ha, but that was my mum... stubborn to the end!

Although we were always close, as Mum aged the dynamics of our relationship changed towards the end of her life. Mum and I enjoyed a wonderful "different" aspect of our relationship; we loved hanging out as really good friends, enjoying lunches over a bottle of wine, and really that was everything!

Even with our challenges, the trip had been an amazing time for my mum and me. I would never have enjoyed this experience with her had it not been for Josh's accident. Because of our destinies changing, I became best friends with my mum, which as we both grew older was a far more "adult" relationship to have with her.

Josh's healing trip to the USA had been the catalyst of our trip. While we were away we kept in touch with him, through Skype calls most days, hearing his progress, and celebrating his successes.

Josh had several strenuous sessions with Mark, and in each session he made significant progress. The first session Josh had to be carried up the stairs of Mark's Californian home, and by his last session Josh was pushing Mark's wife around their front garden and street with her in his wheel chair.

Josh was walking a little before he commenced his recovery program with Mark, but improved a great deal from Mark's exercises.

Josh has always regarded Mark as being responsible for starting him walking with greater confidence, strength, and energy. Mark worked tirelessly on restoring Josh's Chi energy.

Mark taught Josh so much about the importance of Chi Energy as the life force of his body. This is a topic Josh discusses when doing his motivational talks.

When Josh wasn't working with Mark in California, he and Dana travelled to Colorado in between the sessions. So, in effect, Josh had a break, also!

We are still in touch with Mark after all these years. We will be always grateful to all those who helped us along our journey.

Josh's accident changed all of our destinies. Nearly 15 years later, other than hating what he goes through daily with the various issues he deals with and unrelenting pain, I have to say it's been a remarkable time of learning, faith, new experiences, opportunities, meeting new friends and believing more and more that anything is possible.

Chapter 15.   First Love, Kissing Frogs and then He found His Princess

After such a catastrophic accident, one of the biggest issues you face as a parent is whether your child will be able to enjoy a relationship, marry, and have children. I must admit in those early dark days the thought of anything normal was so remote, but I have to say it was still there, even if totally buried somewhere in the drama of the injury at the time.

As an only child, Josh always loved hanging out with children; he was the ultimate "kid" –"Pied Piper." It was a joy to see how happy he was when he was surrounded by children. There was a side of him that really never grew up. With the grim predictions from his doctors we were left feeling sad that Josh would never be able to father children, yet another devastating prediction in those dark days. Obviously we didn't dwell on this, but especially after Josh and Amelia married there was always the fear they would not be able to conceive a much-wanted baby.

One thing I have learned over all these years is that when suffering an injury such as Josh's, the last thing he needed was a toxic relationship on top of everything else he was dealing with.

I have spoken to many families who are frustrated and angry over friendships, girlfriends, fiancées, and even marriages that have failed through an accident involving in a spinal cord injury to a loved one.

Only from my personal experience with Josh over all these years, I simply say the same thing, "Your loved one is better off on their own, as hard, isolating, scary, and lonely as it seems at the time. It is better to surround themselves with positive, supportive people who are there for them, and who will love and support them unconditionally."

Any recovery from this injury is difficult enough, without having to deal with and manage a close relationship with someone who is angry, bitter, unsupportive, and resentful.

Even in normal circumstances, finishing a relationship is never easy. This injury is so tough that sometimes one's survival goals have to be put first. Tough decisions need to be made, and toxic people need to be exited from their life.

To maintain a recovery program or goals, you need to focus, surrounding yourself with positive, supportive people, so as hard as it is, finishing a

145

negative or toxic relationship will release the negativity, allowing the focus to shift to the positive.

But in finally ending it, all contact, including text messages and other forms of social media should, if possible, be ceased or at least minimized.

I have experienced that in some relationships, by keeping up the contact, even if it's just texting, the relationship is still being "fed" keeping the toxicity seeping into the mindset of the injured person.

As hard as it sounds, totally ceasing all communication is better in the long run, extremely tough in the beginning, but they get over it!

Emerging from a negative relationship, over time, it is my experience that those injured become emotionally stronger, in many cases understanding that they after all, are not the damaged one!

On the positive side of things, many pre injury relationships grow stronger. I have seen many relationships flourish and grow, becoming powerful and fulfilling creating a truly committed recovery/support team.

There are no steadfast rules in life, and like a spinal cord injury, where no one injury is the same, every relationship is different. Depending on the individuals, they will flourish or fail due to the never ending pressure of this cruel savage injury.

On the 25th June 2000, Josh getting married was the last thing on my mind, but as Josh started to improve, you start to wonder what their lives will be like now.

Even at preschool Josh always had a girlfriend. Obviously in those days it was cute and innocent, and as he grew older there always seemed to be girl somewhere in his life. But none of them, you would say, was serious.

He was your typical teenager loving life, hanging out with his mates, and having fun.

First Love

When Josh was 16, he met Bry. They were introduced through mutual friends while snowboarding at our local ski fields. When Josh returned home at the end of the weekend, all he talked about was Bry and how much fun they had snowboarding, and hanging out!

Josh had recently returned from Switzerland. He wasn't interested in school at all, and all he cared about was snowboarding, and now Bry. The following Saturday I drove him to a party. As I dropped him off, he introduced me to Bry. She seemed like a lovely young girl, but to be honest, at the time, I never really took a lot of notice.

Then in a heartbeat, instead of a house full of boys, there were girls everywhere!

Bry would come over to our home, straight from school, still in her school uniform, usually with a bunch of her girlfriends.

Wendy and I would be trying to work and there would be this fun chaos happening around us.

When Bry and the girls where in the house, it was about laughter, fun, and noise from everyone – it was a very happy time!

They were all so young; loving life!

Josh and Bry both shared the passions of snowboarding and travel. They were always chatting about adventures, planning to travel together once they finished school. I remember one day they were saying that they would like to travel around Europe in a van. Josh would drive, and Bry would take photos - both of them would snowboard.

Bry was Josh's first serious girlfriend. They always seemed to be having fun, laughing and not taking life too seriously. At their age it was all so very innocent!

Bry decided to study in France for a year, and while Josh was disappointed, he understood and totally supported her. He missed her terribly; they kept in touch through email, letters, and the occasional phone call.

As part of our trip to Europe (1998) over the school Christmas break, Josh and I planned a week in Paris. We contacted Bry's parents, asking them if she could stay with us for the week. They agreed, so plans were made to meet up with her at our hotel, located near the Louvre.

Josh was so excited! We arrived at the hotel the evening before, and Josh was up early the next morning; he wanted everything to be perfect for Bry's arrival! He left the hotel immediately after breakfast, returning with a bunch of red roses and a card. He prepared everything in readiness for

147

her arrival.

Finally Bry was there with us. It was the beginning of a fabulous, fun week. Bry spoke fluent French, so going anywhere with her, especially to eat, was really easy. Bry knew all the galleries to go too, as well. She was very familiar with Paris.

Josh and Bry would be out most of the day exploring Paris, and I would meet them at night for dinner. Usually Bry and I would be up early (Josh liked to sleep in), and the two of us would walk the city of Paris, exploring the quiet streets before the crowds arrived, and then bringing breakfast back to the hotel.

At the end of the week, Josh and I left for Switzerland. Bry came to the railway station to say good bye, and as the train pulled out, there was Bry running along the platform waving madly.

Just after Bry returned home to Australia, they broke up. It was a very sad time for us all! Looking back, I realize that they were very young and these things are bound to happen! But even now I look back on that week in Paris as a special time in our lives.

After his accident, I was glad Josh had had the opportunity to travel independently, especially to Europe. While he still enjoys travelling, it is not as easy these days for him. Bry is truly my daughter from another mother.

Bry came back into our lives at our most crucial time of need, during those crazy early weeks after his accident. Bringing support and positivity, Bry was very dedicated to ensuring Josh maintained the will to live; importantly his belief in his ability to recover. Our friendship is something I truly treasure!

Just prior to his accident, Josh was more interested in snowboarding, partying, and spending time with his mates, rather than having a girlfriend. True to form though, there were always girls hanging around him, but frankly I wasn't overly concerned with what he was doing, especially as he was living on the mountain.

We caught up by phone often. I was pushing him to get a job and somewhere to live on the mountain, because for the whole month of May he had been up there, all he'd done was snowboard and party hard.

The snow season had started early with large snow falls occurring from

148

early May, which was extremely rare in Australia. On the night before his accident, he had phoned Wendy (I was away in Perth), wishing her happy birthday, and telling her that he would know about a job Sunday night and he thought he'd found an apartment.

After the accident, as Josh started feeling better and more in control of his body (August 2000), he was desperate to get back up to the mountain. He needed closure. He needed to run through in his head just what had gone wrong that fateful day. He needed to smell the snow, to be somewhere he truly loved.

Having my full support, knowing he had unfinished business with the jump, what could he have done to change the outcome?

Everyone thought we were crazy, but I knew Josh and how important this was to him. He pushed me and pushed me, to ask if he could obtain a leave pass from rehab for the weekend.

In late August, we received the go ahead from his medical team for Josh to return to the mountain. I now needed to approach the snow resort for permission, as to get Josh safely up to the village we needed to be able to bring his car directly to the hotel. There was no way Josh could manage over-snow transport, which was the usual way you accessed the village.

Fortunately our request was approved very quickly.

I went ahead and made bookings at the same hotel where Josh had spent his last normal, carefree day before his accident - the rainy day where he had relaxed in the spa with his friends all day.

Mentally, Josh needed to experience the accident setting of the jump and the site; he needed to actually see where the jump was built, allowing himself to go over the process in his head, on the site, so he could work out what had gone wrong!

I knew it was important for him to accept responsibility for what had happened, so he could move forward with his recovery.

Very early in Josh's recovery process, I realized that his injury was as much of a mental injury as it was physical; quite quickly he had started to accept that it was an accident. He had made the decision to do the jump, he accepted responsibility for that, but he had lingering questions about what had gone wrong. The unanswered questions were messing with his wellbeing.

149

As this was Josh's first real taste of freedom, although he had been home some weekends, travelling to the mountain was a long trip. He was still very frail. We took our time, taking around 3 1/2 hours to get there.

We arrived late in the afternoon, just before sunset.

The hotel was beautiful. Our room looked out over the lower snowfields, and even at the end of the season there was still plenty of snow - it was perfect, although a real bittersweet experience for us both.

We had dinner with a few of Josh's friends. Amongst them was a young woman I'll call "Jenny" who seemed to be very concerned and supportive of him. Josh really enjoyed catching up with his friends. He was happy and relaxed. *Tiny steps in getting his old life back!*

After dinner one of his mates, who groomed the mountain's slopes at night, asked Josh if he would like to ride with him in the giant snow grooming machine.

Josh asked me what I thought. Did I think he could manage it? My only concerns were to make sure he didn't get cold. He had to keep warm, and he would have to be strapped safely into the seat.

The night was black as the boys carried Josh to the cabin of the machine, carefully lifting him into the passenger seat.

Some reading this book will shake their heads, saying, yet again, what was I thinking? Well, the one thing that drove me all through the early period of Josh's recovery was that he needed to believe he would get his old life back. Getting involved in something he loved was all part of his recovery process.

I needed to show him that I was confident he could do this!

Josh returned to the hotel after a few hours, very tired yet jubilant. He was so happy; this trip would prove to be the best medicine for him.

Again, it was these little things that in the end added up to getting him to where he is today.

The next day the boys wheeled Josh down to the accident site.

Seeing the site for the first time I was furious as to why he hadn't been stopped from attempting the jump. In my wildest dreams, I couldn't understand why he hadn't been pulled up by someone with authority before he jumped.

Hindsight is amazing, but as much as we wanted too, we couldn't turn back time!

The jump changed Josh's life forever. While I don't regret the past 15 years (it has been an incredible journey), I am sad for Josh. He is constantly battling an uncooperative body, while suffering unrelenting pain.

This just makes me really sad!

Josh, on the other hand, felt real closure, knowing it was an accident. Nothing he did on that fateful day would have changed the outcome.

Saturday night Josh and I enjoyed dinner with his friends at their favorite party hotel in the resort. I looked around and saw how excited everyone was to have Josh back on his home turf. I decided to leave early, feeling confident he was safe with his friends. When Josh finally got back to the room he was excited and full of hope, saying how much fun he had seeing everyone.

That weekend we had made another tiny step!

Jenny was there to say goodbye when we left Sunday afternoon.

Over the next month, she came down a few times to Melbourne on her days off to see Josh in rehab. At the end of the season she returned to Melbourne to stay with friends. By time Josh was released in November, they had started hanging out together. As I was working again, and since Josh couldn't be left on his own, it made sense for Jenny to move in with us to help support Josh, and they became involved.

Although glad to be home, this period proved to be a very difficult time for Josh. His constant therapy was taking great effort, he'd lost a lot of weight, and he was coming to terms with the job of getting his life back.

There was so much going on that he needed to totally focus on achieving his ongoing recovery goals.

Every day we were learning things we didn't know about the injury!

Jenny and Josh decided to go to a motor bike event near our home. It was a very hot day and none of us realized the dangers of dehydration with a spinal cord injury; by time they returned home, Josh was very ill,

151

suffering from extreme dehydration and a migraine.

It took him several days to recover.

There always seemed to be something that we didn't know or hadn't been warned about in relation to the injury. We were constantly on a learning curve; at times it felt like a crazy rollercoaster ride.

Jenny stayed with us for about three months. For various reasons their relationship failed, and Jenny went to the U.S. to work.

In those early hard months there was a lot of pressure on Josh. Frankly, at that early stage, I preferred Josh to be on his own. He needed to focus on himself, rather than have the pressure of a relationship that was difficult at best.

Focusing on his recovery, without the complications of a relationship, was paramount. Nothing was easy, and it was very hard in those early months!

Fortunately, he had some amazing chick friends, so he was never without a group of gals around him.

Over the next nine years Josh had three more long term relationships, and they all lived with Josh and me; fortunately the last two were when I had the church apartment, which was large and allowed them the privacy of their own living space.

All three relationships in my opinion were one sided, and certainly proved very challenging for all of us.

Even though I worked away most weeks, living together under one roof, even in a large apartment, made for difficult and extremely challenging lives.

What I observed was that Josh loved each of these young women unconditionally. Josh, once in a relationship, is totally committed.

Although each of the relationships was different, Josh always seemed to have to try too hard to make up for those things he could no longer do. But on the other hand, he was loving, supportive, and generous to these girls, as was I, paying for holidays, dinners, and providing a generous lifestyle for them all.

I am sure each one of those girls thought they loved Josh at the time, but dealing with this injury day in day out is tough on everyone.

Fortunately, as Josh matured he realized he was lacking nothing in the relationship stakes, and as each relationship ran its course, Josh grew to understand he had nothing to feel inadequate about.

In truth all these girls had their own issues. They were all different, and as they moved on I am sure they would replicate their problems over and over again.

Josh, however, learned from each break-up, and as he moved on, he gained an understanding for what he truly wanted in a future relationship. In the end, he grew and matured a great deal from these relationships. Importantly, he gained more confidence believing he would always contribute equally to the "right" relationship.

These relationships, over a period of years, caused me so much stress. They brought such tough times for all of us, and as much as I tried to be supportive, I felt that all four relationships were going nowhere, each causing Josh more grief than joy.

After the last relationship ended in 2008, there were a series of girls around, but frankly I was over it, and made no attempt to get close to any of them.

One thing I will say about these four girlfriends is that each one contributed in some way to Josh's ongoing recovery, so it wasn't all bad. But as a mum you know when something isn't right, and at times it is very hard not to say what you think!

Though these relationships, Josh would say to me "You always criticize my girlfriends; they are never right in your eyes. Mum, you are so tough!"

I would always say the same thing, "When I see them look at you the way you do to them, then I'll be happy and supportive. I won't be critical, I will celebrate with you both."

I was getting tired of the never-ending group of Josh's friends coming over to drink and hang out in our garden. I always seemed to have a house full of the boys. There was rarely a time when we had our apartment to ourselves.

Josh's friends called our church garden the "Belgian Beer Garden of Port Melbourne." They all thought it was funny. I was less than impressed and felt I could never get away from them. I desperately wanted to enjoy my own space, in my home!

Our apartment was located near the corner of two of Port Melbourne's busiest streets. There was always a constant stream of people walking past our front garden. In the summer our garden was a "pick up location" for the boys. To make matters worse, we were two blocks from the popular "Port" beach, even more reason to come down and hung out!

Every warm weekend I had to endure a house full of boys, sitting in my garden drinking and chatting up the girls who were walking past.

There were nights when as many as five or six would stay over, really wrecking my peace.

Work wise, I had a very high pressure role, running a national sales and marketing team for a financial services company, usually spending 3-4 days a week travelling around Australia. The hours were long, the stress was never ending, and frankly I got tired of having no ability to relax and have some peace and quiet on the few days each week I was home.

While Josh led an exceptionally busy social life, I, on the other hand, had virtually none.

Due to work commitments and the constant party at my apartment I was very frustrated. It got to the stage that Josh and I were constantly arguing. I understood it was difficult for him still living with his mum, but at that stage neither of us had any option.

Even during this party period, Josh was still working out, getting more and more improvement, but it was very subtle.

With no end in sight to Josh's partying, I was getting to the stage I hated where my life was going. All I seemed to be doing was working extreme hours, spending more time in airports than at home, paying the endless bills, and supporting an expensive inner city lifestyle. I had no respite at all.

The constant arguments I was having with Josh were causing me to fast lose my patience with him and with having a house full of his mates every waking hour. I was finally out of patience; something had to change!

I felt I had no alternative. I decided to sell our much loved church apartment, and set Josh up in a home of his own (year 2009).

Finally I would buy my own apartment, where I would have my own space, live the life I wanted to. Basically I would finally be getting on with my life.

I loved the old church. It had been an amazing place to live in, and at the time we needed space, it was perfect, but it was time to move on!

Josh found a large home in Caroline Springs, in the North West suburbs of Melbourne, and after months of searching, I found the perfect apartment in a small boutique block, close to the beach in Port Melbourne.

I finally achieved my dream of uninterrupted sea views. I loved watching the sea from my front balcony and enjoyed the fantastic city views from my bedroom at the rear of the apartment. I had the best of both worlds.

It was an exciting time for us both. I loved my new apartment!

Josh loved it too. He would come over with the doggies, sometimes staying overnight, but the majority of his friends were banned. Don't get me wrong, these were great guys, but I was over them! When they were visiting, the furry grandkids and I enjoyed walks on the beach. They loved looking out from the balcony at the goings on below, and riding in the elevator.

For the first time in years, I had the time to really enjoy my life, and only had me to worry about. On the occasions when Josh and I did catch up, we were more relaxed and happy together. For the first time in months, we were actually enjoying hanging out.

Josh's house was large, comprising of four bedrooms, an office, a living room, and a large open plan kitchen, dining, and family room. Our plan was to get a few mates to move in with him to help around the house, walk our furry kids, and pay a nominal rent to help pay off the mortgage.

Well there are no surprises. Josh's home became party central. Frankly I was beyond caring and what I couldn't see didn't worry me!

As long as Josh looked after our dogs and kept up his training, that was all I cared about! I was still supporting Josh financially, but he had started his public speaking so he was earning a little money.

Josh started talking about a girl he had met on one of his Sydney weekends away. Frankly, I truly had no interest.

I was working really hard, trying to reduce the mortgages on both properties, importantly getting on with my life!

All I wanted him to do was focus on his health and fitness. The only joy for me was that when he had a girlfriend he tended to settle down and curtail his party lifestyle.

I finally met Amelia. It is no secret that I totally messed up our first meeting, and in fairness at that stage, I wasn't really interested in getting close to yet another girlfriend unless I knew they were serious.

With Josh living in Caroline Springs, I really didn't see Josh and Amelia often, so I wasn't aware of how serious they were until the 16th March 2011, my birthday.

Josh arranged a talk for some of his friends and Simon's clients to hear his recovery story. Most of Josh's friends had no idea he was a quadriplegic. They thought his injury had to do with an accident that had damaged his legs.

Amelia, her mother Jude, and her sister Laura came along to support him.

For the first time, I saw Amelia really loved Josh, for who he was. His injury was just part of who he was to her. She "looked at him the way he looked at her" and actually appeared really devoted to him.

I realized that night that these two would be together forever...they were soul mates. From that evening I have totally supported their relationship!

Receiving some money from our mother's estate, my sisters and I decided to take a holiday to Europe for five weeks (October 2011). Part of our journey was to take some of our mother's ashes to Ireland. We planned to replicate as much as possible the trip Mum and I had done in 2001.

We flew from Melbourne, via London, to Shannon, commencing our journey in Ireland. We stayed with Dom and her family in their home in Salt Hill.

Arriving back to the house after a late lunch, my phone rang. It was Josh. I immediately thought what's wrong? But this was to be a very different call from Josh. He was so excited, saying he had something to ask me. He wanted my blessing for him asking Amelia to be his wife.

I was so excited for them both, there were happy tears over that long distance phone call, and of course I gave him my blessing.

He planned to surprise Amelia by proposing to her on his 30th birthday, at a party they were organizing.

Over the next five weeks the surprise proposal would become the worst kept secret ever, and until this day I am surprised that Amelia didn't hear about it.

Josh arranged for our old family friends, Antonia and Robert, (who have a fine jewelry store in Beaumaris) to make the engagement ring, which he had designed. They were excited to be a part of Josh's journey; they had known him since he was a little boy.

I arrived back from my trip on November 11th; from the airport, I was whisked off to Beaumaris to collect the precious ring. I became the custodian of it until it was time to hand it to Josh just before the big moment.

Josh was so excited. He wanted everything to be perfect.

To add to the drama of the day, Channel 7, a local television station, was producing a feature on Josh's journey of recovery. They had not finalized the story, as they were waiting for me to return home, and once they found out about the proposal, they decided they wanted to include the big moment in the feature.

Along with all the excitement involved with the party, we were dealing with the television crew waiting for Josh's birthday speech. Everyone except Amelia knew what was going to happen. Amelia was oblivious to Josh's plans, thinking the TV crew was there because of Josh's 30th.

Finally the big announcement was near. Josh called Amelia up to join him. I could tell he was nervous, and then he said "I'd like to ask Amelia"... then he lost it, emotions took the better of him, and amid all the cheering from the party goers, Amelia said YES!

There were happy tears all around...and we now we had a double celebration.

Momentarily I thought back to 12 years earlier, when I was pleading and praying for my son's life, with doctors and God. Oh my God, what an emotional journey this has been!

Although Josh always appears "out there", he is a very traditional man. He is extremely protective and loving, and will be an excellent father as Amelia will be a fabulous mother.

Happy son, happy Mum!

16th February 2013...The biggest day

Josh had achieved his goal of walking without his stick in October 2012, while attending PW Carlsbad for four months. Returning home from the USA, in December 2012, he had maintained a rigorous training program. He was determined, even though the wedding was on the beach (his least favorite walking surface), he was adamant he would not to use or see his walking stick on this very special day.

Saturday was an emotional, memorable day for all of us. Josh had finally found his soul mate, best friend, lover, and future mother of his children.

I know in my heart and soul that every day Josh will continue to drive his battered body further than anyone ever thought possible, achieving new goals and milestones, because he wants to be a "normal" husband and, hopefully, dad to his children.

I was excited yet calm. I thought back to those dark early days after his accident and I could never have dreamed we would come this far. **Today, my son would be married.**

I had seen Josh on Friday afternoon. He looked so well, extremely happy, and was looking forward to the future with the one he loved.

He spent his last day as a single man with his mates Daniel, Laslo, Chrisso, and a friend Patrick Hammerli, who had flown into Melbourne from Switzerland to attend the wedding. For a wedding treat, I had booked Josh and the boys into a beautiful boutique hotel near where the wedding would take place, so he didn't have to drive home after celebrating with his mates.

I had done the same for Amelia and her bridal party. They were in an apartment hotel nearby, having their own celebrations.

The Wedding

The wedding service and reception were to be held at a beachside restaurant called the Sandbar Beach Cafe situated on the beautiful Middle Park beach, near the City of Melbourne.

The afternoon was stunning, the weather was hot, the day was clear, and there was a light breeze blowing off the bay, which would hopefully provide a slight cooling effect for our afternoon celebrations.

Wendy had booked a hotel for us all to get ready in and stay the night.

Susan, Wendy, Asri, family friend Ray, cousin Richard and grandniece Ivy, and I travelled by maxi cab to the venue.

On arriving at Sandbar around 4:00 PM, the staff was putting the finishing touches on the venue. It looked just as Josh and Amelia had planned: casual, friendly, and with a relaxed beach theme. We could have been in Bali.

It was a truly beautiful day, perfect for a beach wedding!

I texted to Josh and Amelia that "everything was perfect beachside."

The beach was crowded with "sun worshipers" enjoying another beautiful Melbourne summer day. They were lying on the sand, some right up to the edge of the deck of the restaurant.

Momentarily, I thought this could be a problem when they are trying to pose the photos. Anyway, there was nothing we could do.

In the end it was better to have a hot summer's day, than experience a cooler windier one.

Josh asked me to meet and greet the guests as they arrived. It made sense, as I knew most of them. I hadn't seen his father for some time, and I was wondering what sort of reaction I would get from him. I didn't have to wait long. He and his wife Chris were walking toward the restaurant. I welcomed and hugged them both saying "Let's just enjoy our son's wedding, today will be so special, it will be a wonderful day!" Success!

Everyone seemed to arrive at once. All were so excited; many had been part of Josh's recovery journey.

In the distance, I could hear the motorcycles rumbling down Beach Road. Josh riding a Harley, was escorted by his mates Wicksie, Paul (aka Dutchy), Sean, and Lazlo, all on their own Harleys.

Their entrance was dramatic, with the bikes taking center stage for a few minutes prior to the bridal party arriving. Everyone was taking pictures on their cameras and smart phones. Josh's team of Chrisso, Daniel, and Lazlo, looked fantastic, all in black - everyone looked amazing and fresh considering the searing heat.

I had known most of the boys since they were very young. Now seeing them all grown up and still the best of mates was truly heart-warming.

Josh made his way over to me, and said "I was nearly off to hospital this morning. Thought I was having another seizure. The boys have been great." Talk about drop a bomb on Mum!

This was the last thing I wanted to hear on his wedding day, and in a state of shock, I asked him if he was okay. He said yes, but needed to really hydrate himself, as he was still not 100%. I rushed inside the Sandbar and grabbed iced bottled water for him and the boys.

In an instant emotionally, I hovered between joy and panic. Josh said he was sorry to have to tell me, but didn't want to tell Amelia, so rightfully I got the gong.

I guess he needed to prepare one of us in case something went wrong! Before Josh took his place on the deck, we had a couple of lovely photos taken together.

We were all patiently waiting for the gals to arrive!

And arrive they did, the bridesmaids all looking beautiful, in different pastel colors and Amelia, stunning in her beautiful handcrafted gown.

Amelia's bridal party danced down the makeshift aisle of guests on either side to Rihanna's song, *We Found Love in a Hopeless Place.*

The wedding party looked amazing; so beautiful, so handsome, the children in the bridal party were really cute, stealing the show from the fabulous bridesmaids.

Malcolm and Amelia entered the restaurant and together they "bopped" down the aisle to the deck, where the ceremony was to be held.

Still meeting and greeting, I finally managed to get into the restaurant moving through to where the marriage vows were taking place.

The seating area was quite small. I found a spare seat next to Michelle (Handgrenade) and Andrew (Josh's step brother); after Josh's bombshell I was feeling a mixture of emotions; scared, nervous and excited.

The celebrant officiating the wedding service was Josh's old high school principal Lynton, who, on retiring from teaching, became a Marriage Celebrant.

160

It meant a lot to us having Lynton officiate, as he had known Josh for all those years. It made the marriage ceremony more personal for all of us!

The service began, and we all strained forward to listen to what was being said. The breeze had come up slightly, making it a little difficult to hear, yet the sun was blazing hot.

The sun was shining directly onto the bridal party. Knowing Josh's situation, I just watched him and frankly prayed for the service to be over. I was in between fear, joy, and happiness.

I watched Josh's every movement, looking for a tell-tale sign. He seemed happy, yet a few times he really looked like he was struggling to focus. In hindsight he was probably fine, but at that moment, I was so scared that something would go wrong.

Josh was holding Amelia's hands, and at one stage he asked for water. I was praying all would be okay! I was trying to figure out what I would do if he had a seizure. Ugh, too much stress!

Josh managed to get through the service. I was so relieved, yeah!

The service was the most vulnerable time for Josh, as he was standing in the direct sun, dressed in black. From now on I was positive he would be fine!

And he was!

Finally it was time for me to have some fun, enjoy the day and catch up with all of our family and friends. Marie had flown in from Perth, saying this was one wedding she would not miss!

Everything was fantastic!

Our furry kids and grandkids made a starring appearance, so they could be part of the celebrations even if only for a short time.

They immediately stole the show, dressed in their new wedding collars. Montana, never wanting to be left out, put her front paws on the table when Josh was signing their marriage certificate. It was almost like she was making sure all was completed, all was official.

The formal part of the afternoon over, and it was time for photos and enjoying the celebrations. The beach was still very crowded - it was such a hot evening, with only a little breeze off the water.

161

The photographer was posing the wedding party on the beach, between the sun lovers. It was so much fun.

Josh's most hated surface to walk on is beach sand, because it is such a random surface.

Josh really needed to focus on his every step, so going onto the sand for photos was potentially stressful for him. Yet he was so happy he took it all in his stride until the photographer asked him to "stroll" towards the pier. Josh turned around saying, "Sorry, no can do, these legs can only take me so far today and it's going to be a huge day. They are not all-terrain legs." Everyone laughed.

The remainder of the night was spent catching up with guests, lots of photos, and lots of love and hugs. Importantly, Josh and Amelia were ecstatic!

Everyone was in fine form. Collectively, we all wanted the day to go off perfectly, and it did!

The Sandbar team was amazing, professional, and easy to work with. They orchestrated the evening with no fuss and with total professionalism.

All our friends and family came together as one, all with the same goal: to join with us in celebrating a memorable day for us all.

There were several friends at the wedding who had been with us on our journey those past 12 1/2 years. For us all it was such a marvelous day!

My sisters, brother, nieces, nephews, new and old friends, all coming together to celebrate with Josh and Amelia on their very special day; it was such a wonderful wedding!

Josh and Amelia created a Memorial Table with photos of all Josh's mates who had passed. Holding pride of place was a beautiful photo of his grandma. He wanted them all with us all in spirit. They would enjoy the day, along with the boy's parents, who were honored guests.

Special thanks to the Greedy, McMillan, and Holland families. We will always love you, will always miss your beautiful sons, but I am sure they were there, standing behind Josh, making sure nothing went wrong.

The boys and his grandma always have his back!

There was a funny ending to the night

As usual in Melbourne, taxis are at a premium on Saturday nights, especially for venues near the City. Josh didn't drink much alcohol, choosing water instead to keep himself hydrated.

Around midnight, as everything came to a close at the Sandbar, it became apparent there were several friends who needed taxis.

The illusive taxis were proving to be increasingly harder to hail down. Josh decided to drive some of his guests back to their respective hotels.

He needed his car keys, but his groomsman who had been looking after them, was nowhere to be found. Calls were made, and Josh finally located him and arranged to have the keys returned to the Sandbar.

Once Josh got his keys back, he spent the next two hours ferrying friends back to their various hotels in shifts.

Finally, Josh and Amelia arrived at their hotel around 2:30 AM.

We met in Port Melbourne the next morning for a combined family breakfast. Josh joked that it had not been the first night he had planned, but he couldn't have thought of a better way to have spent it, making sure their precious friends found their way safely to their respective hotels. LOVE IT!

So now I am the "B Plan" and will always be happy to be there.

My son has found his life partner. They are both so very happy that I know their lives will be amazing, because the love they have for each other will get them through any problems they may have! Happy son, happy mum!

For all you parents wondering what the future holds for your children who have been struck down with this injury, keep positive, keep moving forward. No matter how slowly, always believe that positive is the only way, and have faith the right person will be there for your loved one when the time is right!

Chapter 16. Josh's Furry Kids

Montana, aka "Little Miss"

As Josh approached the 3rd anniversary of his injury, he was going through a very tough time physically and emotionally. Realization had hit him that his injury was a life injury, and frankly I think he was tired of constantly fighting with his body every waking hour. I also think mentally he was beyond exhaustion, so much of his recovery was mind driven, and he really had not stopped in those first three years!

Through this time Josh and I were arguing nonstop. I really believed we had both hit the wall emotionally. I had never grieved for my son, and Josh was realizing that this rollercoaster life of constant rehab and recovery programs was going to continue. There was no end in sight for either of us!

It probably didn't help that I was totally focused on getting a bonus, so we could finally get our own place. I had hardly been home, except for weekends, for nearly five months. My life revolved around airports, hotels, and endless presentations to financial planners.

To add to this, Josh was involved in a relationship that was slowly undermining his confidence and challenging his self-esteem. I think he felt he always had to try so hard to stay with this young woman. They were living with me at the time.

I found her selfish and self-centered, too immature to deal with someone like Josh who was trying to hold their relationship together, on top of maintaining his grueling recovery program.

I was fully engaged in my business, trying to rebuild our financial security after the first year's expenses of Josh's injury, plus our stint in the USA (2001-2002). I was working away from home so much through the week, totally relying on Josh, to hold everything together in Melbourne, while I worked in every state of Australia.

My goal for 2003 was to finally be able to get enough money together to buy an apartment for us in Port Melbourne. To achieve this, I had to rely on Josh to keep himself committed and focused.

Dutchy had recently bought an English Staffordshire Bull Terrier, Tilly, and the two of them would come around to visit us. Josh and I fell in love with her.

We had always had dogs, but since my marriage break up and with my crazy hours, I decided it was too hard to get another furry kid!

Seeing Josh with Tilly made me realize that he really needed someone to love, who would love him unconditionally.

We talked it over and decided to look for a puppy. It would be Josh's dog; he would choose her!

It would be good for him, give him someone to love, someone who would need him, would love him unconditionally, and importantly he would have a loyal companion, someone for Josh to care and be responsible for.

We researched various breeds and decided on an American Staffie. (In the U.S. usually referred to as a pit-bull. In Australia, American Staffordshire Bull Terriers are a separate breed.)

So then the fun began!

In those days it was rare to adopt a rescue dog or puppy. I came from the school that encouraged buying a dog for breeding, temperament, and character.

All our past furry kids had all been well researched before we brought them into our family. In those days I saw no need to change from what had worked for us in the past.

Over the years I have now come to realize the importance of rescuing and adopting furry friends.

We found a litter of American Staffie pups advertised through a registered breeder. Josh rang them and made arrangements for us to visit them.

Our strategy, decided on before we arrived, was to play it cool not get too enthusiastic!

Under no circumstances should we rush into anything!

We rang the doorbell, and immediately heard the scratching of little paws racing towards us. The door opened, and we were hit with a wall of puppies.

Josh picked up a cute red colored pup with a prominent white flash. He carried her into the room and put her down.

There were puppies coming at us in all directions! It wasn't a matter of playing it cool, it was how do you choose? Which is exactly what Josh said to me. I will fess up there was a little blue colored furry kid I fell in love with. Josh sat down, and without hesitation the tiny red pup Josh had carried in raced to Josh and sat on his foot. Nothing could budge her. And that's how we were found by Montana, she chose Josh. He actually had no choice in the matter!

I honestly believe Montana was chosen for Josh by a higher power. There was no way we would have ever looked at another puppy after she parked herself on Josh's foot!

At that early stage we had no idea of the importance this tiny little roly-poly puppy would have on not just Josh's and my lives, but anyone who came in contact with her.

As I write this, my eyes fill with tears - happy tears, for the joy she has brought us over the years, her intelligence, her unconditional love, her loyalty... she just knows!

Montana is more human than most humans; she has the best attitude!

Montana was loved by all who ever came in contact with her. She didn't have an angry bone in her body, and even though she had never been around children, she was totally gentle and loving to them.

She had the most wonderful personality. Her eyes at times mirrored the worries of the world, very knowing, very aware of everything.

Montana instinctively understood Josh's injury. Even as a puppy, she knew when he was struggling with his body or the mental darkness that overwhelmed him at times. On those days she never left his side.

When Josh was struggling physically and emotionally she was there, resting her head on him, putting a paw on his leg or climbing onto his lap.

When she walks with Josh, she turns her head and watches him every so often.

Montana loved riding shot gun in Josh's or my car, proudly sitting in the front seat like a little person. On a long trip she will curl up on the seat resting her head on your hand, at times making it really difficult to change gears.

Relegated to the back seat, she sits where she can rest her paws on the front center console, usually trying to put her head there as well.

The beach was a favorite place for Montana. She has spent most of her life in Port Melbourne - being so close to the beach, it was her playground, swimming and playing in the sand all her life. After moving to the Basin in the Dandenong Ranges, Montana quickly embraced her new life of space, bush and huge garden to play in becoming Dora the explorer, frolicking around the garden, and then later when Josh and Amelia got their own place, enjoying her new home in Point Cook.

Gardens provided a new activity for Montana, since she was raised in apartments. Mind you, one of my apartments, the old Church, had a large ornamental garden which Montana claimed as hers. She loved it, lying on the artificial grass and watching people walk by.

While living in the church, Melbourne had suffered a prolonged drought. A local television station wanted to do a story on an inner city property with a drought proof garden. They were particularly interested in how dogs dealt with fake grass, and our apartment was chosen.

The TV crew was surprised at how much Montana loved the grass. She really played up to the camera. So that night, when it was featured on the evening news, nearly the entire segment featured Montana showing off in her garden.

Montana is a very social, friendly dog. She loves to hang out, so it's not unusual when visitors arrive and sit down that she jumps up on the sofa and sits with them.

Our attitude with Montana was that this was her home. She could sit where she liked, and if someone doesn't like that then it's their problem.

There were very few people Montana didn't like, so it was rare for her not to be friendly and welcoming towards everyone she met.

Our homes have always been dog friendly, so if you didn't like dogs or were stressed about some dog hair on your clothes, you didn't usually return.

Don't get me wrong, our apartments were always clean and tidy, but they were her homes and she had all the same rights the two legged ones had.

Montana was as comfortable in an elevator as taking the stairs. In fact she loved running up and down stairs - great exercise for her on a rainy day.

With me being away so much, Josh and I had a set up a full gym in a large enclosed area that I rented in our apartment complex.

Josh taught Montana to run on the treadmill, which allowed her to get her exercise when I wasn't around to walk her.

She never was tied onto the treadmill, she just ran on it like a human. For fun we would coach her slowly increasing the speed, encouraging her to pick up her pace. She just took everything in her stride and ran faster.

Someone once asked me "How many beds does Montana have?" The answer was always the same - at home "However many she wants."

When we all lived together, she would share herself at night between Josh's bed and mine.

Montana was a very clean dog. Living in an apartment she was always getting bathed, her red coat always glistening shiny.

While in Port Melbourne, she was walked once or twice a day. She was fascinated with cats, and she knew where every pussy cat lived.

As we walked by their houses, she would stand on her two rear legs looking over the fence for those pesky cats. In fairness, she never hurt any, but if a cat ever strayed into our yard in Port Melbourne they didn't stay long.

Montana also loved chasing the pigeons that drank from her water bowls.

Montana, although never trained, would have been a fantastic service dog. She had a natural perception for those experiencing a trauma or illness.

In 2010, just before my mother passed away from cancer, whenever Montana would visit Mum with Josh, she would sit beside her or try and get on the chair with her. While around Mum, she would be really calm, and would watch her with real sadness in her eyes.

The day before Mum passed, Montana came in to visit her in hospice. Montana just lay quietly beside her bed, and no matter who came in, she never left Mum's bed.

When Mum passed, all Josh wanted were her old lady floral recliners. When Josh isn't well or having a bad day, you will find Montana sitting on his lap, in one of the precious old recliners.

Montana has been a huge part of Josh's recovery. During those dark times for about 3-4 years after the accident, she gave him focus and a reason to keep improving. Her love was unconditional, her intelligence - super human. She does talk, and most of all she just gets it! I love you bubby girl and thank you so much for coming into our lives. I have had many dogs over the years, but I have never had a dog like Montana. She is truly my best little buddy and a wonderful, loyal loving "furry kid" to Josh!

Something to look forward to - Montana has asked me to help her write her story about "her dad" - I have promised her it will be my next project!

Montana was so precious to us. We loved her so dearly, and one evening while I was stroking her neck I found a lump. The next day we took her to the vet, and he did a biopsy. It was an early stage cancer, and we were totally devastated.

Montana was operated on immediately, and the cancer was removed.

Fortunately after all these years, Montana has maintained excellent health, with the cancer being successfully treated.

Thor

And then there was Thor, aka Biggest or Buddies.

All Josh's life, up until my divorce, we always had two dogs. We decided it was time to bring in a furry friend for Montana and another furry companion for Josh. We had a very large garden in the old church, so it would be a perfect time.

I was thinking French bulldog, a cute little lap dog, but my son, as usual, was thinking something else!

Josh's friend bred American Bulldogs. When they heard we were looking for another furry friend, they offered to give Josh one of their puppies.

Yet again I did my research. Such a practical work dog when you live in an apartment? NOT!

For fun and recreation American Bulldogs love to pull trailers, so it's not a sensible dog for someone with a spinal cord injury -- but!

Not to be put off, Josh took me to see the puppies, we were greeted by the dad, a friendly giant standing wagging his tail with a truck tire in his mouth.

Now I am a reasonable person, but I exploded. There was no room for a giant dog, whose choice of toys would likely be a truck tire, living in a luxury apartment in Port Melbourne.

So that was that. I wouldn't even look at the puppies. We went home, and Josh was so disappointed, but he understood the truck tire couldn't be argued with. But with Josh there is always more to the story.

Two weeks later Josh visited Paula. He wanted her to do a psychic reading for him, and he returned home beaming.

Paula, saw a little white puppy, living in a shed, waiting for Josh to give him a forever home.

Josh knew immediately that it was the last puppy from the American Bulldog litter. He said, "Paula, there is no way Mum will let me have him." Paula answered "He is waiting for you. Bring him home, give it a few weeks, and your mum will love him."

So here was Josh, beaming, full of confidence, telling me what Paula had said, and the rest is history.

Josh contacted his friends let them know the good news, and the new bed and blankets were purchased. Thor had a new dad.

After meeting Thor, we all realized, yet again, that the Universe had chosen a very special, unique furry kid for Josh.

Thor was brought into the apartment in Josh's arms. He was black from living in the shed, but he was beautiful, so healthy, and in great condition. His legs were long and his paws were huge. This dog was going to grow into a giant.

A tradition we have always followed when introducing a new dog to our family is that we leave the new puppy in the garden and let the older dog find them on their own, and we did the same with Thor. From the moment Montana found Thor in our garden, their relationship grew. Montana loved him. She was like a mother to him, always cleaning him. They quickly became great mates. In those early days, Thor used to walk under Montana. Now he towers over her, but she is the boss and he knows it!

Josh bathed Thor three times to restore his white coat, dried him with my hair dryer, and then put him on his bed.

From the moment he came out of the bathroom clean that first afternoon, Thor belonged with us!

Because of his potential adult size, he was trained from a puppy that when he was inside the apartment, he had to be on his bed. Outside was play and sunbaking, inside was bed.

Thor was never allowed on the furniture, although we knew he would sneak on the sofas from time to time when there was no one around.

Thor toilet trained really easily, always telling Josh or me when he needed to go out. He quickly developed into a beautiful loving dog, who really saw himself as a small dog. He is like a gentle giant. He has the best disposition, and his goal in life is to give love.

I walk both Montana and Thor, and together they weigh nearly 200 pounds. They are walked on harnesses. I managed them really well, but everyone else had to walk them separately, except of course, Josh and Amelia.

When Josh walks them, they are both so gentle, and neither pull hard. They just walk calmly beside him.

They know that with dad they have to be good, and do as they are told; with their dad they are always extremely obedient and well behaved.

Not long after we brought Thor into our family, Montana had to have an operation on her leg. After her surgery she went to doggie rehab, so we decided Thor should go, too!

Thor had come to us in the winter, and living near the beach, Josh was wondering how Thor would do swimming.

There was a pool at Montana's rehab, and it was there that Thor was introduced to water.

Once in the pool, Thor was so funny. He had no idea how to swim; he just stood there.

This was so unusual. Of all the dogs we have had over the years, Thor was the first of our doggies that didn't swim naturally. We found a doggie life jacket for him, which he wore until he mastered the water.

172

It didn't take long before he figured it out. Once he started swimming confidently (his swimming style is very different from any dog we have ever had) there was no stopping him.

Taking him to the beach (there were dog beaches where we lived), he bounded straight into the water, and basically wouldn't come out. We would have to bribe him to come back to the beach. Montana is the opposite. She races into the water, has a quick swim, and then she's out.

Thor is happy to stay in the water for hours.

One early morning, I walked them down to Dog Beach in Port Melbourne.

As usual, Thor bounded into the water and then he saw someone paddling a canoe way in the distance. Umm, he thought this is something new. Next thing I see him swimming after the canoe. He was fascinated by it.

The guy in the canoe could not believe it. Thor stayed with him for ages, keeping up with the canoe, swimming around and around it.

Most of Josh's cars over the years have been pick-ups.

Thor, like Montana, loves the truck. When he is inside the cabin, he is well behaved, curling up and sleeping most of the time. In the back of the truck, Thor enjoys the wind in his eyes and hanging his head out over the side of truck, entertaining everyone who sees him.

Thor has the most beautiful nature. Both he and Montana were very popular when we had the old church apartment. During the day the furry kids would be in the garden. It was nothing to see people stopping to pat them most times of the day. They were both social butterflies.

One afternoon, I was phoned by one of our neighbors, saying I needed to come home. She said there is nothing serious but something is going on and I needed to see it. Fortunately my office was close by, and I raced home. When I arrived, I saw a crowd of people at my gate laughing. Thor had pulled one of the large cushions off one of the seats in the yard and had totally destroyed it. Montana was sitting back, overlooking the carnage like the little miss she is, looking innocent, and there was Thor entertaining his audience, sitting in the middle of the white kapok that was scattered everywhere.

On the artificial lawn, you can imagine the mess; white cushion stuffing everywhere.

When Thor saw me, he knew he was in trouble, and he tried hiding. As he was white and the mess was white he thought he blended in well...NOT... his size gave him away! It appears that he had been amusing our neighbors and his audience for a few hours. Everyone was laughing so hard, I couldn't be mad at him!

One Christmas Josh bought Thor a skateboard. It wasn't too long before he mastered it, skating around our garden paths. Thor was fascinated with toys and things that moved, playing with them and moving them around until he understands them.

Unfortunately, one of Josh's mates was messing with his skateboard and broke it.

What makes Thor such a special dog is that he is extremely intuitive to Josh's emotional and health state. He just gets it. When Josh is down or struggling, he will wander over to Josh and place his huge paw on his leg and sit there; he is hard to resist. Usually Josh's demeanor instantly improves. Yet again Thor proved to be the perfect furry friend and companion for Josh and Montana.

He loves birds, sometime watching them for ages, and if given the chance will play with them without hurting them.

He watches television, and you often find him fully engrossed in something on the TV. He really loves playing with the ball, but once he fetches it and brings it back he won't drop it, so you have to bribe him to get it from him. Thor never wanders away; in fact he is a real home body. He has and is given so much love.

He loved living in the Basin with Amelia's family. Both furry kids fitted in really well with their change of living arrangements.

Amelia's brother Tom has autism, and initially there were concerns as to how he would react to the dogs. Well no surprises, he loved them both, as they did him! When Tom was overly stressed, both Montana and Thor would sit with him until he calmed down, proving yet again how special they both were! Love and support knows no bounds with them.

For me, the most amazing thing occurs when Josh is not well or feeling flat, they become friendly guards. They shadow him, staying with him until he brightens up.

These two beautiful dogs were certainly chosen to get Josh through the bad days, and give him a reason to continue with his recovery. I know they have been the catalyst, several times, in Josh getting back on track again. On those really tough days they don't leave him and if he ignores them they use their paws and eyes to make contact happen, and then Josh finds it hard to stay sad.

Once Montana and Thor met Amelia, it was instant love. They knew this lady, even in those early days, would be their mum. The attraction was instant, just like their dad's was!

We have been blessed with Montana and Thor. Montana is like a solid tank, strong and youthful and amazingly healthy, Thor has grown into such a powerful, huge dog, and yet he is so gentle, kind and playful! He has no idea of his size. In fact, we think he sees himself as small. Thor and Montana are a credit to the time Josh has put into them over the years, they are great buddies, and they love each other, although Montana is the boss.

Over the years we have had many dogs, but by far the two best at getting on and loving each other has been Montana and Thor.

As I have mentioned before, both these furry kids, have been gifts from the Universe.

It has been well documented through Josh's book how he went through his "dark times." I honestly believe it was the love of Montana and Thor who kept him wanting to keep going. When everything failed in 2010, if it wasn't for his loyal dedicated furry kids, I know Josh would never have survived. It was only them that brought him out of the darkness.

Part 3 - The Light - Nothing is I'Mpossible Where the Will Is Strong

Chapter 17.   An Exciting New Direction

The 16th of March 2011 I celebrated my birthday - A new year and a new beginning.

2010 had been such a difficult, sad time for Josh and me. We had experienced 12 months of losses (the passing of my mum, Josh tragically losing four close friends, and my previously successful business was unexpectedly destroyed in a heartbeat, taking with it our financial security).

I needed to do something positive to start my new year.

In my mind, my birthday commences my new year, so it was important for me to have a very positive start to it.

By accident Josh had scheduled a talk for the 16th. When he realized it was my birthday, he wanted to cancel it and reschedule. I could not have thought of a more positive way to start my year, so we went ahead with it and didn't cancel.

The night was to discuss his recovery and to raise money for spinal cord injury research. The venue was Simon's Vitality Chiropractic practice in Middle Park.

We blasted Facebook, and emailed friends and Melbourne families we were mentoring; basically anyone who was local saw the promos for the night.

We ended up with over 60 people! This was exciting for us both; the crowd was huge, the room was full.

Josh and Simon presented together; their joint approach was well received, and you could have heard a pin drop. The surprise most of Josh's friends had was that Josh was still medically a complete quadriplegic. Many of his friends attending had only known Josh for 5 - 6 years, and they had no idea of the extent of his injury. They had experienced him partying hard, riding motor bikes full on, snowboarding, and basically attacking life like an able bodied male; after this revelation many of his friends looked at Josh in a new light.

It was interesting looking at the "Oh My God" expressions of their faces. No one uttered a sound, even though Josh and Simon spoke for over an hour.

In fact hardly anyone moved!

At the conclusion we opened it up to questions.

The question that stood out in my mind was from Josh's acupuncturist, who asked "Given Josh has rewired his nervous system and brain, had anyone thought of brain mapping Josh?"

Simon answered this with a simple "He would have to be dead to gain a true picture of what he has achieved." This really took everyone aback!

A young woman and her partner attended Josh's talk. She had become a quadriplegic through a diving accident and had just returned from a recovery facility in the USA called PW in Carlsbad, California. At the conclusion of Josh's talk, they stayed around to chat and meet Josh.

Josh's mate Bronte had mentioned PW to Josh, as it had been his goal to attend it, but Josh had never really followed it up for himself, especially after Bronte had passed away. Personally, I had never heard of it. As previously mentioned, neither of us had ever researched spinal cord injury.

The more they told us about the recovery program, the more interested I became. The facility sounded fantastic, but we had heard of lots of "fantastic" places in the past, so while it all sounded great, we curbed our enthusiasm.

When I finally reached home, everything changed. I checked out the website and I knew immediately Josh had to go there. I felt that we finally had a solution for all those families that came to us for help. I called Josh asking him to take a look at the website. Josh being Josh, it took him about two weeks to finally look at it!

When he finally did open the website, he rang me immediately. He agreed, he had to go to the USA.

Very quickly we decided that Josh would attend PW in September 2011 for 4 – 6 weeks. It appeared all the negativity of the past 12 months had started to evaporate. Josh had a new focus, which would hopefully see him improve his gait and walk without his cane.

Once Amelia heard about PW, she too was committed in supporting Josh attending this seemingly amazing facility. It was decided that she would go to the USA with Josh for the planned six weeks. I was happy that Amelia wanted to travel with Josh, as at the time I was working part time and couldn't afford to go there myself for an extended period.

After my mother had died (June 2010) and Josh had lost a 4th friend from a motor bike accident, after an extended period of him mourning their loss and him going off the rails, Josh made a goal to "ditch his walking stick" which had been his constant companion for the past nine years. Since August 2010, Josh had embarked on a fitness campaign; he had his goal and was determined to achieve it.

The fitness program was totally supported by Simon and team at Vitality, including Jenny their acupuncturist. Simon secured Josh a sponsorship with his local gym, Sweat, which had offered Josh cardio workouts whenever he wanted to attend.

For Josh, hearing about PW gave his fitness program a whole new meaning. Knowing this was a huge opportunity to finally get rid his walking stick, Josh pushed his fitness program to a whole new level. I loved seeing him so committed after all our months of sadness.

Josh's friend Colin (aka Silver Fox) arranged a sponsorship with the Bell Street Gym in Coburg; he commenced working with Josh four nights a week on a weight and strength training program.

Everyone who knew Josh was committed to helping him. Amelia started Josh on a more healthful diet. With Colin they designed an additive program to compliment Josh's strict training regime and diet.

For the first time in many years, money (or lack of money) was a real issue for me, so Amelia and some of Josh's friends got together and arranged a fund raiser to help raise the money necessary for the trip to the USA.

We had budgeted for expenses including everything of about $25,000 to $30,000.

At US$110 per hour for training, the cost for the rehab was around

US$7,000, but if Josh achieved the results it would be worth it.

In all the years since Josh's accident we had never held a fund raiser for him. I always managed to find money from somewhere, but this time it was different. I reluctantly agreed that we had to hold an event to fund or partially fund the trip. With my circumstances changing so dramatically in 2010, I realized we had no choice!

For the first time in many years Josh started to bulk up in a healthy way. He looked strong and was becoming extremely fit. He started going to bed early, a huge thing for Josh as he was a real night owl, but now his life was disciplined and focused on the goals of ditching the stick and being in peak physical condition, allowing him to get as much improvement as possible from his six weeks at PW.

By time Josh and Amelia left for Southern California, I could honestly say I have never seen Josh so fit (pre or post-accident) and so committed to achieving the goal to "ditch his stick".

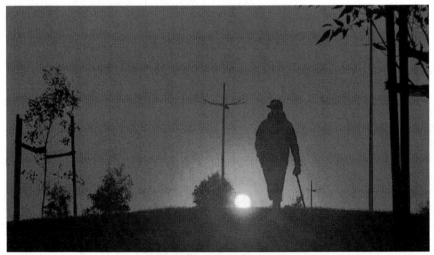

Josh Walking into the Sunrise

There were two other families from Australia attending Project Walk at the same time as Josh and Amelia, so together they rented a four bedroom house in Oceanside, near Carlsbad, not far from where PW was located.

When Josh and Amelia reached the house, they found it nothing like the brochure, but they didn't care, they were there for one reason, PW. So as long as they had somewhere to sleep they were fine.

They chose a room that had a private bathroom, with stairs leading down to the large garden swimming pool. The pool would prove to be a huge bonus for them, after hours of tough training!

Josh was pumped about commencing his program at PW, feeling that at last he had a proven system that, given time, would give him more of his old life back.

Arriving at PW on Monday, he and Amelia immediately threw themselves into his recovery program. They weren't disappointed!

The center was very positive, with music pumping, and clients high fiving and punching fists celebrating an achievement with laughter and encouragement. The only difference between a normal gym and PW's was that there were people in wheel chairs, although they did their recovery program out of their chairs.

Everyone there was focused on getting their lives back, or as much of it as possible. All clients trained with 2 -3 dedicated trainers, who were equally committed to them achieving their goals.

Initially Josh was taken aback, as for the past 11 ½ years he had not been around wheel chairs or many people with spinal cord injuries. It took him a couple of days to work through those mind challenges, but he diligently worked through it, concentrating on his trainers and taking on board everything they said.

There had been a huge build up between Josh and his trainers prior to him leaving Australia, with Josh challenging them to give him their best. He would not fail, and he was fit, focused and ready for anything!

Before leaving Australia the message Josh sent to his trainers at PW was simply, "Bring it on, I am up to anything you throw at me."

Amelia was amazing. Filming Josh, making sure he was hydrated, ensuring that he was eating the right food; it was a real team effort!

From day one Josh felt his body waking up. It was so exciting for him and all of those who loved and supported him.

Even though Josh had continually experienced recovery for the previous 11 ½ years, this program was more accelerated and more intensively focused. Josh was experiencing more recovery post injury! His body was truly waking up. Josh's medical team would be shocked, telling us in those first weeks of his injury that recovery after two years was impossible. What is important to understand, however, is that even in Josh's darkest period he had learned to maintain a certain level of fitness, always attending Simon's practice for adjustments, as well as keeping up his acupuncture.

Josh rang me after his first day's training, asking me to come to Carlsbad. He said "Mum, we've been on this journey together, and now as I feel I can achieve my final goals. I want you to experience PW, and see the amazing recovery results they are getting for their clients. Mum, you have to come here, you'll love it."

After speaking to my sisters about taking a possible trip to Carlsbad, I worked out that I could go for two weeks.

Little did I know those two weeks would change my life!

His PW program saw Josh work out for four days a week, for three hours a day. Also, he and Amelia joined a local gym to concentrate on a weights program.

Their day consisted of PW in the morning, followed by a healthful lunch, and then the local gym for a weights session. Weather permitting, they would enjoy a swim after all the hard work outs as an added bonus.

I arrived at PW two weeks into Josh's training. The first time I walked into the gym in September 2011 I cried happy tears, tears of relief. At last we had an answer for the many families who had contacted us over the years.

The overriding emotion for me the moment I entered the facility was HOPE!

Importantly for me, for the first time since being catapulted into this crazy world of SCI I saw parents smiling, happily watching their injured loved ones fight to get their lives back.

For an injury, where even today NO HOPE is given by many in the medical profession, it was finally a relief for me to experience injured people gaining recovery below-injury!

(There were many times over the ensuring months that I ended up in tears, happy tears, especially when I saw someone up on the walking machine for the first time, or achieving one of their other goals.)

Finally, I met Josh's dedicated and talented trainers. I was immediately blown away by the enthusiasm and positivity of all concerned.

The facility looked like a gym, felt like a gym, and was so positive. Everyone was happy, everyone was committed, and I loved it!

The first morning I asked Josh's trainer Jason if he thought Josh would ever run again, and without hesitation he answered "absolutely."

I was amazed at his confidence!

I loved my first visit to PW, but the bonus for me was the city of Carlsbad. I truly fell in love with this beautiful place.

Through the Internet I had found accommodation directly opposite the stunning Carlsbad beach, at the Best Western on Carlsbad Boulevard.

Although it was an older style hotel, you couldn't fault it. It was very clean and fresh, the staff was amazing, and the location was perfect, close to everything, restaurants, shops, walking paths. It was perfect!

Josh, Amelia, and I set up a routine. They would come to the hotel for breakfast, and while Josh was sorting out his daily routine Amelia and I would go for an hour walk along the shore. On our return, we would have breakfast and go to PW. I offered to pay for their breakfasts, but the hotel's restaurant staff would never take anything from me. They loved meeting Josh and Amelia and hearing their stories about PW.

I really enjoyed my early morning walks with Amelia. Sometimes we saw dolphins frolicking in the ocean, and every day there seemed to be a new experience!

Both Josh and Amelia really enjoyed the Carlsbad lifestyle. They spent a lot of time with me while I was there. We enjoyed eating out at many of the Mexican and seafood restaurants, and enjoyed the magnificent Carlsbad sunrises and sunsets.

Personally, I was particularly fascinated with the Agua Hedionda Lagoon. I thought it was a magnificent body of water, something totally unique in its ability to blend the city, the environment, and the many businesses small and large that dotted the lagoon, offering the community a fantastic natural resource to enjoy!

(Little did I know in those early days, before I left Carlsbad in 2014, I would end up consulting to the Lagoon's Foundation in a development role.)

Even though I could only afford to stay in the USA for two weeks, we still managed a few days in Sonoma. It was terrific to introduce Amelia to Lesli, Curtis, and the Sonoma crew, and for Josh and me to catch up with everyone.

While we were in Sonoma, we attended the Red and White Ball, held outdoors in Sonoma Square. The square was beautifully decorated, and at one stage during the evening Amelia said to me "It's so beautiful, it's like a movie set." And it was! This was a night we would always remember, hanging out with our Sonoma pals, enjoying magnificent wines and yummy food.

Together we enjoyed a fun time that allowed Josh and Amelia a short break from their intensive training routine. The following Tuesday they were back at PW.

For the first time since 2010, I personally felt everything was going to be all right, not just for me but Josh and Amelia.

After months of sadness I felt full of hope and energy. I had fallen in love with Carlsbad and PW.

Returning home, Amelia and Josh kept me up to date with his ongoing progress, which although at times was very subtle, was amazing and inspiring to me.

What was truly mind-blowing was that after 11 1/2 years Josh was continuing to wake up his body. He could feel it responding in nearly every session he did.

On his last day, Josh rang me in tears. In his final PW session in the last five minutes, he ran! It wasn't the prettiest run, but for someone who was told categorically he would never get out of bed, it was everything!

Importantly, his "feral" right leg commenced integrating itself back into Josh's body.

I cried happy tears, and thought to myself, thank God we didn't listen to his doctors, and thank God we backed each other!

Josh really wanted to stay longer, but unfortunately financially it wasn't possible.

184

For Josh, running was not the end. It was simply another step in achieving his final goal of walking down the street without any assistance and with no one having to wait for him.

Chapter 18. A New Life, a New Beginning

Although Josh no longer attends the recovery facility (for personal reasons) there was no way this book or Josh's book *Relentless: Walking against All Odds* could have been written without the inclusion of our experience there because of the **positive** effect it had on Josh's rehabilitation and recovery.

Over the years since 2011, Josh and I have introduced several clients to the recovery center. Many are now repeat clients, and some having returned more than three times. We have been and remain strong advocates of its recovery program.

Our commitment has brought in significant revenue to the center since 2011. Neither Josh nor I have ever sought, charged, or received any commissions or payments for the referrals we made to the recovery center, and when Josh attended the facility we paid the full hourly rate. I charged them a modest consultancy fee for my services for the period June 2012 - April 2013. Additionally, I paid all my own relocation costs, visa, and legal fees.

During the two weeks I was at the recovery center in 2011 with Josh and Amelia, I had several conversations with the senior executive regarding a position he was creating. The facility needed a Development and Marketing Executive; someone who was a self-starter, who understood that below-injury recovery was possible for those suffering a spinal cord injury, and who was confident and able to generate greater support in the local community for the center and its scholarship fund.

A second problem concerning the center was that there were very few local clients attending, even though there were approximately 120 new spinal cord injuries every year in San Diego County.

(At the time I commenced consulting to the center, there were fewer than 10 local clients attending on a regular basis.)

The recovery center had determined that they needed someone to build their brand, while promoting the recovery options locally. I was asked if I would be interested in the position. The senior executive wasn't quite ready to offer it, but he was hopeful it would be created early 2012.

With all the sadness Josh and I had experienced with this injury, I felt I would have an opportunity to really be able to help families in getting the word out about below-injury recovery options for spinal cord injury. I rationalized that if the message was strong and powerful in the USA, it would eventually filter through to Australia. The bottom line for me was that I would be able to help families deal with this devastating injury, and offer hope! An opportunity like this was a godsend; the timing was perfect.

At the time, I was looking for something meaningful to do as far as work was concerned. I was tired of my previous corporate life. My happiest times and where I experienced my greatest joy and fulfillment was in helping families dealing with the SCI of a child or loved one. I still believe (even with the situation I find myself in today) the decision I made to move to the USA was the right one.

From when I commenced discussions with the recovery center until I started there in June 2012, I was unable to accept additional consulting contracts in Australia, as my work was of a long term nature. My skill set was not suited to short term projects, so I was not earning any income from October 2011 until June 2012.

To support Josh and myself through this period, I relied on some public speaking income, my savings, and my precious retirement funds. I was confident all would be fine once I settled in the USA with my new role.

Before my eventual move to Southern California I made three trips to the recovery center (where I volunteered in the facility), trying to learn as much as possible about the business before making a final decision to leave my life in Australia for a new life in the USA.

After each visit, I felt more confident that I was heading in the right direction!

Before committing to a role with the center, I had to be sure I would qualify for the necessary visa I would need. The senior executive recommended a lawyer in Los Angeles. The recovery center had used him in the past, and my thoughts were that this man knew the center and what was being achieved there, so I would therefore be better off appointing him, I knew my visa application would need a "strong" case study to be built to justify the approval.

I met with the lawyer on one of my trips to the USA. We discussed my unique situation in great detail, especially my financial position. He recommended that I should apply for an E2 business visa. He was confident that although I wouldn't meet the business investment criteria, because of the uniqueness of my experience with below-injury recovery, coupled with my 14 years management consulting in Australia, he was very confident I would gain the necessary visa approval.

However, he agreed that he would have to build a strong case to get it accepted.

The recovery center did not want to sponsor me for an employment visa. They had done so in the past with another employee and didn't want to go through that process and expense again. While it was annoying and disappointing, since this would have been the easiest and quickest option, I let it go. I was on a mission to help families and grow their business of hope and recovery.

To move to the USA, I had to sell everything I owned except my furniture and my art collection. I even had to give away, sell, or drink my extensive wine collection, only being allowed to bring 72 bottles with me to the USA. Anyway, none of this was important in the long run. It was just "stuff."

I sold down my remaining retirement funds, liquidated my investments, and sold my car. In my mind, I was moving from Australia forever. I would spend the rest of my working life with the recovery center, building their business and helping families. I would be living in the most beautiful city - Carlsbad, making a new life for myself. That was my mindset. I felt so happy and relieved that finally after all these years I was starting to do things for me again!

And to quote the senior executive, repeated several times during my time there ~ "Kay, you will always be a part of my recovery center team."

I believed the commitment of the center to work with Josh and I was genuine and real!

In the months to come, I was saddened by the level I was misled, and the broken promises regarding the role and the relationship.

The lawyer, even though I was referred to him by the recovery center, was another huge mistake which was not only costly, but emotionally devastating.

In Australia, my expertise, experience, and reputation was as a business builder and relationship manager, working with corporations, introducing their senior executive teams and their boards to centers of influence in the financial services sector of Australia. To achieve the success needed, I worked closely with senior executive teams and their boards. My role was to coordinate the meetings as well as their facilitation. Once the relationship was established, my role was to manage the relationship, further develop it, and ensuring that it was strong and productive. I had successfully run my consulting business specializing in this area for over 15 years. From 1997 up until leaving Australia in June 2012, I had been involved in recruiting, building, and managing national sales and marketing teams in the financial services sector.

I felt my past experience and accomplishments would set me up for a successful transition for the Development and Marketing role at the recovery center.

As previously mentioned, I arrived at the center in June of 2012, full of hope. My personal goals were simple:

1. Speak to as many people, organizations, groups, and clubs about the possibility of below-injury recovery through the recovery center (building solid foundations in the community).

2. Help families in whatever way I could (this part I would truly enjoy).

3. Create multiple funding sources for the recovery center scholarship program (offering a lifeline for those who desired recovery, but couldn't afford to attend the center).

4. Seek strategic relationships to secure scholarship funds (securing ongoing revenue streams and ongoing income streams for the facility).

My past experience told me it would take me approximately three years, the first year hard work creating the relationships, building awareness, working with any early supporters, year 2 consolidating the work in year 1 gaining more supporters, and in year 3 it should all come together. In the past I have adopted this approach and it has always worked, I didn't see I needed to change what had previously been successful. To achieve results would be hard work, putting massive hours into my role, but that's how I had always worked. I was truly ready!

It was hard saying good bye to my family and friends in Australia, but I felt I had no choice. Now I had a recovery solution for families; I wasn't going to let anything stand in my way.

Once moving to Southern California, I can honestly say that I truly loved walking into the center's gym every morning, witnessing the positive atmosphere and the smiling faces of the clients doing whatever it took to get their lives back, and of course the enthusiasm of the wonderful, dedicated trainers.

I always knew when one of the children with an SCI would be attending the gym for their recovery training. Games were set up in readiness for their arrival. It was so hard for the young children to understand the importance of their recovery training. In reality, many never knew a life out of the chair, but their parents understood the importance of reconnecting those tiny injured bodies to movement. The children were all very cute. They would speed around the center in their chairs, with everyone encouraging them. At times it was hard for the parents. Often their child would be tired, and yet the therapy had to continue.

Whenever I was in the center, I would always make a habit of walking through the gym two or three times a day, offering encouragement and support. Sometimes I would help film a milestone, or just stop by and hang out, offering some encouragement, especially if the client was there without family support. Often I would take those clients out for dinner or a tour of local sights, trying to make their time at the facility not so lonely without their loved ones. I always tried to attend client farewells, as that was always a bittersweet time for the client, the trainers, and those who were hands on in the center. Sadly, many left because they couldn't afford the fees any longer, I truly hope one day soon the medical insurance companies start to see the positive healthful effect those suffering SCI attending below injury recovery facilities.

In my spare time, I enjoyed chatting to the parents or loved ones. It was so tough on them. Their lives had dramatically changed too, and they were there to support their loved ones giving them their personal cheer squads.

Something that always made my heart happy was seeing the parents or loved ones supporting each other. They would gather in the lounge or the kitchen area, supporting each other and comparing notes. It was our own very special caring community.

I know lifelong friendships were made by many attending the center, with Facebook and other social media enabling them to keep in touch, once they had returned to their communities/countries. There were periods you experienced a mini "United Nations" as families from all over the world and all over the USA congregated with the single purpose of recovery.

I too made lifelong friends, sometimes with families I only ever met through social media, being constantly in touch with them. Within our community there was the safety of understanding what we were are going through.

I am fortunate to be in touch with friends and families throughout the world. Our one common link is that we have a child or loved one with an SCI.

Although many clients attending the recovery center may not walk, for me there is joy in seeing any improvement, no matter how slight. Any improvement below injury level should be celebrated.

Allowing someone the ability to feed themselves, move from a power chair to a manual chair, sit up unaided, all improvements towards getting some aspect of their lives back, were exciting to me! I always encouraged and celebrated improvement at any level. The walking part, I believe, was between God and the individual. As I said too many parents, sometimes it's harder for the individual who walks, especially someone like Josh. Josh cannot feel his legs properly, and for him nothing is automatic. He lives in a manually-operated body. He has to calculate every move, every step, and most people don't understand this about him.

An important aspect the facility provided to their clients was the normality of some of the recovery activities. Many a time you would see a client throwing a football or baseball to one of the trainers. It's the simple things most of the clients miss; the "normal" act of throwing a ball is great therapy.

The community was very important. Often someone with a spinal cord injury feels isolated from their old community. Once they attended the recovery center, they created a network of friends, supporters and mentors through this experience, which on those dark days was a wonderful, powerful resource.

I had the dream role; what went wrong?

From the moment I arrived, I was initially supported by the senior executive and most of the management team. They all saw Josh and me as a formidable team that was totally committed to helping the center build their brand, which obviously equated to more success for them.

192

In my first meeting with the senior executive (the week I arrived), I was blindsided by a facility associate. I didn't see it coming and I was frankly confused and disappointed. I had flown half way across the world, I had left my family to help others, I had sold everything I had to help in building the recovery center business, and here I was being undermined in my first meeting. To say I was confused was an understatement. This sadly was a pattern replicated on many occasions, causing me even more disappointment and confusion.

Having no network in Southern California other than through the recovery center team, I wanted to "hit the ground running". I rationalized that the most effective way to do this was to pick the brains of the executive and management team, since they were all living locally.

Before arriving to take up my role, I developed a document which was emailed to the senior executive and his team. It was simply a "Who do you know?" "Where do your kids go to school" "What clubs do you belong to?" questionnaire. I was hoping their answers would give me a "kick start" allowing me to start achieving some early results for them.

Of the team of six, I received one completed survey (from the CFO).

I asked on several occasions for the others to complete their surveys. It never happened. No one had time, apparently!

The facility was a member of the local Chamber of Commerce, and in early July, I attended a Sundowner at a local Carlsbad location. I loved the event. It was very impressive, especially with the number of people attending. All I could think of was how will I meet and get to know all these people?

In my initial remuneration discussions with the senior executive, before accepting the position, he initially offered me 30 - 40% of what I raised in donations. I immediately rejected this, since being a parent there was no way I would ethically work in this way, taking a percentage of my fundraising efforts. I felt it was misleading for me to be remunerated in this way.

I advised him I would need to be paid at least an amount equivalent to 1/3 of my Australian earnings per month as a retainer. For that figure I would work unlimited hours. I was still assisting Josh in Australia and paying for all my visa fees, furniture storage, and my airfares (to the date I relocated to the USA the amount was in excess of $30,000).

I was led to believe by the senior executive that I would receive the figure I had requested.

In late May, after my unit was sold, my furniture packed up for removal to the USA, and just a few weeks before I was to leave Australia, I received an email from him, stating that the recovery center could only afford to pay me approximately 20% of what I would earn in Australia, and he was only prepared to give me a three month contract. The much lower retainer would barely cover my rent, food and fuel; everything else would have to come from my savings.

Totally devastated, not knowing what to do, I contacted him. He said the three months was a formality, and after this period the contract would be renewed. He promised the consultancy fee would be reviewed in September, to an amount more like I had been initially promised.

While I was disappointed, I trusted him. My main concern at that time was getting the word out there in the community about the recovery center.

The one issue that was confusing to me was that someone had been doing a part of the position before me on a salary plus benefits. I was sure she would have been on a far greater salary than what they were now offering me. As a consultant, I never received any benefits from the center.

So here I was barely covering my living expenses, but I didn't care; I was happy feeling I was making a difference! I had faith all would be okay. I was on a mission to spread the word of hope and recovery, and nothing would stop me! Personally, I didn't want to dwell on the negatives. All through my time at the center, Josh and I were continuing to refer clients there.

In fact, I was advised by the Center Manager that Josh and I referred over 8% of the clients to the facility during 2011-2013.

Josh spent a total of 5 1/2 months at the recovery center. Through two visits we paid the same hourly rate everyone paid for the training. Our only benefit was that Josh was trained by his preferred trainers in every session.

It made it easy for me when I was chatting to loved ones knowing I paid the same as them.

Up until recently we still referred clients to the facility. We loved the work and recovery process in the gym and will always be supportive of the work of Eric Harness, Director of Research, and the talented facility trainers (Eric has since left the Center).

I consulted to the recovery center from June 9th 2012 until April 2013, taking three weeks out for Josh's wedding. I was never given the promised increase, even though I was assured almost monthly it would happen. Not being focused on money, I always believed it would happen.

With no network and little support from the center's management team in the 10 months I represented them, these were some of the current and ongoing events I was working on. All these initiatives came through my endeavors. Remember, when I started there I knew no one.

I knew I had to meet people, influencers, but how? In the past I had always relied on my old networks, but here in the USA I had no real networks. But I quickly realized the community was heavily involved with the Chamber of Commerce and Rotary. Although not a Rotarian in Australia, I was a friend of Rotary with two clubs, one in Melbourne and one in Bali. My sister Wendy, a long time Rotarian, researched the local clubs. We discussed them and decided I should join Carlsbad Hi Noon.

1. I became heavily involved with the local Chamber of Commerce attending all significant Chamber functions (usually at my cost), representing the recovery center at the majority of Sundowners, Chamber Breakfasts, and Coffee Connections from July 2012, as well as meeting many new people at every event I attended. I started to make friends; this was a truly added benefit for all my hard work.

2. I went on to be involved in three Chamber committees: Ambassador, Military Affairs, and Education.

3. Organized, coordinated, and was the emcee at a local business luncheon within six weeks of my arrival. Successfully introduced the recovery facility and the The Ekso robotic exo skeleton to selected invited local business people, city council members, and local influencers.

4. Member of the Carlsbad High Noon Rotary since July 2012, winning Rookie of the Year 2012-13.

5. Developed the relationship with a local Business Association; my role was to represent the recovery center within this association.

They planned to hold community events with a percentage of proceeds from some of these events in 2013 going to the facility's scholarship fund.

6. Member of committee for a music festival, May 2014 – The recovery center was to benefit from selling tickets for this event. Once I left, this initiative did not progress even though I had put a significant effort into developing it.

7. Local non-profit invited the recovery center to enter a team in their Fun Run in June 2013, with monies raised by the center's team going directly to their scholarship fund.

8. I was invited to join a professional women's network. This group was an invitation-only women's network with member groups in Orange County, North County, and San Diego. I met several of the members who ran successful businesses, small/ medium/ large (to listed corporations). They held regular forums and business breakfasts. You had to be a business owner to join. One of the members offered to hold a function for the recovery center. I was confident once relationships were further developed it would result in a lot more support for the center's Scholarship Program.

9. The recovery center was to be the beneficiary of a golf day organized through a local tavern. I was involved on the committee, coordinating the volunteers and much of the logistics for the event.

10. Developed relationship with the local Tourism Authority, and arranged for the center's senior executive and me to speak to their board.

11. Arranged and hosted in conjunction with the Center Manager several VIP tours for awareness and gaining support for the recovery center from community leaders, business people, organizations, and potential donors.

12. Developed the concept, "Wheel in My Wheel Tracks Corporate Program" to encourage local corporations to get involved through an employee challenge program, which would have encompassed potential partnerships with annual fund raising events. All corporate participants were to gain external sponsorship of their event, with all proceeds to the center's scholarship fund. At the time of my leaving, I had one major local corporation in the

process of committing to participation. (It is my understanding that this initiative never progressed.)

13. Developed speaking opportunities with service organizations. The center's senior executive and I spoke at two local groups, and there were more in the pipeline.

14. Hosted a "lunch and learn" at the Center with my Rotary Club in April 2013 for 15 Rotarians and young leaders.

15. Liaison and organization of the recovery center's 1/2 Marathon Team for North County non-profit 1/2 Marathon.

16. Organized Corporate Tables for Facility's major Corporate Initiative 2012, selling 10 tables, introducing many new potential supporters to the recovery center.

17. I spoke to countless parents on a nearly daily basis about their loved ones progress, and interacted with the new families through social media. My relationship with Michelle, a triage nurse from Montana, regarding her son resulted in him having three visits to the recovery center. In April 2013, through my relationship with Michelle, I was invited to speak to physiotherapy students and lecturers at the University of Montana focusing on my experience with below-injury recovery.

18. Developed a relationship with the inventor of an adaptive paddle board for people in wheel chairs to use, that saw the recovery center's clients involved in the worldwide launch of the first adaptive paddle board on the city's Agua Hedionda Lagoon. I coordinated the launch with the Lagoon Foundation, who ensured the support of the City Officials. It was an extremely successful event for the Center and its clients.

19. Josh continues to promote his recovery center experience in his motivational presentations.

From the moment I arrived in Southern California I researched the various foundations established (community/ corporate/ businesses) that could possibly support the center's scholarship fund or assist with the gym's equipment purchases.

The problem was that the incidence of spinal cord injury is relatively low. The recovery center was therefore competing in a very crowded market,

197

against programs that were offering broad based community benefits. It became apparent to me that we needed to look wider as to where our fundraising and sponsorship activities needed to focus.

The more research I did, I realized that the one market segment that constantly received significant support from our facility was the local business community. There were several standout areas, especially in "health tourism" with the majority of the center's clients coming from out of state and out of country. I discussed my research with several people I knew in the Chamber. One of the members recommended I approach a local college's business department that volunteered to work with non-profits in assisting with specific projects. I contacted the department head and presented the case for the recovery center. After a follow-up meeting, my proposition was accepted. There was normally a fee of $1,500, but I was able to negotiate the report to be completed pro bono. Basically, I wanted a *qualitative* survey done in conjunction with our clients and staff. The report was to be focused on three segments.

- Local

- Rest of California and the USA

- Overseas

Each client segment was to be interviewed to allow the report to be produced. The outcome would demonstrate the economic impact of the recovery center on the local business community. The data focus would be on tourism, transportation, living expenses, entertainment, and so forth. Additionally, I wanted to include the economic effect of the center's staff on the community, since at the time there were 40 staff members, and many had relocated to work for the local facility.

My objective was to create a survey methodology for not only the local recovery center, but all the related facilities throughout the USA, to enable them to evaluate the effects of their facilities on their local communities, opening up significant opportunities for their individual foundations and scholarship programs, and to be able to supply qualitative data to their local business communities, thus allowing them to build a case for receiving financial support.

Armed with an independent survey from a respected college would give me the data I needed to approach the benefiting businesses for sponsorship dollars. If it worked locally it would work for the other centers.

I was clear in my parameters with the college's team that it had to be a "drill-down qualitative document." We had three meetings, and the final document was to be signed off by the three recovery center colleagues who had attended all the meetings and were fully aware of the objectives of my survey.

I had to return to Australia for Josh's wedding, and while there I was stunned to receive the final survey document which had been approved by the recovery center. The team had turned my *qualitative* survey into a *quantitative* document, which for what I wanted to achieve was useless. I was extremely disappointed!

Having left the recovery center by the time the survey was presented, I was in disbelief at one of recommendations, which was to align with local nursing homes; a total no-no to the majority of young people suffering this injury. To quote an executive no longer with the center who was privy to the final document "You would have been devastated with the results." I don't blame the college in any way; their survey was signed off by three recovery center executives who had obviously failed to grasp the significance of what I was trying to achieve, even though they attended all the meetings with me.

Returning to Australia for Josh's wedding my first priority was to attend an appointment to have my visa finalized with the US Embassy in Melbourne. After what I can only describe as a disastrous hearing at the Embassy, where I was advised that my visa would not be granted due to their concerns on the viability of my business (see Chapter 23, *Making a Living; The Art of Patience 2010-2014*).

After confirming with the Embassy I could travel to the USA on an existing tourist visa, I decided to keep the scheduled flight return to Carlsbad, to give notice on my apartment, sell everything, and return to Australia.

I felt totally lost, disillusioned, and unbelievably sad! My heart ached!

I advised the facility's senior executive that my visa application had been denied. The plan, after talking to him, was to work through until I had to leave, as I had several projects that needed to be finalized.

On my return to Southern California, and hearing about my visa issues, several community leaders, fellow Rotarians, approached me to re-apply, offering their support. I advised the recovery center of this. Two weeks before I was due to return to Australia, I was referred to an immigration lawyer in San Diego, who agreed to lodge an emergency visa application for me.

The cost was $11,000, and he assured me he had never lost a case! I was torn; with little money left, could I take the risk? My family in Australia wanted me home. They did not support me staying in the U.S., and in their view I was wasting what remained of my precious funds.

In my heart I loved what I did. I loved the interaction with the recovery center's families. I loved being able to give hope, but mostly I was happy living in Southern California. I was gaining my independence back for the first time since Josh's accident and I reveled in it.

The application was lodged two days before I was due to leave. I telephoned the facility's senior executive, advising him I would be staying. He wasn't available, so I left a message for him.

He phoned me the next day saying my position was no longer available, and they had decided to make other plans. But if I wanted to I could buy a franchise. They would be happy to sell me one. He emailed the paper work and details to me, saying "because of who I was, he would give me a deal"!

My answer to this "deal of a lifetime" was a resounding *NO*. Even if I had wanted to purchase one, my money was nearly gone!

I returned to my office at 7 AM the next morning, clearing my desk and that was it. The dream was over, and to this day I have never heard from anyone in the executive team.

With all my past expertise with working with boards and senior management teams, in the time I was with the recovery center I never met the entire board, and I never attended any senior management meetings. In hindsight I was set up to fail!

For what I achieved, while there, my time was not wasted; however at times I still shake my head and wonder why I was ever offered the position in the first place!

For me though, the time I spent working in such an amazing place of "hope" was not wasted, I met so many wonderful families, the lives I touched and the friendships I made. I will always be grateful for that.

Most importantly, it gave me a chance to meet and enjoy the caring, supportive Carlsbad community. I have made lifelong friendships and Carlsbad will always have a huge place in my heart.

Chapter 19. Money, Money, Money - Learning to Survive on a Wing and a Prayer

Quick Overview

In 2000, my management consulting business was three years old, all the hard work had been done, and I was receiving the rewards. Nine months earlier I established a second business with Wendy, and life was great! My plans moving forward included at least three months a year travel. I had turned 50 earlier in the year, and being single, with Josh getting on with his life, I was planning to semi retire at 55 and retire completely at 60, to pursue my goals to work with rescuing and working with exotic animals.

Wendy and I were planning with a group of friends to build a townhouse development in Port Melbourne. Life was great!

And then the phone rang, and from the moment I picked it up, my life as I knew it was over. I had a whole new life that would take me into near bankruptcy twice in the following 14 years, into a financial world I could never have imagined in my wildest dreams. Not one of my pre-accident goals ever came to fruition. *Knowing what I know now, I have no regrets. In fact I don't even recognize my old life these days.*

Josh and I speak at seminars in financial services. After I finish, Josh always commences his talk by saying how bad he feels that he has caused me so much financial pain. My answer is always the same: "That you had an accident, I was the parent, and I should have had you protected better financially. You didn't mess up, I did!" Hopefully those reading my book will understand the importance of insuring their children, either through a child trauma cover or as they turn 18 years of age look for a comprehensive insurance protection package that will cover them no matter what happens. From my past life as a financial planner, I knew all this. I should have taken out the necessary insurance on Josh, but like most families I just didn't think about it!

The emotional and financial cost of a catastrophic spinal cord injury dramatically affects those suffering the injury and their loved ones on many levels.

All Lives Change in a Heartbeat!

There is the abrupt and total change of everyone's future whom are close to the person who is injured.

In many cases, family homes need to be renovated or sold, new homes purchased to accommodate wheel chairs, bathrooms need to be altered to accommodate a wheel chair, changes made to showers, etc., sleeping requirements - sometimes new beds need to be purchased and bedrooms modified, motor vehicles have to be adapted or a new user friendly vehicle purchased, and, at the far extreme, jobs and careers are abandoned!

Nothing Is Ever the Same!

In Victoria, Australia, if you have a motor vehicle accident you are covered to a certain extent through Transport Accident Commission (TAC). There was definitely a difference in how the TAC patients were treated, especially when Josh was in the rehabilitation unit.

In those days there was almost a "them and us" attitude - from the medical staff, not the patients!

The type of accident Josh had was not covered by any traditional insurance (i.e., TAC), it was simply an accident. Fortunately, at the time, Josh did have some insurance coverage.

1. Total Permanent Death Policy through HostPlus underwritten by AXA.

2. Insurance for Personal Loan through Westpac Bank (Josh had taken a small personal loan to purchase a motorcycle. I had encouraged him to purchase the small loan insurance policy in case anything happened to him, more as a learning exercise for the future, to teach him the importance of responsible borrowing).

3. Accident Policy through an American Insurance Company, value $480,000.

It is compulsory in Australia for all citizens who work to contribute towards their retirement. Even at the age Josh was, he had a small retirement fund through his employer, and this allowed him access to a

Total Permanent Death Policy through Host Plus underwritten by AXA.

When we had time to breathe, those first 6-8 weeks were beyond horrendous. We contacted, through our lawyer, the three insurers involved, and the outcome was:

- TPD Host Plus SETTLED almost $50,000 within 12 months of the accident. This allowed Josh to purchase a new car. (Those reading this book in other countries need to understand that motor vehicles are a lot more expensive in Australia, and in all honestly, Josh did buy a sports model car, but for his hard work he deserved it.)

- Westpac loan SETTLED immediately through their insurance coverage, because of this, Josh owned his motorcycle.

Precedence was established through the successful settlement of the two policies, so we were therefore confident Josh would eventually be awarded the settlement of $480,000.

The Accident Policy settlement dragged on for nearly three years. During that time I had personally funded Josh's recovery.

The policy was never paid out. The American Insurance Company offered $1,200 on a $480,000 settlement - we never settled.

Comment regarding the Insurance Policy:

My son's medical practitioners were as one - Josh would never walk again, much less get out of bed. Josh did walk out of hospital, and in fact within 2 1/2 years he no longer used his wheel chair. But here was the sting for Josh and me: 14 years on, Josh still *presents medically as a complete quadriplegic,* because, against all odds, he walked. He regained some of his old life back, but the insurance company refused to pay because he "improved"; he regained movement in his limbs.

This was something we never understood. Any medical practitioner in the world who viewed Josh's MRI's today would say confidently that they were viewing the MRI of a "complete quadriplegic", and yet the insurance company failed to pay on the basis of physical evidence alone. The medical evidence confirms complete quadriplegia. Josh *never* recovered internally. He deals with issues on a daily basis that every quadriplegic endures. Yet against all odds he recovered enough to maintain a reasonably positive lifestyle. For that, the insurance company

205

penalized him.

We now understand the recovery regime we did consistently on Josh through those early days set him up to live the life he has today. But for Josh, although he lives a fairly active life, nothing is automatic for him. He has to "manually" drive every body movement. We never think about walking, picking something up, or sitting, etc. Josh has to direct his body into action. Nothing in Josh's life and movement is automatic. In Josh's and my eyes, he paid a huge penalty for fighting to get his life back, by the insurance company looking at the physical evidence against the expert medical prognosis. In my opinion, this needs to change, and I will be discussing these issues with insurance companies as opportunities arise. When we trust an insurance company with our future, they need to pay out from the medical prognosis, not rely on the physical.

To reiterate something I have already written, it was NOT an Australian insurance company. It was an American insurance company.

One of the most devastating effects of this injury is financial - as a loved one, it's the last thing you need to worry about when you are facing a battle such as we had. Nevertheless it is the extra layer of worry you can't ignore; it's terrifying and it doesn't go away!

In those early days, I had to focus on Josh and myself. I had just sold my home in Port Melbourne. I therefore didn't have a mortgage. I was renting a house with Wendy, so I only had to pay half the rent. I still had to find the money to pay my car lease, which was part of my business, 50% of the household bills, petrol, food, and fund Josh's alternative recovery team. Wendy was fantastic, but she was also working for herself in a business we had set up nine months earlier; a business I basically walked away from after Josh's accident.

Just before his accident in May 2000, being an empty nester I had leased a Mazda Miatta sports car, not the most practical car for transporting a wheel chair. Being a new lease I would have had to pay huge fees to unwind it, so this was yet another worry I had to deal with. But in the immediate future, it was one of those things I simply put to one side.

For the record, a wheel chair *does* fit into the boot of an MX5, as long as it is secured with straps.

Fortunately, Josh owned a car that was reliable, so in the short term we used his car for transporting him around.

I quickly realized that due to the nature of my business (it required a lot of travel throughout Australia, and most weeks I was away from home) I couldn't work. In fact it would be nearly 12 months before I could return to full time work.

I worked for myself, so basically there was little money coming in for nearly 12 months. Josh's father had made it clear he couldn't or wouldn't help me financially, so there were no expectations there!

So how did we survive? I look back on it now and in truth I have no idea.

My mother and Wendy helped as much as they could! It was so tough!

We always managed to get through somehow - you could say "we lived on a wing and a prayer!"

Josh was flown into the hospital by air ambulance - we had insurance cover for that; if he hadn't been covered, it would have cost me several thousand dollars. Fortunately that was one bill I never had to pay!

Josh was admitted to the Melbourne public hospital as a private patient. Having top Private Health Insurance, this enabled us to have the best doctors operating on him. I am sure we would have had the same doctors had he been Public patient; the catch was that as a Private patient, the hospital could charge more than the "common fee."

Even with Top Private Cover in the first week I was out of pocket several thousand dollars. This was paid out from my precious savings.

I quickly had to change things, and after speaking to the hospital's finance department, they agreed to "discharge" (on paper) Josh as a Private patient and re admit him as a Public patient. As Josh had had his operation by then, I thought we had seen the worst of it; in reality I had no option.

Paula had already warned me in those crazy first few days that it would be impossible for me to work for at least 4 - 6 months. At the time I had said to her "I don't know how we will manage," and she just said "have faith, you will!"

Fortunately, I had set up a Self-Managed Superannuation Fund in 1997, and I had some cash in that!

I also had the proceeds from the sale of my home. Not a lot, but they had been invested in long term investments. Well, they had to be sold!

Due to my previous high earnings as an employee I had three credit cards basically with little on them, that gave me access to nearly $60,000 of expensive credit, but at least that was available.

It was not long before my precious available savings evaporated into thin air. In those days there was a little flexibility in regard to investments in Self-Managed Super Funds. In a desperate effort to get some cash, I sold four of my artworks into my super fund that gave me another $12,000.

In today's environment you would never get away with transactions such as this, but I was desperate, and frankly I did what I had to do!

Several people offered to hold fund raisers for us, but I was too busy to deal with this as was Wendy, so they never happened.

Josh's father's motorcycle club held a fund raiser which raised enough to purchase a new wheelchair for Josh. This was the only help I received from his father. But we were grateful to not have to find the nearly $7,000 the wheelchair cost.

By the end of the 18 months I had maxed out my credit cards to the extent of nearly $60,000, but fortunately I was working again, so by the September of 2001 I was able to start paying them down.

Through all this, I was adamant that Josh's lifestyle would not change. I had to buy him a lot of new clothes. Due to the risk of pressure sores, jeans weren't suitable to wear in those early days, so track pants became the clothes of choice, but not just any old track pants.

Hoodies with zips, the track pants, new shoes, all were a cost. I was funding many of the alternative therapists, not being able to claim them through Josh's Health Insurance, but I never complained as I could see the results and Josh was positive; that was all that mattered!

I was buying health additives and vitamins to help Josh's body recover and put on weight. Josh had lost nearly half of his original pre-accident weight. It was so scary.

Looking back over nearly 14 years, I calculated I had personally spent in excess of A$1.6 million on Josh's recovery and lifestyle needs.

You see, Josh's job for all those years was to recover as much as he could. My side of the bargain we made in those frightening first few days was to fund it. I was fortunate that I had a very successful business until September 2010, when in the space of a morning, I lost nearly everything I had invested, and my three year contract was never paid out! - But that's another story.

We never held a fundraiser until 2011, but by then we had no choice; there was no way I could fund Josh and Amelia's six week trip to PW. I just couldn't

It was decided to hold a fundraiser, and they decided to call it the "Woody Ditch the Stick Campaign". Thanks to Josh's friends, Amelia's organizational prowess, and Michelle "Handgrenade's" auctioneering skills, we raised about $18,000 towards the costs associated with the first trip. The actual costs were around $30,000. Expensive, but necessary. That six weeks in the USA at PW (2011) gave Josh a new lease on his recovery. It was worth every cent we spent.

I funded the remaining costs of $12,000.

The second fundraiser was a totally random event, after Josh and I spoke at the MLC Risk Retreat in Western Australia 2012. The delegates, hearing Josh had become ill, immediately after his inspiring talk passed the hat around to those delegates attending the final dinner, and in the space of an hour had pledged $14,000 towards his four month trip back to California. Again, I funded the remainder of that trip.

Where I am today!

My decision to reapply for my visa (2013/2014) was not a mistake. The last 12 months I spent in Carlsbad was a time where I truly commenced my healing and, more important, gained the confidence I needed to move on with the next phase of my life.

I was in Carlsbad for nearly two years. The first year I was totally committed to getting the word out about below-injury recovery. It was this first 12 months that put my financial security under so much pressure, spending so much on my relocation, setting up an apartment with furniture (my own furniture couldn't be brought over without my visa), my normal living expenses, and expenses involved in my role.

All of this was based on the commitment that I had a long term permanent future in the role I was offered by the senior executive of the Recovery Center.

During my first 12 months in the USA, financially, I was actually going backwards by $5,000 a month. I was still financially supporting Josh, although not as much as in the past, and I had left a few commitments that still needed to be financed in Australia, including my furniture storage.

While I was waiting for the visa to be approved, I couldn't seek any other work in the USA. It was so challenging; I couldn't even get a Social Security number.

Obviously this monthly drain on my savings wasn't sustainable!

The last 12 months I was in the US, I shared apartments, and significantly reduced my living expenses. I hunkered down, living on little and reduced my expenses in Australia.

If I had thought about what had happened in my life, I would have become depressed. My life from 2010 to now was a total "Riches to Rags" story.

When I returned to Australia, I joked that if it wasn't for Wendy offering me a room free of charge in her home, I would have been the best dressed street person in Melbourne.

My one regret was not leaving on December 21st (2013) as I had originally planned. Staying on until February cost me financially, and I lost a lot of time in commencing the re-establishment of my life in Australia.

The last 12 months in the Carlsbad allowed me to recover and grow as a person, personally and professionally. I have an amazing group of friends and contacts from my time in Carlsbad. I do not regret staying on!

I now accept that, barring some miracle, I will never live permanently in the USA. As sad as this is to me, I have to be realistic!

However, the one serious problem I have that at the age of 64 I have no financial backing, security, or any savings at all. My American experience has cost me everything I had, other than my furniture, which is in storage.

I did however, achieve an important goal. I have helped many families, and through Warrior Momz I continue to do this!

I cannot put a price on health and happiness, and if asked, I would do it all again!

I am not sure what the future holds for me, other than finishing this book and continuing my goal of helping families globally dealing with spinal cord injuries and the potential recovery options.

In the meantime, I will live with my sister and learn to use public transport.

My Background and What I've Learned!

My career was in senior management and consulting positions in the Australian Financial Services Sector. I had actually developed financial strategies for families who had children that were disabled. I had extensively researched this area two years before Josh's accident.

I should have known. I should have been better prepared for an event such as his accident. The reality was that I never thought it would happen to us; in fact I never even considered it.

Sadly, that is the one thing every family I have spoken to in regard to their loved ones' injury. They all say the same thing: *we never thought it would happen to us!"*

Whether it is a catastrophic accident or a life threatening illness of a child or other loved one, it affects the whole family, and in some cases the ability for that family to function at most levels.

The situation is made dramatically worse in the USA due to a dysfunctional health insurance system.

In Australia, there is a Medicare safety net which guarantees our citizens hospital coverage in a public hospital in the event of an accident or devastating illness. There are still out of pocket expenses, but at least you have a bed, and care while you need it.

In Josh's case he was in ICU for about six days. He was then transferred to the Acute Spinal Unit within the hospital, where he stayed for approximately 5-6 weeks. From there he was admitted to the Rehabilitation Facility, which was part of the hospital, but external to it. Josh was in rehab for around three months before *we* discharged him...on the 11th of November 2000.

Private Health Insurance, (which Josh had) gave us options in case further surgery or ongoing hospitalization was needed.

What *wasn't* covered by my Risk Personal Insurances was my loss of income earning potential, when I, as a single working parent, had to stop work to support my long term injured child.

There are insurances in Australia that allow cover for "child trauma". In my opinion, all children should have this coverage at a minimum. Radical you say? Well, walk in my shoes and you will have a better understanding of why I make this statement.

Our society is geared to both parents working, so financial pressure adds a huge dimension to stress levels. While income protection insurance covers the breadwinner against injury or illness, it does not cover them for the sudden illness or accident occurring to a child, which can prevent one's ability to work.

If we think it's tough in Australia, I can assure you it is unbelievably tragic in the USA.

I moved to the USA 2012, to focus on spreading the word about below-injury recovery for those with spinal cord injury. Over this period, I was dismayed at the fragmented medical system in the USA. Families through no fault of their own are thrust into the unknown frightening world of spinal cord injury without the lifeline I had in Australia of a stable medical system.

(What was not covered in Australia, were the alternative costs of my son's recovery in excess of AUD$1.6 million as previously mentioned).

Sadly, while in the USA I heard horror stories on a daily basis. I am in contact with families in most parts of the world who are struggling to deal with the costs of rehabilitation and recovery needed when a loved one suffers a spinal cord injury.

Health insurance companies worldwide have to accept that below-injury recovery from a spinal cord injury is possible. The more who accept and support the payment thereof, will have the effect of providing families with a valuable life line. Recovery, in the long term, will possibly give the option for the injured person the ability to re-enter the workforce, overall reducing the costs of their long term care.

Over nearly 14 years I have mentored many families, spending the past two years in the USA working with those who have suffered this debilitating injury. Frankly, I am horrified at the situation so many families are thrust into.

I have set up a network called Warrior Momz that reaches out to the world through social media.

As I mentioned earlier, the one thing that is said by everyone I have mentored is "we never thought it could happen to us". Well, sadly, it does, and the financial ramifications for families are devastating. Retirement plans are put on hold, savings are decimated, and families are forced to run countless fundraisings to support their injured loved one. All this while trying to physically support their loved one's recovery goals, maintaining their family commitments, and maybe still be working.

With my background in financial services, I know there is an answer. Are the insurance products there already? I am not sure.

We can't give up, we have to keep researching!

Relationships and Care!

I have learned that many relationships fail or experience significant stress once a partner suffers a spinal cord injury. It's not just the injured person who has to make huge adjustments to their lives. It's their partners as well, and as I have previously discussed everything changes; everything and everyone are under pressure!

It's a Whole New World!

If there is a marriage or partnership involved, the injury brings with it a totally different set of financial issues that again have the capacity to cause significant emotional grief and relationship stress. There are no rights or wrongs here; I don't intend to make judgements!

From experience, I can say a stressed relationship does great damage mentally to someone who has a spinal cord injury, and frankly they are better off out of it! The injury is hard enough psychologically without overlaying a toxic relationship into the mix. Depending on the circumstances of the accident, it can cause anger, blame, and extreme guilt. There are so many ramifications from this injury that are difficult to manage while trying to gain recovery.

There are additional difficulties when there are children involved.

In my experience, in many cases if a relationship breaks down the injured

213

person usually returns home to live with their own parents, who will always be there for them no matter what. Often, sadly, it is a single parent.

This is beyond tragic, as their parents have potentially been on their own, and "the kids are off their hands", in some cases for several years. In the blink of an eye, they assume the role of caregivers for their injured adult child.

This is very common! Recovery from this injury requires focus, a clear healthy mind, money, loving support and encouragement, correct diet, and medication only for health issues. There are so many things to consider.

A family with insurance that covers even part of the costs of this injury, or replaces an income, will be much better off financially.

As much as you love someone, financial pressure, constantly having to watch or find every dollar, puts so much stress on relationships.

In my view, anyone setting up their long term financial goals must firstly get their "Family Protection Insurance" sorted out as the basis of building a strong financial foundation for the family's long term security.

Financial Planners worldwide need to spend more time with families who come to them for advice discussing the importance of getting the financial foundations in place before worrying about investing their dollars.

Without financial foundations in place, the investment dollars are irrelevant, because a catastrophic injury or illness will see all those plans thrown out the window. Personally, I had significant coverage on myself and my income, but none of this helped me, because the injury was to my son. Had I considered him as part of my financial security it would have been a totally different outcome for me. As I have already stated, I didn't think it would happen to us!

BIGGEST MISTAKE OF OUR LIVES!

I thought it would be interesting to look at some statistics.

USA

There are approximately 200,000 people living with spinal cord injury (SCI) in the USA. Annually there are 12,000 - 20,000 new cases. Every

48 minutes someone in the U.S. is paralyzed from a spinal cord injury.

Males account for 80% of all SCI.

50%-70% of injuries occur in the *15-35 year old* age group.

Causes: 46% motor vehicles, falls 22%, violence 16%, sports 12%, other 4%. The estimated lifetime costs to care for a 25 year old who becomes a quadriplegic is more than $4.5 million, and costs for a paraplegic exceed $2.25 million. (Stats are from the U.S. Center for Disease and Prevention.)

Personally, I think these numbers are on the low side.

Australia

Unfortunately, the most up to date statistics released in 2013 apply to 2007-2008.

There are approximately 12,000 Australians living with SCI. Annually there are between 360 - 420 new cases

Males account for 86% of all SCI. Most at risk is the 15 - 24 year age group.

Causes   : 23% motor vehicle, 23% road users - motor bikes, cyclists, pedestrians, 28% from falls, 9% resulted from being hit or struck, 9% water related, 8% other causes. (Data are from the Australian Government - Australian Institute of health & Welfare.)

Chapter 20. The Son and the Mum

This chapter is probably one of the more important for parents. There have been some intensely personal issues that I have decided not to discuss, but I have left out little, as I felt I had to be honest; if nothing else this chapter is about the love and trust we had for each other. This epic saga of recovery would never have been possible without the strong bond we shared.

The greatest news of all is that we are surviving! And it's been nearly 15 years!

On the 25th of June 2000, up until 3:25 PM that fateful afternoon, Josh and I enjoyed a typical mother and son relationship. I had been divorced from his father since he was 12 years old, but we enjoyed a strong and positive joint parenting relationship, seeing each other regularly to discuss Josh's wellbeing and progress.

After my marriage break up, Josh became very protective of me, and still is.

Just after my marriage failed in 1992, I decided to take Josh overseas to Bali. I knew if I could manage Bali, I could manage travelling anywhere. In the past when we had all travelled together as a family, I always felt we were safe with Garry. He was tall, strong, and protective, so it was a huge challenge for me to travel with Josh as a lone parent. I guess Josh picked up on this, because as we were walking through the hotel on the first day Josh out of nowhere said "Don't worry Mum, I will always look after you." We ended up having a fabulous trip together; it was to be the first of many we would enjoy together.

We enjoyed a positive relationship, and I always encouraged his independence. We loved each other and we laughed together, and as he grew older we continued to "hang out." We enjoyed all the experiences people normally have with their children, including travel (Josh shared my passion for international travel). At times we argued, but I can honestly say although we "banged heads" with each other, no matter how bad it got, we never went to bed angry!

One of the activities I really enjoyed with Josh was eating out. Living in Port Melbourne, there were a few favorite restaurants we ate at regularly. Many nights we would chat casually about whatever was on our minds, and every so often something would trigger a really in-depth conversation where everything was discussed as true friends, equals, who respected each other's opinions.

Those were the nights I treasured! Even after all these years I still fondly remember those nights out with my son! Unfortunately, these days those dinners are few and far between.

Josh's injury changed everything. He went from being totally *independent*, to being totally *dependent*. Our strong relationship, the trust we shared, gave him confidence in me. In those crucial early days, where I was literally fighting for my son's life in a world that was totally foreign; beyond frightening to all of us, his trust and belief in me was critical to his belief that he could recover!!

I was always confident he would walk. I believe my confidence in those early days gave him the courage to believe, to dream that anything was possible!

Important note: I want to say that even though I was confident he would walk, I never pushed Josh in any way. For him to walk was *his* journey, and if at any time had he said to me, "Mum, this is too hard, I'll stay in the chair," I would have totally supported his decision!

As he was growing up, Josh enjoyed a much closer relationship with his father than with me. They had many activities in common, motorcycles and hunting being two of them, neither of which held any interest for me.

After the accident, the opposite occurred in his relationship with his father. I can honestly say his father, in my opinion, never really took the time to understand the injury. Maybe he felt overwhelmed with the sadness of what had happened to his son; we never really discussed the accident. For me, I didn't have the time to deal with what his father was going through, I was only concerned with keeping Josh fit, and focused on his recovery.

In his father's eyes, it seemed his son Josh had died.

Josh and his dad still have a father and son relationship, but sadly, it has totally changed since the night of his accident.

To this day I have never discussed with Garry how he felt about Josh's accident, the immediate aftermath of his words to me the night of the accident and his total lack of financial support even when we were desperate, is something I will never understand, forget, or comprehend.

The change in the relationship between Josh and his dad was something I stayed out of, not offering a comment either way, except on rare occasions. But it saddened me to see the deterioration of their previously strong bond.

Josh still says "I love my dad" and I am glad, because a son needs his dad!

Personally, up until the night of the accident, I maintained a reasonable relationship with Garry. We shared many happy memories over the nearly 30 years we were together, and we did raise an amazing son together for his first 12 years!

While the memories are still there, I no longer have any level of a relationship with Garry.

Josh knew I was confident in the strength of his mind and his ability to recover from the many injuries we had dealt with together over the years.

He trusted me!

In those early days after the accident, everything I did for Josh was driven by my love for him and FEAR. In those crazy early days, I felt I was failing him, feeling totally inadequate, not being able to understand what he was going through as much as I tried, and most of all, not being able to make it easier for him!

The first month, I lived in an internal state of overwhelming fear, combined with a state of constant panic, yet at all times outwardly putting forward the message of positivity, confidence and faith in Josh's ability to recover.

Still to this day, I feel like I let him down as a parent, since no matter what I did I couldn't "cure" him. Parents are meant to protect their kids; we are meant to know the answers. Obviously I know and understand a lot more now, but it is a constantly changing injury and complacency is your worst enemy.

And sadly the doctors, those who we looked to for help and education, didn't understand the recovery opportunities of the injury, and especially didn't understand someone who, in Josh's case, defied the medical prognosis, fighting every day to get his life back - this defies any medical logic or understanding.

Even today, going to any hospital is a nightmare for us. Every time we have had to attend one, it is a potentially life threatening experience for Josh. Basically, a poorly prescribed drug could kill him!

This is not an isolated experience and emotion to us. To this day I have never met a parent in a similar situation who hasn't experienced exactly what we have.

In those crazy first days, it was imperative for me to control my emotions around Josh as much as possible. I wanted him to see me as being strong and confident, but below the surface I was terrified.

As I look back over the years, Josh and I have been to hell and back so many times; we are truly survivors, and neither of us will ever give up on our bond, although there have been times our relationship has been stretched to the breaking point! But our great love for each other always saved a total breakdown. Neither of us would say it's been easy!

I quickly realized in those first few days that I was no longer just Josh's Mum, I had to become his performance coach, his mentor, his advocate, and, in short, the one who kicked his butt!

One thing I refused to be labelled was his "carer". I have heard parents say I am my son's or daughter's carer or caregiver now. Personally, I hate hearing this (sorry to offend you all). Being a carer totally changes the dynamics of the parent/child relationship.

I understand the parent role is very much that of a carer; just don't call yourself one!

In my mind, a parent labelling themselves as being a carer creates a mindset of a long term activity that can stifle recovery.

Obviously you are there for your loved one 24/7, but please refrain from using the term carer. Also, our loved one is injured, not disabled. Disability is another word I don't like associating with spinal cord injury – it is an injury.

We were very careful, mindful of the words we used around Josh when describing his injury.

I was totally focused on maintaining Josh's lifestyle and self-esteem no matter what. It was important for him to believe that although he was badly injured he was still Josh, and nothing had really changed accept that now he was dealing with this unrelenting injury in a body that fought him every step of his journey!

We had our fair share of tough times. Financially the first year was so challenging for us all, including Wendy, I really don't know how we managed, but somehow we did!

Moving to Sonoma, California in September 2001, for me to take up the management position at the winery added a level of stress to Josh's recovery that we didn't factor in at the time. But we both agreed I should accept the position; it was the right thing to do, giving us both new lives after so much sadness. Josh was tired of seeing the sadness in our family's and friend's eyes, and he felt the move would give us both a second chance to establish ourselves in a new community, and to make new friends that didn't know us before the accident.

We quickly commenced building a new social life in Sonoma; it wasn't too hard. Being involved with the winery, there was no shortage of dinners, and wine tastings to attend. We both developed a love for the sensational Sonoma wines and eateries.

Although he had a fun time there living and riding his bike around the area, and working in the winery as the weekend concierge, he left behind his support network healers, family, and friends in Australia. He found that side of his life really tough.

After his father's heart problems, Josh returned to Australia in December 2001.

On returning to Australia, he moved back in with Wendy. Naturally she had rules, but as is usual with Josh he pushed her too hard!

His behavior and lack of respect toward her really upset Wendy to the point she didn't want him around. As much as they loved each other, they both butted heads once too often. Josh's failure to abide by her rules in her house (they were not unreasonable in any way) was just too much for her.

Finally Josh really just pushed Wendy too hard, and she said enough (and she was totally entitled to)!

Wendy asked him to leave.

With no support from his father, he was totally out of control, partying, drinking too much, and sleeping on a mattress on the floor at a friend's house. I was receiving almost daily phone calls from either Wendy or Josh as to what was going on. I didn't know what to do. Josh and I had made the move to Sonoma together, now I was thousands of miles away, and Josh was totally out of control!

The crazy lifestyle he had fallen into ended when he crashed his car.

Fortunately no one was hurt. With Josh now without a car, my brother felt he had no alternative than to broker a peace deal between Josh and Wendy, and against her better judgement she let him return to her home.

She set the rules, to which he readily agreed, and of course not surprisingly, Josh broke the main rule the first weekend he was back with her!

In my heart I wanted to stay in the USA, but things hadn't gone according to plan there (my first day of starting at the winery was September 11, 2001). So much had changed in the USA because of that, and with the issues I was now experiencing with Josh, I knew I had no alternative but to return back to Australia.

Back home I rented a house in Port Melbourne and we settled into a routine. Almost immediately I was offered a lucrative contract for my consulting business, so I hit the ground running, starting work almost immediately.

Before long Josh asked me if his girlfriend could move in with us.

I felt I had no option to agree as most of all I wanted Josh living with me so I could make sure he kept up his rehab and training.

To say their relationship was challenging to Josh and my relationship was an understatement. It wasn't a large house, so there was never enough room to get away from each other.

Unfortunately, Josh brought his girlfriend with him, so to say it was challenging to our relationship was an understatement. It wasn't a large house, so there was never enough room to get away from each other.

And they used to argue; this I truly hated.

I agreed to let Josh get a "furry kid", so once he had Montana, he had someone to love and she loved him unconditionally. The girlfriend was superseded - gone - Montana ruled!

I was working long hours in an extremely stressful role. I was determined to make bonus so I could buy an apartment. The first year to achieve the results I needed, I missed by only a small amount – I was devastated. It was heartbreaking, but the second year I worked harder than ever before, and I made the bonus!

Boy, oh boy, did we celebrate!

Josh, Montana and I moved into a good sized second floor three bedroom apartment two blocks from the beach in Port Melbourne. It had a large balcony for Montana to sun herself on.

It was the 3rd year after Josh's accident. We were constantly arguing, and his attitude to me was aggressive and hurtful. For two years he had gone flat out on his recovery, but as he approached the 3rd year anniversary, I guess he became discouraged. He finally understood he faced a lifetime of recovery, watching his diet, and not drinking. I truly believe he just got over it and let go!

I was at a stage where I was totally over him and frankly if he didn't start focusing on his recovery I was done! It was the hardest of times!

My fears of him going backwards didn't help the situation, but something in him had changed and he wouldn't talk to me about it!

Reality had hit home. Josh understood this was a life injury!

Over the years we have both learned so much. We both agree; year three is probably the hardest to get through.

Since he was a little boy, we always had a saying, "ALWAYS TELL THE TRUTH EVEN IF IT COULD HURT; THE TRUTH OVERRODE EVERYTHING!"

Late one evening, I returned home from two days working in Sydney. I was totally stressed with work and more than stressed with Josh. Something was going on with him and I had to find out what it was. We had been arguing constantly, and life for both of us was miserable!

On the flight back, I was thinking about Josh, trying to figure out what was causing his aggression towards me - my heart ached so much, I felt it would break. As the plane landed, I thought I was having a heart attack, such was my pain.

Finally, I arrived home. We immediately got into a heated argument. It was out of control. I threatened to kick him out, sell his car, and then he said – "Mum I guess I have to tell you the truth and I don't think you'll be happy."

Josh suffers from neurogenic pain, 24/7. I knew this and also knew of his decision not to take any medication.

He told me he had experimenting with some non-prescription drugs to try and manage his pain. He had taken the drugs in his step brother's apartment, so he was in a controlled environment. In his mind he was "safe".

This had happened over two or three weekends.

I was disappointed in him and furious with his step brother, but I had been told the truth, so I had to accept it.

We previously had an agreement about drugs, and he had broken it! Josh knew that was part of our pact we made on the Thursday morning after his accident. I had been very clear I would help him, spend whatever it took, towards his recovery, but he had to stay away from non-prescription and illegal drugs.

I went to my room totally devastated. He had broken his agreement. I hate drugs and here was my greatest fear manifesting.

At least I knew what the problem was!

The next morning he said "Mum, I will stop taking the drugs because I love you and don't want to hurt you anymore." I answered that he needed to stop them for himself, not for me.

He didn't experiment with drugs again until the year the boys died in 2009-2010 - our year in HELL!

After this "come to God" moment, we settled into repairing our relationship, and continued our partnership in his recovery.

After a year of seeing him struggle up the three flights of stairs to our apartment, I decided to look for a small ground floor apartment for Josh.

Almost immediately I found the church. It was a huge apartment, probably double the size of the apartment we were currently living in. Well, it really wasn't an apartment. Actually it was an office space. It had a kitchen, a bathroom, two offices, and two huge open plan areas. The minute I saw it I saw the potential. Josh's father and I had renovated and built three homes, so I had a good idea on design and what I could do. I called Josh to come see the apartment. He walked in and said "Mum this place is perfect." Our immediate problem was whether we afford it.

We chatted with the real estate agent, coming up with a firm offer, and making it subject to selling my apartment. This condition I knew was pushing our luck.

I truly believe the apartment had been waiting for us, a gift, if you like, from the Universe!

Our offer was made and accepted. Josh and I were ecstatic! My apartment sold two days before the contract would have fallen over, and our financing was approved. We were so excited! Not only did we have a large spacious apartment, we had a huge yard for Montana; something she had never had.

Our lives set off in a whole new direction!

My cousin's husband Paul was a builder, and we had him come around to give us a quote for the work. We had roughly sketched a plan on the concrete floor after we pulled up the newly laid horrible teal colored carpet. In hindsight the carpet color made the apartment appear very dark, which we think put a lot of people off buying it.

I had a budget in mind to get everything completed. Paul didn't know my figure, and his quote for everything we wanted, including a new light colored carpet came in just below my budget. Yeah!

Our ambitious "fit out" gave Josh a bedroom with his own bath and living room. We included an additional bedroom, office, and dining room.

Fortunately for me, I was working away most of the time during the construction period. Josh coordinated the project with Paul and his team. All the work was completed while Josh was there. They worked while he slept, and while he watched TV. He hardly left the site; I don't know how he endured the dust and the mess.

On completion, we had a large apartment with our own areas, our own spaces. It was a happy time for us all! Not long after a second furry kid Thor joined our family.

For the first six months Josh's friend Chrisso lived with us. He left at Christmas, and for the first time since finishing the remodel we enjoyed having the apartment on our own.

I enjoyed my peace for a year or so, and then as sure as life goes on, it all changed again when a new girlfriend moved in, creating another set of challenges.

My work was increasingly demanding. I was working out of town most of the week so I only had to put up with her on weekends; that was bad enough!

She stayed around for nearly 18 months, and for me, it was 18 months of hell! It was a time of me walking on egg shells, in my own apartment, while paying most of their bills. It was not a good scene!

The final straw was when she tidied my office while I was on one of my trips overseas. To say I was furious was an understatement. Josh thought I was ungrateful; he always thought I was against all his girlfriends!

Yet again we argued. It was such a tough time. It was my home, yet I felt at times like a visitor.

Their relationship continued to deteriorate, and finally she was gone. I had the pleasure of packing up her stuff and putting it along the wall in our hallway, and then departing the apartment to visit my mother not returning till all was removed. Yay! We were finally on our own again, with the doggies.

Happy days!

Summer was on us. Overnight our church yard became the "Belgian Beer Garden of Port Melbourne" or so Josh's friends called it.

Now that Josh was single again his friends were at our apartment 24/7, drinking beer, chatting up the many girls that walked passed our property.

Within the apartment complex, I leased a large interior space next to our apartment. It was over seven square meters in size, and housed our personal gym purposely set up for Josh and me. It also became a spare room for Josh's multitude of friends, where they could sleep over when they had enjoyed late nights in the City. At times I felt like my home was a halfway home for Josh's many friends. It's fair to say there were many times that Josh tested me at every level.

226

One night Josh hosted a surprise party for one of his friends in the gym room. The party included a stripper and pole dancers, and I was far from happy when I found out. But by then the damage was done! Fortunately the residents in our complex loved Josh and the furry kids so they all allowed him a fair amount of latitude.

No matter how bad it got between us, our love always reigned supreme and we always got over it!

Towards the end of our time in the church, I realized that for Josh to continue to improve he needed his own place away from me. We were in another "live-in girlfriend" phase, and frankly I was tired of it. I desperately wanted to get my own life back on track!

This last girlfriend was just too much, and I was tested at every level by her. In her defense she was only 18. At that time I was truly done!

After nearly eight years of living in our dream home, I put the apartment on the market. Everyone thought I was crazy, but I knew for our relationship to survive, and for Josh to continue to improve, we had to live apart.

The church had been such a great place to live. I really never regretted selling any of my properties, but this was one place I would have given anything to have kept. It had many happy memories, and one very sad one -- Bronte.

Josh's world started to fall apart after Bronte died suddenly from complications from his spinal cord injury.

Josh and Bronte had been casual friends before Bronte's injury.

Bronte suffered a spinal cord injury while training on his motor bike; a random crash, turning into a lifelong injury, seeing him become a quadriplegic.

Josh didn't go to visit Bronte in the hospital until he wanted to see Josh. Once they caught up they both quickly became a huge support to each other.

Josh never had a mentor. He was always on his own with his injury. He would often say the injury is the loneliest injury you can ever suffer, as no injury is the same!

When Bronte was injured, Josh had a friend for the first time who totally understood. Bronte's injury level was very similar to Josh's, so Josh was able to really help Bronte understand the injury and what to expect.

Bronte followed a lot of what Josh had done through his recovery. There were sessions with Paula, Isabel, and off course Simon. Bronte went to Simon for almost a year, and during that time he stood unaided and walked a little. Bronte and Josh supported each other through the 40 days diet, where they ate "pulse" food three times a day for 40 days and 40 nights, only drinking water between meals. While they both felt fantastic after it, they decided it was too radical for them.

They had a lot of fun times together, with neither of them worrying about boundaries!

Bronte used to spend a lot of time at the church with us. He was really part of our family. The dogs loved him, and it was fun having him there. Being around Bronte, Josh was relaxed and very happy; they had their "unique world" which few understood.

One wintery May morning, Josh rang me at work. He was devastated. He told me Bront had died suddenly, and I raced home! In the five minutes it took me to get there, Josh had been phoned by friends saying that Bront was alive, but on life support. He had been admitted to Frankston hospital (about 45 kilometers from our home) so we had a chance to say goodbye!

Bront was an organ donor, so the hospital was keeping him on life support while those receiving Bront's precious organs were either flown in to the hospital, or hospitalized in anticipation of the transplant.

I followed Josh's car to the hospital; bringing his girlfriend with me.

Josh drove his car like a man possessed, I couldn't keep up with him; the 45 minute drive to the hospital was a nightmare! I still wonder why Josh wasn't pulled over for speeding.

Arriving a few minutes apart we rushed to the ward Bront was in.

If I thought I had had bad days before, that day was beyond anything I could imagine. Bront was half sitting up in bed, looking so normal you would think he would wake up at any time. But we all knew he wouldn't. It was a sad, devastating time for all us. Even now as I write this, the memory of that day is as vivid as if it was yesterday. The grief I feel is still overwhelming, even after all these years.

The youth of today are often criticized as detached and uncaring, and yet on that horrific day I witnessed a group of young men, some openly crying, being supported by their friends. They were all there for their mates. It was tragic, yet uplifting seeing these amazing guys. They were like a tribe that took care of each other, along with taking care of Bront's parents and his brother.

By 5 PM I was done. I was emotionally devastated. I was no support to anyone feeling like this, so Josh's girlfriend and I left the hospital. Josh stayed with Bront's family until his life support was turned off, around midnight!

I cannot adequately articulate the devastation I felt losing Bronte. Oh how more than ever, I hated this cruel vicious injury!

Josh didn't return home that night. He actually disappeared for about four days. I knew where he was, and although I was concerned, I knew he was with his mates. They all mourned and celebrated Bront's life together, men supporting each other! The tribe was coming together to mutually support each other in this time of devastating sadness.

It is very difficult for Josh and me to talk about Bront even today, so great was the pain of losing him so tragically! As I write this my eyes are full of tears. Bront's death was one of the major reasons I decided to go to America to spread the word about below injury recovery. I didn't want other families having to go through this devastation! It had been Bront's goal to attend PW!

If we thought we had gone through a tough time there was worse to come, because in the space of just over 12 months from Bront's passing, Josh lost three close mates and my mother died.

Josh was so close to my mum. Their relationship was a model for all grandson/grandmother relationships. One day I would want that relationship with my grandchildren when they arrive. I have a beautiful example with my son and my mum.

After a year of tragedy, I really think Josh thought "What's the point of keeping fit, trying to keep positive, trying to do the right thing?" He went on a partying binge, which included drugs and alcohol - it was as though life was all too hard and he was finally over it!

I was just hanging in there, terrified and worried for Josh's future, truly expecting a dreaded phone call. My mobile phone never left me.

Josh was living in his own home away from me. He had the dogs with him, so if all else failed I knew he loved those dogs so much they would at least give him some reason to keep going. Frankly, they were my only hope! After all we had gone through I really think, through this period, I really lost my son for a time, knowing that after all we had been through, it could end in tragedy. It was such a tough time for us all!

About October 2009, he seemed to pull himself out of it. His furry kids loved him so much. He was totally devoted to them, and once again he decided to lead a clean life.

We talked at length one afternoon. I said to him "Maybe you're the one to tell the boys' stories, to be a surrogate son to their parents."

It was such a tough time for him that he had gotten to the stage he didn't want to answer his phone anymore!

I was so relieved and in awe of my son's strength and courage!

Josh has a chapter in his booked called *"If strength is born from heartbreak, then mountains I could move."* He also has these words tattooed on his side torso. It truly articulates this terrible period of our lives.

After a year of sadness, Amelia "danced" into Josh's life. From their first meeting it was apparent that they would be together. Our lives changed yet again, and this time, for the first time in months, life was so positive. For the first time in months my heart was happy. I no longer dreaded the mobile ringing.

The first time I saw the way Amelia looked at Josh, I was relieved and happy. Finally I knew in my heart that he had found his soul mate!

Josh found a renewed passion to live and cleaned up his life. They say they saved each other, and together they had a future! And the furry kids welcomed their new mum!

The horrors of early 2012 will live with me forever and will always manage to rekindle the fear I have of this injury.

You can never be complacent about this injury!

After all these years I did become complacent in regard to Josh's health. He was so happy, and in a great place mentally with Amelia in his life. Everything was going well, life was good!

230

And then this vicious cruel injury came back with a vengeance, nearly costing Josh his life!

For Christmas 2011, I gave Josh and Amelia a three week holiday in Bali. I was going too, which would allow me to spend some time relaxing with them in a fun environment we all loved.

The first week they stayed at Asri's home with me, celebrating New Year with fireworks, an abundance of fresh seafood, and stunning views of the partying in Kuta.

Once the crowded streets cleared just after New Year's they moved down to a five star hotel on Kuta Beach. The hotel had only been recently completed, with a roof top swimming pool and bar. Josh and Amelia were in 7th heaven!

Five days before they were due to return to Australia, Josh took a bite of a piece of bacon, and he knew instantly the food was bad. Within a few hours, he was suffering from severe food poisoning. He was extremely ill; Amelia had to call a doctor for him.

Josh was severely dehydrated. He needed to go on an intravenous drip for a day to rehydrate him. The food poisoning took a lot out of Josh, and it curtailed his activity for the remainder of their trip.

I was really disappointed this had occurred at a supposedly five star hotel, managed by a prestigious hotel group. In all the years we had travelled to Bali we had never experienced food poisoning there. I had selected that particular hotel because I thought its standards would be high. How disappointing!

Through their holiday Josh had been having several intense healing sessions with Afron, a Timorese Sharman. Once he suffered from food poisoning, he had no further sessions with Afron, as they were so intense Josh didn't feel physically able to deal with them any longer, so he never received his final treatment with him.

On returning home, Josh suffered a series of health problems. He just was not in a good place health-wise. The side effects of SCI are never far away; once the body is weakened it can take several months of hard work to restore its health.

These problems went on for several months, getting progressively worse with time. Josh was feeling really out of kilter. He was having problems

231

with his sleeping, his urethra, and in general his overall health.

Our world crashed when he suffered a near fatal seizure in front of me.

The doctors explained if he had been in his car or on his own he would have died.

Josh's seizure challenged him and me at a level we had never experienced. My confidence was at rock bottom; both Josh and I always tried to project positivity in regard to his injury. During this period the darkness that enveloped us was all encompassing. No matter what, being positive was the last thing on our minds.

Neither of us would have blamed Amelia for walking away, as the seizure set off a series of hospital admissions, and for about six weeks there never appeared to be any good news!

Amelia took it in her stride, showing strength well beyond her years.

But for Josh and me the seizure very nearly destroyed our world and we both realized, for the first time in years, how vulnerable he was! It further reiterated our view that the medical profession does not understand this injury other than the mending of the shattered bones.

Slowly over several months Josh's health returned thanks in part to the wonderful healing work of Uschi and Doug in Encinitas, California. We will be forever grateful to this amazing, caring couple.

The relationship between a son and his mum, when it works, is strong, positive and rewarding. Over the years we have banged heads more times that I can remember, but the one thing we both knew, no matter how tough it got, we loved each other and always had each other's backs! And we always will -- something I know will never change!

Here's a quote from Josh on Face Book Post, he wrote on my last birthday (2014):

"Happy birthday to the most amazing, committed mother, if I didn't have you in my corner 13 years ago to get me out of giving up, I wouldn't be here today because of your strong determination in not only myself but you, we butt heads a lot but that's how a strong bonds roll... You've helped make me the man I'm finally becoming, love u KZE x x."

For me now, I just want to be Josh's mum again - it's time for me to resume that precious relationship and allow Josh and Amelia to build their lives together.

Chapter 21.   Uschi & Doug - Working from Friendship and Love!

Anyone who has read Josh's book will know that we have left no stone unturned in seeking recovery options for him. We have travelled to the USA on several occasions and to Bali, where Josh has worked with many healers. It has been and continues to be an amazing journey of faith; every time we seemed to hit a brick wall with Josh's recovery, out of nowhere someone would suggest another healer/practitioner to us. Some worked and were amazing, and others were a waste of time.

We had the view if it made sense there was nothing to lose, unless it was outright ridiculous or dangerous.

Josh became very good at deciding what was helping him and what wasn't.

After suffering his near fatal seizure in early 2012, and then having ongoing issues with his scarred and torn urethra, we all experienced a very difficult, stressful, scary time.

Oh, how I hated the injury. Just when everything was going well, BAM!

All through 2012 there seemed to be always something going wrong with Josh's health and wellbeing!

Mostly we worked through it, but his seizure totally rocked our confidence, and made me hate the injury and the randomness of its issues more and more!

Just when he seemed to be on top of the world, something would trip him up. It was frustrating and unfair, but I guess that's the nature of this vicious cruel unrelenting injury.

Josh and Amelia had planned to attend PW for four months in August 2012. Josh's goal was to finally Ditch his Stick.

I was already in the US, but I was sick with worry; for the first time since his accident, we were unable to purchase travel insurance for him.

Knowing the cost of medical procedures in the USA, I was terrified if anything went wrong with Josh. He would have to get on the first plane home, and there would be no alternative.

I was excited to see Josh and Amelia again. I had worked really hard getting the apartment ready for them, but I underneath it all, I was quietly terrified; extremely worried something could go wrong with Josh's health while they were staying with me.

Finally Josh and Amelia arrived safely in the US. I had stayed in a hotel at Los Angeles International Airport the night before to make sure I was there in plenty of time to collect them from the early flight.

They were on a direct flight out of Melbourne. The plane arrived about 6 AM.

The moment I saw Josh, I was quietly devastated. He didn't look well at all. He was still suffering from the effects of the seizure with periodical "jolts".

Even after almost five months since the seizure, it was as though, his body retained the memory of the jolts, so when he was tired or stressed, they returned, with a vengeance! I was so sad and so very scared! I hadn't seen him in two months. I couldn't believe how much he had deteriorated.

I remember our first night together in Carlsbad. We went out for dinner to a local Italian-Seafood restaurant, opposite the beach. I wanted to have a special evening to celebrate the beginning of their four months of intensive recovery; a night where we could relax and have some fun!

Both Josh and Amelia were tired from the long flight and the drive back to Carlsbad. We decided to eat early, so we would not be too late getting home. Josh ordered "Surf and Turf" a favorite of his. With no warning, the jolts started. They triggered the memory for me of the morning he suffered the seizure in front of me. I was inwardly terrified, but trying to keep calm.

They started to become more frequent, and I kept asking Josh if he was okay.

Wrong! I was obviously making him worse with my concerns!

Amelia calmly sat there. She didn't want to make an issue, which was the right thing to do, but I was beside myself with fear.

The restaurant was very crowded. Josh was starving, and he needed to eat then and there, but the food took far too long to come! In the end, as his food was being served, he said we'd have to leave, as he felt very un-well.

We asked for our food to be packaged up and left.

Arriving back in the apartment, I was terrified Josh was going to have another seizure, but Amelia remained calm, taking Josh's deteriorating condition in her stride. She was amazing. They told me to go to bed, they'd be okay. I asked Amelia to come get me if she needed any help. I don't think any of us got much sleep that night!

The first weekend they arrived, Josh and Amelia went to Temecula to visit his old friend Robbie M. It was an extremely hot day. Josh, a sun lover, stayed in the shade trying to keep cool, as he was worried about the heat triggering dehydration and possibly another seizure. Robbie noticed Josh wasn't himself, and asked him what was going on. Robbie had suffered many injuries himself in his career, and, like Josh, he also believed in alternative recovery.

After a recent accident he had been recommended to a couple in Encinitas - Uschi and Doug. They were situated not far from where we were living.

Robbie suggested that Josh and Amelia should contact them. He recommended that Josh have treatments with both of them.

Little did we realize the effect these two loving, caring, talented people would have on all our lives!

Uschi practiced Cranial Sacral Therapy, as well as physiotherapy. Doug was a chiropractor.

Very quickly Josh and Amelia discovered that individually these two amazing healers were fabulous, and together they were brilliant!

Uschi and Doug would work on Josh for about two hours each session. Doug would complete his adjustments on Josh, and then Uschi would take over. They collaborated with their work on Josh, each deferring to the each other's skills.

They say there is no gain without pain, and yet Uschi worked her magic quietly and effectively with no pain but with significant gain to Josh's overall wellbeing!

Josh loved them working on him. He could feel the energy coursing through his body. Uschi's work with Josh was so subtle, and yet she just knew exactly where the issues were in his body.

After one of his sessions with her, Josh told me he could feel the spinal fluid flowing freely through the injured section of his spinal cord, such was the effect of Uschi's talent.

Josh referred to Uschi as "golden hands." He said she was the second best healer to ever work with him, the best being Isobel.

Josh and Amelia were both enjoying healing sessions with Uschi and Doug as often as was possible, trying to get at least one in a week.

Through Uschi's skills, Josh really started to feel a lot more in control of his body. Since his accident, he felt it was constantly at odds with him.

The jolts became less frequent. Finally, as the regular sessions progressed, Josh experienced calmness in his body he hadn't had since the accident. The jolts slowly disappeared.

We all finally allowed ourselves to relax. At last, Josh and Amelia were able to focus on the reason they had come to the USA: to attend PW, focusing on him "ditching the stick."

The regular sessions with Doug and Uschi fine tuning his body allowed him fast recovery time. He was achieving some fantastic results in his recovery training sessions at PW.

I was really busy at PW, so it took me some time before I was able to meet Doug and Uschi. We immediately hit it off. They were such an amazing couple, so committed to the wellbeing of Josh and Amelia, along with their other clients.

Uschi told me she had never experienced anyone like Josh before. She said he totally understood his inner body, using the energy she produced. While working on him, he totally maximized the effects of her work.

Eventually, I had several healings with Doug and Uschi, especially after Josh and Amelia returned home.

For Christmas 20132, Josh gave me a session with Uschi.

I had been going through a really tough time financially and emotionally with the recovery center, and I knew I needed to see Uschi. When I arrived at her practice I was mentally and physically exhausted. I lay on the treatment bed in her facility, and she created her magic on me.

For most of the healing session I was so relaxed I slept.

I can honestly say I didn't feel her working on my body, so subtle was her touch. After the session, we caught up for dinner, discussing some of the stresses I was experiencing. I always knew that Uschi would "say it as it was" giving me practical, sincere advice, seemingly always able to bring everything into perspective for me.

The next morning, I woke up after a solid sleep. I felt as though I had been in a full on two hour gym session. I was stiff and sore all over. I called Uschi, and she laughed, saying "I did a lot of work on you yesterday; there was much to adjust and align!"

Mostly, I always tried to make my appointments with them late in the day. Once my session was finished, I would either have dinner with Uschi or them both. I really loved hanging out with them because they were so sincere; their love and counsel always coming from wisdom, love and care.

Doug and Uschi became a great support to me, through the issues around my visa and lack of work.

I referred several friends to them and many of the PW families, so confident I was in their healing abilities. They never let me down!

Their friendship and guidance became very important to me as the year progressed. With them, I knew their care and advice was always from their hearts; they didn't mind giving their opinions, even if it was something I didn't want to hear.

In the end, when I met them for the last time before I left Carlsbad, I was feeling totally devastated, so incredibly sad. Uschi calmly said to me, "Look, Kay, you have to believe returning to Australia is the right thing for you. You have been swimming against the tide for so long, maybe you are not meant to be here!"

I knew she was right. As much as I hated to admit it, Uschi *was* totally right!

One thing I do know is that Doug and Uschi will always be part of our ongoing journey, even in the short term, if it's only being able to keep in touch via email.

Chapter 22. Warrior Momz

PW had a dedicated social media page that allowed people with SCI's and their loved ones to connect with others on their journey. While I was in the PW network, I connected with many of the families who used the site. My connection was coming from that of a parent not someone who consulted to PW.

I was on the site most days answering questions, supporting families, offering hope in some way, and many a time mentoring someone through a tough time or a bad day! It was an important online community for those suffering SCI, as the injury can be very isolating.

Primarily, as a parent, I was connecting with the injured person's support team, whether it was their parents, family, loved ones or friends.

Being a regular to the site, I felt I was helping. I truly loved the connecting with our little community.

With my experience with the injury, I was one that could really help them and provide a light at the end of the dark tunnel.

One of the moms I connected with was Michelle Cole from Montana. She was an ER/Trauma Nurse, and her son Kolter had sustained an injury in a car accident that left him a paraplegic.

Michelle's nursing background was telling her one thing about what she should expect from Kolter's injury, yet her "mom" emotions were telling her there must be another way and she was determined to find it.

Michelle and I instantly connected. She became a sponge for my knowledge and experience, which from her medical background made sense to her.

Our relationship was not one-way. From Michelle I learned a lot about the medical side of the injury, especially the potential negative effects of certain prescription drugs that were administered to those with SCI. She was also able to explain in detail the various medical issues that needed to be monitored for someone with an SCI. You have to remember that up until then I had little exposure to the medical profession since Josh's accident other than our family doctor, so I became a sponge soaking up Michelle's knowledge - it was a win-win friendship.

Having someone with Michelle's experience proved a huge help for someone on the PW online Connect Page who had a question about medication or medical procedures. Very quickly Michelle became my "go to person" when I or one of our community was faced with a medical issue.

As with anyone I mentor, I only ever told her what had worked for Josh, but to her it made sense, so she ran with it. Over the following months Michelle brought Kolter to PW two or three times, at my encouragement.

The first time Michelle came with Kolter we finally met, having the chance to hang out after hours. Michelle filmed everything Kolter did at PW. She was an avid learner, taking in and integrating the knowledge of the talented trainers.

Over a very short time, Michelle's and my friendship grew and blossomed into one of "sistas"; we both loved our sons, and we were united together through two tragedies. We were both determined to learn and experience all we could to help our sons and others travelling this journey.

After her first PW visit, Michelle returned to her home near Missoula. On her return, she and Kolter connected with the Physiotherapy Department at the University of Montana. The University had a Wellness Center where they were involved with ground-breaking work in the area of below-injury recovery from spinal cord injury, along with treating other injuries and ailments.

Kolter commenced attending their wellness center; through his PW experience he and Michelle were able to integrate what they learned in the recovery process with some of the center's programs.

Another mom I connected very strongly with was Jeannie Pickard. Her son Chris suffered a "C" level injury in a car accident leaving him a quadriplegic. As a result of his injury Chris and his parents Paul and Jeannie established PW Atlanta. Jeannie and I met through my role at PW. We chatted often, giving each other mutual support with the various issues we went through with our sons.

Over a period of months Jeannie and I became very close, bouncing ideas off each other, giving each other support, and together helping families. Jeanie is an integral part of the Warrior Momz sisterhood.

More important, Jeannie and I share the bond of loving our sons, (they both have similar injuries) and we are passionate advocates for below-injury recovery.

Another mom who was an important part of the initial support for the Warrior Momz network was Liza Perla. After her daughter Amanda's accident when she became a quadriplegic, they established PW Orlando. Liza and Amanda are a powerful team, pushing for recognition to the possibilities of below injury recovery. They are committed and go over and above with helping families through their facility and the greater SCI community.

Liza, Michelle, and Jeannie became fantastic friends and resources for me, especially when we find someone who needs help on the East Coast.

Due to my initial visa issues in April 2013, I decided to go visit Michelle and Jeannie. It was on my flight to Missoula when the concept of forming Warrior Momz came to me.

The idea was to establish a central resource where sharing information and fielding questions providing answers and support could be achieved under the one umbrella. I spoke to Jeannie and Michelle; they loved the idea.

During my visit with Michelle, I was asked to speak to the physiotherapy students and some of the faculty of the University of Montana. I presented Josh's story to a captivated audience. The head of the facility Sue O., also presented, it was very exciting for me to have this opportunity. It was a true meeting of the mum and science; a very humbling experience for me.

On returning to Carlsbad, I registered a business name, web address, and Facebook page ... and so Warrior Momz was born.

Through Warrior Momz I commenced a blog radio program, where I interviewed people relevant to our audience. It was an efficient way to get the word out about what's happening in below-injury recovery, stem cell or robotics, or really anything that was relevant to spinal cord injury. (Currently I have suspended my radio program due to logistical issues. Since returning to Australia I am considering whether I have the time to recommence the program.)

Used positively, social media is a valuable asset to those suffering spinal cord injuries by connecting them with likeminded people all over the World. I manage two Facebook Warrior Momz pages. One lists the members, allowing them to make comments or ask questions. On the other one, I post updates daily.

From small beginnings, the Warrior Momz network continues to grow, offering support to families in many parts of the USA, Australia and the Globe. Really, this is what we are about; offering support, a light of hope and encouragement.

Knowing you are not alone is so important, as a spinal cord injury is extremely isolating, especially in those early scary days.

I think back now nearly 15 years, and as a family we had nothing, no one, to offer us encouragement or support. No one to offer us any hope. There wasn't anyone who understood what we were going through as a family.

We didn't have the instant information network that Facebook and Instagram now provide us.

Social media was non-existent!

Something I really love - if one of our Momz hears of someone suffering a new spinal cord injury, you know there will be private messages made to the family and their loved ones. Slowly we filter information through to them, only making actual contact with them when they are ready. Sometimes it takes a year for a family to connect with us; it makes no difference how long we are there for them when they are ready.

I feel blessed to have met these amazing women; they are all so committed. The really amazing outcome is that all these Momz were thrown into this crazy world and they all want to give back help others.

I have made many friends from our Warrior Momz network; we all share a unique bond. We all just get it, and we will never give up!

Our network is small, about 100 active Momz, and they are so caring and powerful in their belief to help – nothing is too much for them. Since moving back to Australia it is not as easy for me to keep in touch, but I usually manage 2/3 Skype calls every week or so to Moms mainly in the USA. Obviously I am also active on social media.

Chapter 23. Making a Living - The Art of Patience - Waiting 2010-14

Since September 2010, I had been searching for the next phase/challenge of my life! I needed to earn money, and I was desperate to leave Australia due to the sadness that never left me while living here. I lost everything I had accumulated when the company I had helped build for nine years was suddenly placed into administration. I personally lost everything: my financial security and all that I had worked so hard for, was gone in basically a few hours one morning. And worst of all, no matter what I did, how hard I fought, I couldn't do anything about it!

Prior to going into administration, for some months the company executives and outside business consultants had been working towards a total restructure plan. Working with several major groups, a package had been brought to the table, and I was advised it had been approved and signed off.

As part of the Company's restructure plan I had been offered a three year contract. They needed me to stay to offer continuity to our clients. Initially, I didn't want to stay. I wanted to move on with my life, but I was convinced I was needed, so I reluctantly agreed to stay to ensure there was stability and continuity with the Relationship Management, Sales and Marketing Team.

Although I was tired from nearly nine years of the nonstop building of the business, I knew I could re build our network or at least part of it, thus ensuring the success of the company into the future, as well as the protection of the investor's capital!

My contract couldn't be formalized until the restructure was approved.

Arriving at the office on Monday morning September 7th, I was advised the restructure had been signed off the previous Friday. It was "go ahead full steam."

Although relieved that finally the company was "good to go," I knew my life for the next three years would be lived totally committed to the rebuild, so basically there would be no time for anything else. As physically, mentally, and emotionally tired as I was, somehow I had to find the strength needed to keep going; there was so much resting on my shoulders! I had no alternative.

Later in the morning, I left the office to attend a chiropractic appointment. While there I was called back, and on my arrival I was advised that "Administrators" had been called in. It was unexpected and sudden!

All Management and staff were to receive their entitlements. I was devastated to find out, although I had my three year contract in place valued in excess of $450,000, it was never signed by the Senior Management Team. I therefore was not entitled to be paid out. For all my work and commitment I received nothing, even though my continued employment for the next three years was an important part of the restructure package that had been approved.

For me though, the worst was yet to come! For several months after the company collapsed, I worked tirelessly trying to retain and protect the value of the investments. Volunteering to work with the "Rescue" group for months receiving no payment, my obligation was to my clients and the investors who had invested several million dollars over the nine years I was working with the company.

I felt totally disappointed and devastated by the treatment I received from some of my clients, business associates, and old friends, many of whom I had known through my working career spanning over 45 years. Basically they turned their backs on me.

Totally disillusioned at what had occurred, I struggled, as I was still supporting Josh financially. No matter what, I had made my son a promise and I would not back down from that.

Yet I felt for his relationship to progress with Amelia, I needed to be less available to him, feeling our relationship would be better as well.

Josh and I had lived together for nearly 10 years after his accident. While we loved and supported each other, we were both looking to get on with our own lives.

I really needed a break, having not stopped for a breather since 25th June 2000. It had been a long tough road, and frankly I needed to find out who I wanted to be!

My sisters and Josh were extremely worried about me, my health, my anger, my total despair, my sadness, and my lack of not knowing what I wanted to do next! This coming from a person who in the past had never left anything to chance, always having a B Plan; since the collapse of the Company in September 2010 I was totally directionless! I did not have any plan at all for my future.

During this tough financial time I had no alternative but to sell Josh's home. The only upside was that he was back in Port Melbourne, renting a small flat with Amelia and the furry kids. Selling his house was so hard. It had always been my dream to make sure he had his own home, and now he had to rent again. I was devastated. I felt I had totally failed him! He was fantastic, understanding everything had changed. He never complained once.

We talked about me going to Bali, to set up a business with my sister Asri, but in my mind I wanted to do something totally different. So as much as I loved Bali it wasn't something new to me!

I needed a challenge; something totally out of left field!

The Christmas of 2010 I went to Bali for six weeks, staying with the ever supportive Asri. I was searching for something; answers that never seemed to materialize. I needed to clear my head, rid myself of the sadness, so I walked and walked every day, sometimes up to 16 kilometers. Even in the monsoonal rain, I walked, much to the amusement of the locals. They would call from their shops or houses "madam it's raining", I would return their concerns saying, "jalan jalan" which is Balinese for walking! They would laugh, nodding their heads, understanding I wasn't crazy!

This period became a time of great reflection for me. I looked back on my life and realized that at some stage I had lost ME. I had worked full time since I was 16 years old. I always gained promotions way beyond my years, because of my skills, and each new position came with more money and more responsibility.

Having Josh in 1981, and being the major breadwinner in our family for several years, I had just kept ploughing on, balancing trying to be a good mom, loving wife and successful executive.

Here I was in 2010, and I had never applied for a job. Since my first position in 1966, I had always been "approached" or "head hunted". I didn't even have a CV. I had never needed one, yet the phone stopped ringing after September 2010.

The sadness enveloped me. Every day I woke up with the same feeling. I truly felt if I stayed in Australia I would die. I am not exaggerating or over dramatizing my state of mind - it was that simple!

247

In the space of just over three months (June 5th - September 13th 2010) I lost my mother, I had to make redundant my Sales and Marketing team, a team we had meticulously built over eight years, and the company was gone, along with my financial future.

Every morning I would wake up, feeling a little less alive. I couldn't break myself out of it. It wasn't a depression, it was simply I was over it, not on life, just over all that had happened!

My entire life, I had lived by the mantra of "always doing the right thing," strongly believing in Karma, always trying to learn from my mistakes, turning a tragedy such as Josh's accident into a learning experience, for not just Josh and me, but for other families as well. Yet here I was in this predicament. I felt my belief system was seriously challenged. I spent hours questioning the Universe and my faith in it!

On my 61st birthday everything changed - I finally had a mission, a direction, something totally different; something I could throw my passion into, something I could use to help families dealing with Spinal Cord Injury. We heard about PW.

PW was based in the City of Carlsbad, California, and once I actually discovered the beautiful city, I knew I wanted to live there forever!

PW was keen to have me assist them in growing their outreach in the Spinal Cord Injury Recovery community, so it seemed to be a match made in heaven.

My U.S. lawyer had been confident of my visa application. He had seen no problems, so I was confident in my move to Carlsbad, into my new consultancy position at PW. With everything finally sold, for the first time in two years I was truly confident about my future. I was heading in the right direction.

Prior to arriving, my lawyer set up a U.S. Corporation for me, and a long term family friend Shirley arranged my bank accounts, so on the 8th June 2012, I was able to hit the ground running. Shirley was amazing, collecting me from Los Angeles airport, taking me to the bank, and making sure all was in readiness for me to commence my new life in the USA.

Friends and family wondered how I would manage relocating to a new country, city life, but I waved aside their concerns confidently asserting I would be fine. Truthfully I was excited, the last years in Australia were filled with so much sadness and loss I wanted a new clean page created in my life story.

Moving to Carlsbad, I quickly realized the task ahead of me was daunting. PW had done very little marketing in the community. Very few locals knew of them, so knowing no one, I plunged myself into the networking engine of the city, the Chamber of Commerce and Rotary.

Many of the Chamber members I met were interested in why I was there. They had heard about PW, but most had no idea of the work being done there; importantly, what was being achieved with for their clients.

They had great support for Josh; they loved to hear his story. In fact Chamber President Ted became particularly supportive of Josh and me, once he met Josh during one of his visits to PW.

To understand and learn more about the Carlsbad community, I attended everything, including dinners and lunches. I used every chance to meet new people to tell the PW story to! I was always very positive.

Things were really tight, as the money I was earning was nowhere near covering my basic expenses. Without a visa it was difficult to find more consulting work. Most of my past clients in Australia had been very long term in nature (I was a builder of businesses, nothing short term in that), so I held off looking for additional work in the States in anticipation of getting my visa. In my mind, I was confident that everything would work out. I simply had to be patient. I was beginning to create momentum, and I was where I needed to be!

I was so happy, I felt this was the work I was meant to be doing!

In a climate where I was continually nervous about my visa, by December, I was having difficulties with the lack of support or any feedback from the senior executive. I was beginning to feel totally isolated when I was in the facility, having no discussion with the senior executive at any level. I had reached a stage where I actually dreaded going into the PW headquarters, which was really sad! I was so confused by my treatment, but without any feedback from the senior executive, I had no idea what the problem was, or even if there was a problem. It certainly wasn't my performance, as things were really coming together. The saving grace was that I loved the interaction with the clients and their families, and this was my greatest joy!

So here I was departing from Los Angeles on the 9th February, leaving

249

my car, my clothes, my furniture and apartment with no guarantee of getting the elusive visa. I was excited about the wedding, but the dread and fear of the visa issue loomed over me!

The appointment at the Embassy was made for the day after I arrived back in Melbourne. I had wanted to leave as much time as possible for my application's evaluation before I returned to the USA in three weeks' time. Arriving at the Embassy in plenty of time, I truly wanted the interview over and done with so I could get on with the more exciting wedding week celebrations.

To say the interview was a disaster was an understatement! The Chief of Staff was aggressive, even sarcastic. The worse thing was, I was standing at the counter having to put up with my life being discussed in full hearing of everyone in the waiting room. I felt extremely embarrassed; he made me feel like a total failure! I left the interview in tears, totally devastated. I really felt like a criminal. Emotionally I was a wreck, yet I had to pull myself together for the wedding, so leaving the building I "filed my grief" as "pending" and threw myself into the celebrations of the wedding week.

Ten days later I was advised my visa application had been refused. Devastating news! Yet I was still at a loss to understand the treatment I had received at the Embassy. I soon received my answer.

My application was returned by the mail, and reading it I finally understood why I had been refused. In all honesty, when reading it, the file was so amateurish and poorly presented I would have refused it myself. The lawyer was supposed to format in an acceptable form the Business Plan I had sent through (July 2012) in "draft" form. But the document hadn't been touched; it was my original draft.

No case had been made for my"special" circumstances, and none of the references I supplied were included, not even PW's reference. In fact, the document was distressing to read. There were typos, spelling mistakes, and incorrect information. It was nothing short of embarrassing; all errors were carefully circled, noted and highlighted by the Embassy visa team.

I felt totally let down by people I trusted. For what this had cost me, the application was a total waste of money and time. Yet again, I felt the vile feeling of failure. I really thought OMG what do I have to do to get it right? Frankly I didn't know what I would do, I had no "B" plan, all I knew was I wanted to be living and working, making a difference in the

USA, and now this goal had been totally destroyed; there was nothing I could do about it.

Knowing how tough the Immigration/Homeland security officials were in Los Angeles, I contacted the U.S. Embassy (Melbourne) and asked them about returning to the USA to sell all my possessions. They advised me that the B1/2 visa which I already had would allow me to reenter the border. With this knowledge, I decided to return to the U.S. as planned. What was the worst they could do?

Not allow me back in?

I remembered all those Border Control shows I had watched, saying a quick prayer I wasn't going to end up being featured on the show.

My QANTAS flight had arrived early at Los Angeles, and I coached myself to be positive, saying over and over "I can do this. /" I'll quickly get through Homeland Security, grab my bags, breeze through Customs, and I'll be on the road home to Carlsbad in no time. How wrong was I?

Arriving at the Homeland Security check the following occurred:

"Ms. Ledson, when you left the USA you had overstayed your visa."

"No, I applied for an E2."

"Where is it in your Passport?"

"I went to Australia to get it, but they refused it at the U.S. Embassy in Melbourne; I have come back to sell everything and return home."

Umm, nothing is easy; I was referred to an area nearby – "Ms. Ledson, you must stay between the lines, don't move, someone will come for you."

Learning from the Border Patrol television show, I kept saying to myself, keep calm, stay focused, *and don't get mad!*

Three interviews later, (the worst part about it was that I was justifying my case to people who appeared to be no older than 20) I understand they were only doing their job, by sticking to the rigid guidelines imposed, but they made me feel like an illegal alien. It was scary and very frustrating.

Eventually I was admitted for a period of five weeks, after which I had to return to Australia! Time taken nearly three hours!

I rented a car.

Driving to Carlsbad, I truly don't know how I made it back home safely.

I was extremely traumatized by my experience at the Homeland Security check. I was sad at having to leave the USA. I was seriously challenging the Universe, really beating up on myself for trusting the wrong people. How naive I was, always believing everything would be okay!

When does my life get easier? Geez, sometimes it's so hard to be positive!

Overwhelmed, I felt I had failed, failed the families I came to help, failed my family, especially Josh, and failed myself. I really questioned why the Universe had allowed me to have learned all this amazing information, knowledge and understanding regarding below-injury recovery; yet now I would never use it in the USA, due to my lack of a visa.

Back in Carlsbad, I moved quickly, giving notice on my apartment, and making arrangements to sell my furniture and household goods. I rang our friend Graham in Temecula, and he said he would sell my car for me once I left.

On Monday morning, I advised PW, saying I would finish at the end of March. The senior executive didn't say much. I personally felt he was relieved. The others, however, including the Chairwoman of the Board, were extremely disappointed I wouldn't be around to finish my work.

I had two events to host, plus projects I was working on to finalize. I threw myself into getting as much completed as possible.

My one saving grace was that I had still had enough money to pay a deposit on an apartment back in Port Melbourne, so at that stage, even though I wanted to stay in the USA, in my mind I had no alternative. I could still buy myself a home on my return.

And then I went to Rotary! Many of the members encouraged me to reapply for the elusive E2 visa. They all were all supportive, offering to help me!

The problem was that I now didn't have any work after the end of March, but I knew in my heart my work in the USA wasn't over. I really believed Josh would do better in the USA once his planned book was released - I really wanted to stay! In truth I wanted to stay for me more than anything! I loved my life there!

I have always been a fighter for what I believed in, so why should I quit now? Staying in Carlsbad, continuing my work there, was important to me. I would not go down without a fight!

I briefly met with to two local lawyers about my case. One said she didn't have time to process a new application, and the other took nearly three weeks to tell me that I had only a 5 or 10 % chance of being successful with my application.

In any case I was running out of time!

With my lease expired, I had found somewhere temporary to live, and basically at the last moment I was referred to a lawyer who had never lost a case. The catch was it would cost $12,000 up front for an emergency application to be lodged. I had less than a week before I was to leave. I had to make a decision return to Australia or stay, and if I wanted to stay I had no alternative but to agree to the payment.

Briefly, I thought by going back to Australia, I had enough for a deposit on an apartment, but dammit I want to stay, so I paid over the money to my lawyer.

The application was lodged the day before I was to leave the USA. I had a reprieve, at least temporarily. Talk about stress!

My fate was sealed, with the door to PW now firmly slammed closed, I felt sadder than sad!

I had put my heart and soul into helping PW build their brand and achieved my goals in helping so many families. I had come to the USA full of hope, yet now PW was no longer an option.

In the time I was there I had worked so hard and made so many amazing contacts, I really felt it would all be wasted if I walked away from the sector.

I had established Warrior Momz, my blog radio program was gaining momentum, the group managing the marketing for me was very positive they could get me some advertising to help me financially, so I was quietly confident I would be all right.

Soon after I finished with PW, I had been approached to do some consulting for a group in the SCI area. Lindy and Carol really wanted me to be a part of their team. They were confident their funding would be through by July, so I just had to hang in until then. Knowing and respecting them both, I was excited by the prospect of working with them.

They indicated there were exciting things happening with their business, and they wanted both Josh and me involved. We had two meetings, all seemed promising, and I was slowly learning patience was a virtue! My immediate problem was that I still didn't have any work!

Lisa, the Executive Director of a local foundation, asked me to help her with their Annual Gala Fundraiser. I explained that I had no experience in this area, but she was willing to give me a chance. Right from the start, Lisa was honest with me, saying she couldn't pay me much. I, on the other hand, was grateful for the work. It was ironic that I would end up consulting to this foundation, as I had fallen in love with this magnificent Carlsbad waterway on my first visit in 2011.

I always referred to the Agua Hedionda Lagoon as the Jewell in Carlsbad's Crown and now I got to "work" there!

I was slowly feeling more confident I would make it financially!

Josh was furious with me for not returning to Melbourne. As much as I tried to explain, he wouldn't listen and would not understand. Emotionally it was a tough time for me! I had made my decision and I was sticking by it!

For the first time in 13 years, I was putting my needs and what I wanted to do first! I was commencing the journey to get my own life back!

Even though Josh didn't want to hear it, I felt he would be better off in the USA once his book was out, so that was a significant overriding factor in my decision to stay.

My sisters were supportive, but even they couldn't understand my change of plans. Both were worried about me financially and emotionally.

My Bali sister wanted me back. She had a business in Bali she wanted me to establish with her, but I had made my decision and that was it!

Everyone I loved was either mad with me or totally confused by my decision to stay! I seriously thought that I was for the first time in many years totally on my own, isolated, as far as those that I loved were concerned.

Some weeks later, Josh told me both Wendy and he were convinced I had lost my mind. They thought about coming to the USA to "rescue" me. Glad that never happened! That would have been truly embarrassing!

The reality was that once I had made the decision to stay, my Carlsbad network supported me totally. Although my money was running out, I held the unwavering belief that everything would turn around! I was where I was meant to be!

I honestly believed with the work I was still doing with Spinal Cord Injury, something work-wise would come through, if it was meant to!

Always I totally believed I was meant to be in the USA.

Lisa was fantastic, giving me as much work as she could. It was paying my rent, so I was grateful.

Lisa gained the foundation's board's approval to contract my company as a consultant to the foundation in the area of Development.

Additionally, I was also to be involved with fund raising through the various events being held there.

I loved working at the foundation's Discovery Center, and the positive influence of their school program was a delight to see. For someone who proudly had lived in apartments for over 20 years because I was scared of snakes and didn't want to deal with lizards, and wildlife as such, as I gained more confidence, I even enjoyed interacting with the critters, especially Lincoln the Australian Bearded Dragon.

Although working very hard, I didn't feel like I was contributing as quickly as I would have liked. But these things take time, and Lisa was very patient!

I continued talking and meeting with Lindy and Carol. They were still unable to give me a start date, but I kept thinking, be patient I'll be alright, this is meant to be!

Overriding all my efforts was the fact that my money was running out fast. I was determined to stay in the U.S., wanting to keep up my commitment to helping families, but I was getting really nervous.

I had so much faith in everything working out. I just kept telling myself to be positive, just had to hang in there. But finding more work, with all I was doing was becoming frustrating and challenging at every level.

The people running the management of my radio show yet again promised me sponsors. But nothing was happening, no matter how much I berated them.

While working on Josh's book I had to stop my regular radio blogs, which was disappointing, but there was only so much I could do in 24 hours!

Through the foundation, I met Jamie. I immediately loved her energy and passion, and we had so much fun!

Jamie was a positive, inspiring mentor and friend. Jamie's friendship was a beacon, "a bright light" in my life. She was always positive, supportive, and an excellent sounding board for me. We started hanging out together, catching up for regular brain storming sessions. There was never any stress with our friendship. We thought in a similar manner, and I loved spending time with her.

It was a relationship built on the meeting of the minds more than anything, with both of us essentially working on our own; for me it was refreshing to have someone to bounce ideas off.

We also hung out, meeting for lunch or dinner on a regular basis. There were always ideas for social media and marketing discussed at a positive, more often at a "what if" level.

Jamie was also my gym buddy on the days I managed to get there. She was interested in Josh's journey and offered to help me with his book launch.

From only knowing Jamie for a relatively short time I know she and I will be friends forever. We love and support each other! And still do to today; our friendship is only growing stronger since I returned to Australia.

To make my new E2 application stronger, I arranged to lease a corporate office in the very professional Carlsbad's Palomar Airport Executive Office Suites. The guys managing the complex were very helpful. I explained my situation, and they offered me a flexible lease arrangement for six months. It was an expense I could have done without, but I needed the E2 visa. I felt with a corporate office, Homeland Security would take my visa application more seriously.

Finally, after all these months, my E2 was approved in principle. I could finally get my Social Security card, another step in legitimizing my new American life.

A hitch in finalizing the visa was that I had to attend an interview at the very embassy that had refused my application initially in Melbourne, and apparently there was no way around this. So while I was quietly celebrating, I was very nervous about this development. Although I was fast running out of money, already passing "minimum" bank account balance, and if it got to that level I had to go home.

When I altered my return ticket to Australia I had made the date the 21st of December, having calculated that my money would be nearly out by then, so if I hadn't been able to get more work by then, I would have to return home. At the time, I had allowed myself eight months.

It was around September that I began preliminary talks with Jane regarding some consulting work; we had originally started talking conceptually in July, but although we caught up regularly, it was a slow process.

Just after my visa was conditionally approved, she started to get more serious. Jane was prepared to offer me a permanent full time executive position, so I finally had another option!

It was decided I would work from my office, and the other existing team members of Jane's organization would help with the monthly rental. She even discussed looking for a bigger office, but I was nervous about increasing my commitment even though I would be supported with the monthly rental. Until I had pen to paper with a contract, I was reluctant to enter into a larger financial commitment.

It all looked so positive, and it made sense for us to work together. The opportunity of an offer was genuine and exciting. Jane needed me and I needed her. Perfect!

As the role grew, it would be harder to maintain my other work commitments. My concern was the foundation. I made it clear to Jane that I would not desert Lisa or the Board, even if it meant me working longer hours.

By this stage, I had dismissed Lindy and Carol's work potential, as although we talked and wanted it to work out, nothing ever happened.

With Jane's work potential looking extremely promising, I was confident

Warrior Momz would survive. I could still maintain my social media commitments, along with my radio program!

I wanted more than anything the certainty of ongoing work, so I could relax and be confident that I would receive my visa when I returned to Australia on my booked flight the 21st of December.

Although Jane and I were meeting nearly every day trying to finalize the consultancy offer, it was not proving to be easy. It had been a long ongoing process while we discussed development of a totally new "arm" of her current organization. This change had been on her radar for a long time, but she had never found the right person to collaborate with until she met me. Jane understood that for me to remain in the USA the E2 visa required certain levels of income, which she assured me was more than possible. We talked, planned and commenced working on an action plan. I was totally confident all would be alright. Finally, after all these months of battling for work, I could see a light at the end of the tunnel!

We are nearly at the end of November, and Jane and I are still talking, still planning. I am not earning any money except from the foundation. I am so far past my emergency level (moneywise) it is now critical! I still had my flight booked for the 21st December, but I was running out of time and a decision needed to be made. If the decision was to return to Australia, I needed to advise Lisa and the foundation board. I did not want to leave her in the lurch, as I was involved in several projects!

I arranged a meeting with Jane, repeating what I had been telling her all along; I can't stay in the US unless I start earning money. Jane suggested I return to Australia to get on my feet financially, wanting me to return to the USA in six months to commence my work with her. (In hindsight this should have been my first warning.)

I said, "This has been going on since July, in one form or another. Jane, either you want me to work with you or not. If I go home, I won't be back! I have to get on with my life; I can't afford to run two households, which is what I had been doing since I arrived in the U.S. nearly two years ago."

Jane reiterated, "But I need you to progress my planned expansion. I can't develop this other arm unless you are here." The next day we met, and I received a draft contract from her that either worked with an E2 visa, or potentially would be the start of the H1, for which she said she would sponsor me.

The offer was prepared for the position of "Executive of Marketing and Finance", with a list of duties in case my E2 visa was refused at the Melbourne interview. If there was a problem with the E2 at the interview, Jane would sponsor me for a H1 visa as an executive employee of her 501 c 3.

At Jane's request, I contacted my airline and changed my return flight to the 15th February 2014.

Jane and I signed the contract. I was paid an advance of $5,000, which would keep me in the USA with the money I had left for another three months (but only 3 months). I still needed to earn money fast. With our plans pretty well finalized, I didn't see this as a problem. I would hit the ground running in December, January to mid-February. At the time of signing the contract, I actually thought that even if I only earn half of what I was contracted to earn, I'd be fine, and for the first time in two years, I breathed a sigh of relief. At last I was here for good; I was beyond happy!

As part of the new role, I needed to follow up leads, Centers of Influence, but there was always an excuse from Jane that stopped me. The names weren't available, or she didn't have the cards with her, or we have to wait for this person…

Although this was disappointing, Jane was my friend and I trusted her!

Ever optimistic, I'd be fine. I knew I had all of January! Thank goodness for the consultancy at the foundation; it was giving me enough for my food, fuel and few bills.

With the contract in place, Jane and I made an appointment to see my immigration lawyer. The new role changed my original business plan. The lawyer was "mildly" concerned, but felt with the remuneration package that came with the consultancy I should be all right. She wanted me back in Australia finalizing my visa prior to April, when an audit would take place on my U.S. Corporation. With my earnings so low this would have, in her opinion, jeopardized my application, so her advice was to get the visa in February, come back to U.S., and hit the ground running.

I was already involved in research projects for the new business arm, investigating Public Speaking for Jane and Grants for her 501 c 3. While the work was interesting, it was time consuming. I was looking forward to getting into the sponsorship and value adding side of the role.

I spent Christmas with Faye and her family. It was fun, but I had cut the top off my pinkie in an accident on the 23rd December. My reaction of recoiling back suddenly after the accident pulled a muscle in my back, so I was in a lot of pain for several days.

Even with all that, I was looking forward to being busy, once Christmas and the New Year were behind me!

Jane went away for a week, and while she was gone I focused on the research I was doing for her, as well as working with the foundation.

Just after New Year, Jamie and I decided to catch up for lunch. By this time Jane was back and she asked, if she could join us.

Jamie and I arrived early. I was updating her about my various research projects, what I was going to be doing with the marketing and follow up of the public speaking side of the business, as this was to be a huge responsibility of my new role. Over the break, I had developed an extensive contact list for the public speaking gigs. I was just waiting for Jane to give me the go ahead.

Jamie also had some of her business contacts interested in sponsoring an event I was marketing for Jane's new entity. I was excited, and at last I could start bringing some revenue in.

We were having such a fun time when Jane joined us. Her face was grave. She outlined some changes she wanted to make in her life and in the 20 minutes it took her to tell us, I realized my dream of working and living in the USA was gone, dead in the water! Worse for me, Jane was saying that she only put everything together to help me stay in the USA; she really didn't want to expand her business! Now she felt under too much pressure because of worrying about me! With all these months we had been speaking, talking with her team, these changes, this expansion was always on her drawing board, the reality was Jane changed her plans and to save face she put it back on me!

From Day 1 when we first commenced our discussions on her "grand" expansion plan/dream, it was always about her gratitude with finding me to work with her to create her master plan for her 501 c 3.

Totally numbed, in disbelief I said, "Jane, don't worry about me, I am done. I'll return to Australia, you go ahead, get on with your life."

Lunch over! Jane left immediately. Jamie and I stood together outside the restaurant, and we both were dumbfounded, at the same time saying, "What the hell just happened?"

I was devastated, yet again at the very time I had dared to dream finally I could make this place I loved so much my home, in a heartbeat it changed. I said to Jamie, "I am done, I am going home!"

My next stop was to speak to Lisa. She was extremely upset, disappointed with me at not telling her sooner. She said she would do anything I needed to help me stay in the U.S. I simply said it's too late! There is nothing that can be done, my finances were such, and I had nowhere to move. Everything other than what I get for my car will be gone by February 15th. There would be no extra money coming in during January!

It was one of the toughest times of my life. I felt I had failed not just me, but Josh, my family, Lisa, the Board of the foundation, and those who supported me. I was angry, sad, and mentally exhausted. I frankly had no idea how I would get through the next six weeks before I returned to Australia.

I rang my lawyer. She was disappointed, but said rather than cancel my application they would put it on hold.

What I do know is that Jane's offer in wanting me to assist her in expanding her business was genuine, and it would have helped us both. I was the perfect person to help her and she knew it! Contrary to her saying she only did it to help me that was an unfortunate comment to make. We had spent countless hours, days, months, discussing the expansion, exciting new programs; it was just as much about what she wanted as what I wanted. We both would have benefitted in this plan!

But things changed for Jane. I get that, but don't throw it back and blame me!

I had arrived in the USA, June 2012 with around $200,000, which was everything I had! I left some funds in Australia helping Josh financially with some expenses, paying my life insurance, furniture storage, along with some other commitments in Australia. Basically I was running two households.

From day one in the US, I was on a mission to help families, to introduce the opportunities afforded through below-injury recovery. After burying two young men in Australia, and seeing the pain in the faces of their families, in my mind I had no choice!

261

I believed the promises of PW. I was there for a reason! First and foremost, I was a mum, and I understood more than anyone what families have to go through with this horrendous cruel injury. I was the perfect person for the position they offered me, but their motivations changed. It was me that was sacrificed.

Initially my reason in moving to the USA was always for the families. My motivation for this has never altered. Although returning to Australia with less than $15,000 to my name, I have no regrets, other than maybe trusting and believing in the wrong people, but that's me. I always look for the good; somehow I miss the ones who have other ulterior motives.

I can't walk away from Warrior Momz. Today as I write this I think who really cares if I do walk away, and then I think of the Momz that are part of our little group. I think of the work in the mentoring Josh and I constantly do with families caught up in the hideous injury and I can't walk away!

My move to the USA has cost me everything I have financially, but I gained so much as well; my fabulous friends in Carlsbad, the healing I went through there. With everything that has happened, what I haven't lost is my passion for life, helping families and fighting for those who suffer a spinal cord injury. I also haven't lost my unconditional love for the Carlsbad community!

Note: For privacy reasons, I have changed the names of people in this chapter.

Chapter 24.   Carlsbad - A Time for Healing - Learning to Laugh Again!

Just after I moved to Carlsbad, Wendy suggested I join Rotary. She offered to research the local Carlsbad Clubs and together we chose the Carlsbad Hi-Noon Club. Wendy contacted the then-President Yvonne, and she agreed to sponsor me for membership. I have to say at the very first meeting I attended, I had no idea the effect this club and its members would have on me. Over the period of the two years I was a member, Rotary became like a second family to me, offering me enormous friendship, support and encouragement. I loved being part of this club, making many new friends and for the first time in years I was enjoying an active social life through the many volunteering projects and Club activities! I even won the Rookie of the Year 2013, much to my delight!

Something I looked forward to every week at our meeting was our singing. The club sang two and sometimes three songs. Initially I was not sure about the singing, not knowing the words, but I soon joined in and loved it.

You know singing is such food for the soul! It really made my heart happy!

For me, Carlsbad was proving to be the answer to my dreams, a chance for me to rebuild my life, find *me*, and actually commence creating a new life, in a place I loved so much.

What was truly great was that I was nobody special to anyone there - I was just the Aussie, Kay. No one had any expectations of me; just how I wanted it!

In my mind Carlsbad, became my "active living Kay Cave," a place of comfort, friendship and fun times!

I really felt for the first time in 12 years I could get a life for myself.

To better understand the city, I would watch the televised City Council meetings, learning so much from them, and watching the documentaries/news features covering the history and growth of Carlsbad, on the local City television station.

The weather was amazing. For someone who in the past celebrated the change of seasons in Melbourne, I never tired of the beautiful weather in

Carlsbad. Frankly, every day was a little different, and although the sun shone nearly every day, there were times when it was foggy or overcast in the mornings. Very rarely did it rain; the climate really suited me! And the spectacular sunrises and sunsets made your heart radiate!

The beautiful weather allowed me to enjoy driving with the roof down on my car; my one luxury when I arrived was to buy a 2012 Mustang convertible, all optioned up. It was the perfect car to enjoy the amazing weather of San Diego County.

Cruising down the Interstate 5, music blaring, roof down, enjoying the blazing sunshine - I had discovered heaven and I loved it more every day! It was a rare occasion I drove with the roof on the car so beautiful was the weather.

Josh and Amelia were doing fine, and being away from them I was still able to maintain a positive relationship with them both. I was confident in their relationship together, and it was a time of great relief for me as well, knowing Josh had found his soul mate! Through this period I was still assisting Josh financially, although not as much as I had in the past.

My one regret was that I missed my furry grand kids, Montana and Thor. I especially missed Montana. She and I had been through so much together, we had such a strong bond; we loved hanging out!

I loved Thor, but he was really Josh and Amelia's dog. I am sure he didn't miss me like I knew Montana did.

I tried Skyping them, but Montana would get frustrated not being able to physically see me, in the end, when I called she would walk away. OMG, how I missed her.

Initially we had planned to bring them over to live with me, but with my visa delays, it didn't end up being practical, especially due to Montana's age.

The first 12 months I moved around, initially getting a small apartment in Vista, finally settling into a two bedroom unit near the beach in Carlsbad Village. With Josh and Amelia attending PW for four months in early August, I needed to get everything ready for them.

Without my visa, I couldn't bring my furniture from Australia, so I had to buy furniture, appliances, linen etc., for the apartment. I hadn't factored this expense into my budget, but I had no alternative. I was still more than confident that all would be okay; as I knew in my heart, I was meant to live here permanently.

I was starting to make more and more friends, and enjoying an active social life for the first time in many years. I wasn't dating anyone, just enjoying hanging out with friends.

On moving to my new Carlsbad apartment, some friends there introduced me to polo. It was played at the Del Mar Polo Fields every Sunday during the season. Polo quickly became my regular Sunday activity, making friends with some of the regulars. It was a lot of eating, chatting and enjoying a glass of wine or two. I loved it, and we even managed to watch the polo at times!

Volunteering for activities and projects through Rotary was something I really enjoyed. It was a positive, easy way to make even more new friends, as we shared a commitment to helping others through Rotary

One of the projects I had so much fun volunteering for was helping to build the Mexico house. Every year a group of our Rotarians travelled down to Tijuana to build a house for a Mexican family in one day.

It was a long day, an early start from Carlsbad travelling in convoy to the border. Arriving at the location there was no time to relax; we all embraced the task ahead of us working together in a team to create this small family home in a day.

It was very hot down there, but that didn't deter us, the comradeship was brilliant, everyone working for a cause!

You see another side of Rotarians when you volunteer with them. They always made me feel so welcome, even though they had trouble understanding my accent. I learned to speaaaaaaaaakk slowwwwwwwwwllllllly!

Over painting the house and ourselves, Patty J. and I really bonded - talk about laugh nonstop. We worked hard but had so much fun in doing it.

Rotary gave me "community purpose." In Rotary, I felt as I was a part of an amazing community; it had been many years since I had experienced this, and I enjoyed every opportunity to be involved!

Really that was it. I realized that Carlsbad was where I learned to live, laugh, and broaden my world again. Importantly, I was able to commence the building of my very own "new" life!

It had been so long since I really laughed, yet every time I was out with the Carlsbad gals, or a group of friends we laughed! I have so many photos at one dinner or another, we were always laughing.

I'm talking "belly laughs" I was having so much fun!

The Universe hadn't let me down after all!

Josh and Amelia arrived in August. They too enjoyed the lifestyle Carlsbad provided and quickly settled into their beach life and their temporary home. They both loved the location of the unit; we decided to buy bikes to get around town easier. Josh even tried his hand with a Razor scooter, it was a bit short for him, but at least he tried it.

Amelia and I would walk every morning. It was a precious way to get to know each other a little better before the wedding.

Amelia had ordered her wedding gown to be handmade in China, she had it was shipped to my unit, so she could make sure it fitted her. Finally it arrived! It looked so beautiful on her, and after making sure it was a perfect fit the gown was safely stored until they returned home.

It was such an exciting time for us all!

Unfortunately Josh and Amelia didn't meet many of my friends while they were in Carlsbad, as their weekends were usually busy catching up with their own mates who lived in nearby Temecula and Huntington Beach.

During the week they were both devoted to training. When they weren't at PW, they would work out at one of the local gyms. It was during this time Josh went surfing again. Wow, what a day that was!

Josh had caught up with some Aussie friends who were over for Moto Cross competitions. For fun and relaxation, they surfed off Oceanside near the pier area. They invited Josh to join them one Sunday morning. We had only recently discovered Oceanside beach, falling in love with it, especially the boardwalk area and the marina.

It was a cold, windy morning, and the boys had brought a wet suit for Josh. Amelia and I sat on the rear of his car while he pulled the suit on.

The boys went out with him, and before we knew it, Josh was surfing for the first time in over 13 years. *One more activity crossed of his bucket list.*

Amelia and I were so excited for him! It was the little things that made the hard work of his unrelenting training all worthwhile!

Josh and Amelia left Carlsbad at the end of November to prepare for their wedding. I had really enjoyed having them there with me. It was a fun important healing time for us all. Josh was feeling fantastic after all his healings with Uschi and Doug, and with no more jolts he was back to normal, more in control of his body again. Thank you, God!

Once they left, I fell back into my solo lifestyle, keeping busy with PW, and trying to get my visa sorted. I had heaps to do. I was becoming more and more involved with community activities that directly and indirectly were building the PW image and reputation.

A gentle soul named Kawika came into my life. He had designed a "concept" paddle board, for adaptive paddle boarding, allowing those confined to a wheel chair to have access to a water sport.

He planned to launch the board on the Agua Hedionda Lagoon. I loved the concept of someone who had a spinal cord injury being able to get back on the water. Kawika demonstrated the board to Eric Harness, who also loved the concept. So PW was on board with it; exciting and inspiring times.

We spent many hours working on how PW clients could be involved. I saw it as a huge benefit to them, with all the emphasis on water sports in Carlsbad. Once introduced to the concept, our clients loved the idea. When Kawika found out I was returning to Australia for the wedding, he postponed the launch until I was scheduled to return. He wanted me to be part of this amazing happy day!

Before I knew it, I was on my way to Los Angeles to catch the flight home, hopefully finalizing my visa, and being part of a very special celebration -- Josh and Amelia's wedding.

Returning to USA, giving notice at my unit, I was offered the chance to rent a room from a woman I had met through polo. Her home was in Carlsbad, so it really suited me for a short time, as I was scheduled to leave the US the first week of April.

Re-applying for the visa necessitated my need to once again find my own place. My temporary arrangement was not working out on any level, and

267

frankly I felt I needed my own space!

I was lucky to find a spacious one bedroom apartment in Oceanside. I wasn't familiar with the area, but it was safe, near shops and main roads, and I only had to sign a six month lease! Yet again I bought furniture, a meager amount this time, just to get me through until I could bring my own possessions from Australia.

I think you could describe my apartment decorating style as definitely shabby chic, having searched the local Thrift Stores for bits of furniture to make the place livable. I was happy with what I achieved on such a small budget; it was comfortable and warm. I reflected on how much I had changed from my previous "luxury" lifestyle in Port Melbourne surrounded by my beautiful art and furniture. Looking back, I was happier in this tiny apartment, possessions / appearances were no longer important to me.

Finishing up at PW, my last official function was the launch of the adaptive paddle board on the Agua Hedionda Lagoon. It was an important event for Carlsbad. This was an historical launch, a World first. The launch was a celebration for the City, with Mayor Matt Hall officiating, it highlighted the magnificent Agua Hedionda Lagoon, with Lisa representing the foundation, Project Walk was involved; one of their clients paddled the board around the lagoon to the official launch area, and of course the amazing, dedicated Kawika and his partner Lisa, saw his dream come true.

It was truly a community event, a huge celebration, with many Carlsbad locals joining in! Several of the PW clients came down to try out the board. The ever-watchful Kawika, ensuring everyone had their turn. The smiles on their faces showed everyone concerned, this was going to be a truly wonderful activity, to be enjoyed by the PW clients, further enhancing their Carlsbad "recovery" experience.

During this time we started Josh's book. We had partnered with a "writer" so I thought my input would be negligible. Our writer contracted the book to a Canadian publisher; the plan was to launch Josh's book at a major Canadian Women's Conference in October 2013.

In hindsight, as with this book, it was impossible to write *Relentless* chronologically, as every twist and turn of our stories needed to be followed through to a conclusion.

We knew that Josh's story was always going to be difficult to tell, because there were so many twists and turns with it.

It was decided the easiest way would be for Josh to tape each chapter then send the file through to our writer, who would transcribe the file, formulating his words into the story. Sounded easy!

My role was to read each chapter for accuracy, it would then be sent through to the publisher. Initially it was to be written chronologically, but the publisher had other ideas.

Communication between all the parties wasn't easy. Thank goodness for Skype; times for meetings needed to be coordinated with the various time zones of Melbourne, Southern California, and Vancouver, with up to eight people involved.

This understandably was never going to be easy!

As the weeks progressed, I was becoming increasingly nervous about the way the book was coming together. I didn't want to alter it too much, as it wasn't my book; my only changes were on accuracy points, so initially I changed little. The chapters were being sent through, but we heard nothing from the publishers. I was becoming extremely stressed, as the more chapters coming through for me to edit, the more I had the feeling the book wasn't being written as a manuscript. Rather, it was a transcription of Josh's words. Suddenly I received an urgent message to set up a Skype call from the publishers.

They informed us that although they loved the story and believed in the book, and they were confident it would sell and be read, the story in its current form was written as transcript, not any way near a manuscript. Agh - my fears were realized!

I don't want to go into details other than to say there was a great deal of stress involved with getting this book to press. From mid-August through to the night that it was finally signed off I had little more than four hours sleep a night. In fact four hours was good. I worked on the book, editing the manuscript seven days a week in every bit of spare time, taking a little time off each week to hang out with my buddies for a few hours over dinner in the Carlsbad village.

During this period I was still consulting to the foundation. We were also under a lot of pressure because of the number of events we had in the pipeline.

I was exhausted. At one stage Lisa said "Get the book finished, I'll pick up your workload!" Lisa and the Board showed me amazing patience and support through this period. I will always be grateful to them!

My sisters were planning a visit for two weeks in September. I was looking forward to showing them the city I loved so much, to finally introduce them to the Carlsbad crew, and to just hang out with them.

Their first night in town, I volunteered them to help at an event the foundation was holding. Wendy was not pleased to be cooking mussel soup on her first night (she didn't even like mussels), and Susie was kept equally busy cooking and pouring drinks! It was a fun introduction to Carlsbad for them. Umm, well, they did work hard, but they met lots of people including the Wednesday night crew of Kori and Maureen. With anything I am usually involved in, there is potentially a downside. Unfortunately more often than not, and it affected my sisters!

I had planned for Wendy to drive my car while they were there, but she wasn't keen to! I had no idea about public transport, and as I was working for most of their visit, they needed to be able to get themselves around. Somehow between them, they figured out the public transport system. My sisters are true legends! And they are very forgiving of their sometimes out of control "big" sister.

Not only was I working full time, I was totally involved in writing/editing *Relentless* as well as trying to fit in time to hang out with them.

Our days were something like this: I would be writing from about 4 AM in the morning until breakfast. I would drop them at a station or bus stop, and they would go sightseeing around San Diego County using the train or bus sometimes both. We would meet for dinner, and the day would end with us all going home and me disappearing into my room to write. I felt bad, but I had no alternative; the book had taken on a life of its own for us all!

But through all my craziness, we did manage to have some fun! The three of us enjoyed a weekend in Los Angeles. We started our Saturday with breakfast and a long walk and the eclectic Venice beach. Later we ventured to downtown Los Angeles, finding the stars on the pavements and exploring Rodeo Drive. We had a lot of fun and the weather was perfect.

Sunday we enjoyed more sightseeing, returning to Carlsbad via Mission Viejo, where we enjoyed a "family" dinner at a local Mexican Restaurant with our old friends Shirley and Bill Harmon.

Even on this weekend of fun and relaxation, I was involved with the book, and for me there was no downtime.

We planned a trip to San Francisco and Sonoma for five days. I was so excited that finally Wendy and Susan would meet my Sonoma family and friends. There was so much fun to be had, so much to see, and so many amazing wines to taste! This trip was to be a total break for me work-wise, but the book still had to be worked on in my spare time. We drove up to LAX (Los Angeles airport) the night before our early flight to San Francisco, enjoying a lovely Italian dinner at one of my favorite LAX hotel Italian restaurants.

We three sisters enjoyed some authentic Italian food washed down with magnificent Californian wine, and we laughed.

The flight into San Francisco was on time. We collected the rental car, and with all the driving we were going to be doing we decided on an SUV to allow us plenty of room. We drove into San Francisco. There was a Federal Election in Australia, and with voting being compulsory, we all had to vote that weekend. For convenience, we chose the polling booth manned by my Australian mate Dawn, in downtown San Francisco. After voting, we managed a quick coffee with her, before weaving our way through the city traffic to Sonoma.

It was a beautiful day as we drove up through the hilly road into downtown Sonoma.

We parked near the Ledson Hotel on the square. The plan was to have lunch with our cousin Steve Ledson in his hotel's restaurant.

Steve welcomed us to the Ledson Hotel's magnificent restaurant, where we were thoroughly spoiled with sensational dishes of "bespoke" food, washed down with our favorite Ledson wines. The sisters were in 7th heaven!

Finally we said our goodbyes. I drove them to their hotel, the luxurious Macarthur Place Hotel and Spa, and they were very impressed with their suite, so very palatial after "camping" at my Oceanside unit.

For the next three days, my sisters enjoyed being spoiled by my Sonoma "family" Lesli and Curt. Lesli organized a private tour for us, at Repris Winery. Wow, what a mind-blowing experience we all had. We especially loved the treat of champagne on the summit of the winery property mid-morning, finishing with a "cave tour" of the operations. Yet again the sisters were blown away by this truly unique winery experience, and they certainly deserved it after all I had put them through.

I was so happy for Lesli (my sister from another mother). After all her hard work, she had been rewarded with this fabulous position working in the executive team at this magnificent winery.

In the next few days we enjoyed wine tasting at some of my favorite Sonoma wineries. The sisters really loved our special Italian lunch at the new VJB winery in Kenwood, and we were even serenaded while we ate. Everywhere we went in wine country we were really spoiled. Because I knew people working at all the wineries we visited, it was a lot of fun for us all, making the experience even more memorable for my sisters.

Not being able to resist the temptation, Wendy bought some wine to take home to Australia!

I was so happy to finally bring my sisters to Sonoma since it holds a very special place in my heart. Now they totally understood why!

We had two days staying downtown in San Francisco. Wendy and I really wanted to take Susan there, as she hadn't had the chance to enjoy this beautiful city before. Our short trip was spent exploring the City, eating local seafood, having a memorable time.

Back in Carlsbad, they enjoyed two very special dinners Wednesday night at the Aussie Grill, enjoying dinner and wine while experiencing the Carlsbad Farmers Market. It was a huge night with about 12 of us squeezing into the tiny outside eating area in front of the restaurant. Their final dinner was a special treat for them with Terry cooking up a seafood treat for us at Casa Rodman's opposite the beach, with Lisa's special crab cakes. The fantastic location and the memorable sunset, made such a happy night to end their Carlsbad vacation.

Although I hadn't spent as much time with Wendy and Susan as I would have liked, they both had a fabulous time.

It was sad saying good bye to them. I was so glad they got to understand why I had such strong ties to Sonoma and Carlsbad, and more importantly why I wanted to spend the rest of my life living in the USA.

I AM SO LUCKY; I HAVE THE BEST SISTERS!

The book was finally finished two days before the publisher deadlines. I had basically worked 36 out of the 48 hours, and not surprisingly I was exhausted.

In the end everyone pulled together and the book was finally finished!

While we all acknowledge that *Relentless* is no literary masterpiece, it was never meant to be perfect. It is a raw, honest book. The fabulous reviews from those who have read it have been gratifying, humbling and have made it totally worth the effort that we all put into helping Josh bring his story to the world.

Josh was arriving late October. I was so excited to finally see him.

I had hoped Amelia could come with him for the whole trip, as he was always happier with his best friend, lover and wife around. Importantly, I wanted Amelia to be a part of his book celebration. At one stage, Amelia wasn't sure if she would come at all; in the end she decided to come for the last nine days. I wanted her to enjoy the success Josh was experiencing. It was an easy decision for me to use some of my precious remaining savings to fly Amelia over to be a part of this journey.

Relentless was launched in Vancouver at the Women's Conference on the 25/26th of October, 2013. I really wanted to join Josh there, but with my visa problems, I couldn't leave the USA unless I was returning to Australia.

Faye offered to accompany Josh to Vancouver. I was so grateful to her; although she and Josh hadn't met before, they had communicated with each other on Facebook for several months, so I knew they would be great together, both having similar personalities.

Once the Canadian launch was finished, the plans were made for the USA book launches.

On returning to the USA, Josh and I would launch his book at Project Walk Atlanta. This was a huge trip on top of Vancouver, but it was necessary to launch the book with friends who were supportive and involved in SCI recovery.

There would be a Carlsbad Community Launch, along with Project Walk Carlsbad. Kim from PW had asked us to launch there as well. She would make all the arrangements for this event so all we had to do was turn up. Perfect!

My precious savings were evaporating in front of my eyes, but we had worked so hard for this I was confident all would go well, and the money would be well-spent.

I was introduced through a friend, to a "PR Expert." He was prepared to work pro bono, backing himself. He knew he would be part of our long term team, earning fees for his PR company once Josh's presence was established in the USA.

Jamie and I had two very intense meetings with him, fully briefing him on Josh's story. He assured us he could handle all the publicity while Josh was in the USA. He would develop PR opportunities for Josh built around his travel schedule. Jamie offered to assist him, having many media contacts herself, but he would not hear of it, saying he preferred to work alone.

The importance of a focused PR campaign would be critical to Josh's success. I was therefore delighted that he was prepared to take on the role. I was totally confident all would now come together!

With an experienced local running the PR, I was sure we would receive professional coverage, including hopefully some local television.

Josh's story was great, emotional, real, and now it was in the hands of the right person!

Some weeks earlier we had put the "Burning Chair" front book cover on Facebook. There were literately hundreds of positive comments, along with some from the usual critics. They heavily criticized the burning of the chair! Why hadn't we donated it to someone needing a chair? In reality, the hatred of the chair was what gave Josh the will to walk. He lent the chair to Bronte so he had a 2nd chair, which made his life so much easier. Bronte always said he would burn his chair once he walked. Josh thought long and hard about the book cover, finally coming up with the idea of burning the chair. We owned the chair (it was paid for through a fund raising) and, in our view, Josh could do what he liked with it, and that is what we told the critics!

Josh still has the chair. It will remain with him forever as a memory of his journey, and how far he has progressed from the doctors' original prognosis.

At this stage we hadn't seen the finished book, so we all waited anxiously for its delivery, with real sense of excitement and much anticipation!

I arranged for marketing signs and had business cards made in the image of the book's front cover. Everything looked professional.

Finally, the books were delivered to the Discovery Center in Carlsbad the day before Josh arrived. It was so exciting for us all to finally see, touch, and feel the finished book; and we loved it!

Josh flew into Los Angeles two days before he was to leave for Vancouver. The large *Relentless* sign was the first thing he saw as he came through arrival exit. Finally, he had the chance to meet Faye and our PR representative. We had a quick breakfast before returning to our hotel. I had booked a hotel near the airport for two nights. Josh had been in touch with his good friend Dingo, who was coming over to see him and take him back to his apartment in Los Angeles for the night.

Dingo arranged a surprise VIP seating for them to attend the basketball at the Staples Center that evening. Although Josh was very tired, he was excited to be catching up with Dingo, who he hadn't seen for so long. Dingo's apartment was on the opposite block to the Staples Center, so they walked there, which was a feat in itself for Josh.

The next day Dingo arranged for Josh to be a guest of the Jason Ellis Radio Show. Josh loved the experience. He came across really well on the program, and he totally enjoyed the afternoon, having fun with Dingo and Jason.

Josh was very tired when he returned to the hotel late the next afternoon. They had walked not just from Dingo's apartment, but all through the Staples Center the night before. Without his walking stick, a long walk takes on a whole new set of challenges for Josh, but he did it!

We had an early dinner and prepared for his flight to Vancouver early the next morning.

Faye met Josh in Vancouver two days later. I will be forever grateful to Faye supporting Josh while he was there. She made it easy for him; it would have been very difficult for him being up there on his own.

The Women's Conference was disappointing to both Josh and Faye. Our publishers had managed to get Josh a speaking spot on the "stars" stage on the final day. What no one realized was that Josh was speaking at the time the conference break down was commencing. Fortunately, with Faye's help and some muscle men, they managed to drum up a small and attentive audience. Josh and Faye stayed in Vancouver for three extra days as there were special events organized for them by the publishers. The time spent there gave Josh the chance to meet and get to know his publishers and their support team, along with some of the other authors who were part of the publisher's stable.

The downside was that Josh arrived back in Los Angeles exhausted.

I was also concerned we were getting *no* publicity, and yet we had the "PR expert." All I was getting was excuses from him.

Our PR guy and I collected Josh and Faye from the airport, and returned to Carlsbad for the weekend. Josh was fine in the car, but once we arrived at the unit, Josh was very quiet.

Over dinner in a local restaurant, we ended up having a bitter and angry argument which was extremely distressing to me. He made it clear to me that he wanted to get on with his life with Amelia, and although he was grateful for my help, they wanted to do things for themselves in the future. This was something I had been trying to get him to do for some time.

This injury is so tough. In a normal world, Josh would have got on with his life, and me with mine, and we would have caught up every so often and really enjoyed our relationship. His injury caused our lives to change so dramatically; as a parent you never lose the fear of the injury and all the things that can go wrong! I am sure Josh felt we had been too close for too long. He needed to get on with his life with Amelia, and he wanted normality, but at that stage it wasn't possible because our story was so linked together. In reality I was desperate to build my own new life, but being a mother will always come first. I am sure when Josh has his own children he will understand.

That night Josh's angry words over dinner tore my heart into pieces, but no matter how devastated I felt, I knew I would keep supporting him if he needed me to.

The following day we returned to Los Angeles to prepare for an early flight to Atlanta, Georgia. I had flown to Atlanta before, and I warned Josh that it would be a long day, with a stopover in Dallas along the way! Fortunately, Josh decided to use a wheelchair for all the airport transfers, so he was able to rest his legs a little.

I was so excited to be seeing the PW Atlanta team again. Jeannie and Paul, who run PW with their son Chris, are like family to me. Jeannie is a much loved and very valuable Mom in our Warrior Momz network.

Arriving late in the afternoon, Jeannie met us and drove us to a beautiful hotel near the PW Atlanta facility. Jeannie and Paul had booked a lovely room for us, with all the little luxuries southern hospitality affords. That evening, Josh and I enjoyed a fun, entertaining dinner with Jeannie and Paul before we retired for an early night, in anticipation of a huge day at PW Atlanta the next day.

Everyone was excited about the launch. The PW Atlanta team had been extremely busy promoting the event, and they were all committed to Josh speaking to their clients, families and friends of PW Atlanta. The book couldn't have been launched to a more appropriate audience.

The PW Atlanta launch was actually the first time Josh had spoken to a SCI audience and their families. The Atlanta crew did a fantastic job. Jeannie's mom cooked up the most amazing lunch. Yumm, home-made southern food at its very best!

And then everyone started walking or rolling into the facility – they came in wheel chairs, walking frames, and on crutches. There were so many injured people and their families coming to hear Josh's story it was humbling yet amazing! Over 140 attend the launch. As usual Josh was humble, speaking from his heart. I was so proud of him; everyone listened so intently. He was sad, funny, tragic, and happy. Everyone who attended was totally engaged. He spoke for over an hour, and then he took questions, and there was always another question. The questions kept coming. Josh spent nearly an hour answering them. Mind blowing!

The knowledge Josh has for this injury is extremely insightful and astute.

He really understands the way to simplify exercises, set meaningful goals, and gain commitment. It was a wonderful experience for Josh and me to meet the injured and their families. And to be able to give hope is everything!

Josh was able to meet some of his Facebook friends, Sarah, her Mom and Grannie, Erica, who came on a road trip with two friends, travelling for 10 hours to finally meet Josh, Hannah, her mom and grandmother. It was a very humbling experience for Josh.

To say it was a memorable day was an understatement.

I was so proud of Josh; my emotions were on a roller coaster. Publically, he was supportive and loving, but privately he was distant and remote towards me.

I was feeling so confused. After finishing at PW, we joined Jeannie, Paul, their son Chris, friends and family for dinner in their home. It was a truly wonderful end to an amazing day.

We returned to the hotel, totally away blown away with southern hospitality, which if never experienced is a must!

Although tiring, Josh was really happy we made the trip to Atlanta. He was blown away by the reception he received.

We had an early start the next day returning to LA, where we would stay overnight to meet Amelia, who was flying in the following morning.

Once Josh and Amelia returned to Carlsbad, Josh decided to celebrate Amelia's arrival by staying at the Surf Motel, on the beach in Carlsbad for five nights. They both loved that part of Carlsbad, especially the location of the hotel that allowed Josh to walk to most places.

We were up early to meet Amelia. Josh tracked the plane's flight path on his cell phone, he was so excited! Luckily, Amelia came through arrivals very quickly.

Before long we were heading back to Carlsbad, top down on the Mustang, enjoying the beautiful early morning sunshine. I sat in the rear seat of my car for the first time, and loved the experience.

Josh seemed much happier and was back to his old self almost immediately. Personally, I felt a little sad. I had really wanted to have quality time with Josh. I missed our chats. I really felt that all the success we had achieved from the son and mum relationship was all but in tatters, and our precious the time together had been wasted because of Josh's remoteness toward me!

For the first time since Josh arrived in the U.S., I felt relieved. He seemed so much happier having Amelia by his side.

The PW Carlsbad launch was scheduled for that evening. I dropped them off at their hotel so they could get some rest and prepare for another big night.

Kim had really put a lot of effort into organizing the evening. We were surprised to see only a few people in the gym. Given that so much of our history was with PW Carlsbad, with the trainers, and around this gym, but in the end there were fewer than 20 clients and their families there.

But as you know, any group is an exciting group, and the intimacy of this small group allowed Josh to really relax, and be very open to answering the many questions.

I am sure all who attended got so much out of this night; Josh loved being able to help. Really that's what it's all about for him!

The Community *Relentless* launch was fantastic!

Carlsbad is an amazingly supportive community. They initially welcomed "he Aussie" and after they met Josh and Amelia they were embraced, too! Lisa and the Discovery Center team threw themselves into preparing for the event. They quickly transformed the Rotunda to cater for the expected crowd.

Lisa had been a huge help to me, advising me on the catering and the adult beverages. The evening would never have been the success it was, without the team of friends all pitching in. I just love those gals!

My CDM Jamie was in her element, manning the bar, and making everyone smile. Not surprisingly, she did an awesome job!

Over 80 people crowded into the Rotunda. It was the perfect place, with its stunning views, that formed an inspirational setting for Josh's book launch.

Lisa introduced Josh to a room packed full of my friends, and fellow Rotarians. Josh was in great form, and everyone loved him. The cool thing was that many of our guests had never been exposed to someone with a spinal cord injury. The questions at the conclusion were intelligent and insightful, truly showing that Josh had captured their hearts, interest and attention.

Once Josh finished, I thanked everyone for their love and support. My first words were "18 months ago I came to this city and knew no one. As I look around this room, I am so blessed to have found the Community of Carlsbad and to have made lifelong friends."

Josh and Amelia manned a table afterwards to sign and sell copies of *Relentless*. We sold many books that night; the evening was a great success! Finally the community that had been so supportive of me had met Josh and Amelia!

Josh and Amelia left for Australia on the evening of the 15th of November, which was two days after we celebrated his birthday. Josh was no longer concerned about me living in Carlsbad on my own, as he realized I had a caring community to support me.

The last nine days of Josh's visit, once Amelia arrived, were a happy time for us all.

Oh, and for those interested, the PR Guy - the expert - NOTHING, not one thing! This was devastating for us all! He had plenty of excuses, wanting to lay blame on everyone. In the end it was so sad, and we had missed out on any publicity for Josh's visit. Extremely disappointing!

With my lease due for renewing and the landlord increasing the rent substantially, I was at a loss what to do. I was chatting to Maureen and Kori at our usual Wednesday night dinner about my problem with the apartment, and immediately Maureen said "move in with me." I was a little reluctant initially, not wanting to put her out, but she insisted. It would work well for the both of us, so yet again I was moving. I was so glad to be back living in Carlsbad. Maureen and I both enjoyed a good laugh and a glass of wine, so it was a great match. The apartment was walking distance to everything, and it was fun having someone to share things with again. It gave me a chance to really get to know Maureen. What an amazing, outstanding woman; I will love her forever.

With the book launch done, I was back into consulting to the Discovery Center. It was always busy; there was always something happening there. We worked hard, but we had a lot of fun. There were many nights I would stay back with Lisa working on an event or a function that was coming up, and no matter how late is was we never lost our sense of humor. I loved being there.

The Lagoon critters were always up to something. The team was a fun group of gals to work with. I especially loved interacting with our many visitors and course the critters.

Thanksgiving at the Rodman's was an amazing day, filled with yummy food, laughter, and fun conversation. There was even a best dish competition; no surprises everyone was a winner. It was lovely catching up with friends through the day, enjoying outstanding conversations, and lots of laughs. I felt truly happy, thankful for finding such a welcoming group of friends in a fantastic community. Life was truly great!

I was really settling in to my life in Carlsbad, making many friends along the way.

December was a busy month at the Discovery Center. We had so much going on, and by the 23rd we were glad to have a few days off.

As a Christmas surprise, Lisa had arranged for us all to be treated to massages and pedicures - for a few hours the Discovery Center was transformed into a private Spa. We enjoyed tasty treats and presents. Life here for me was so different to the one I had in Australia, so much simpler and to be honest, I was the happiest I had been in years.

Just after New Year's, everything had changed in a heartbeat and I was heading home.

I was devastated to have to formally resign from the Foundation and my much loved Rotary Club.

Poor Lisa, I forwarded her two resignations the same day, one for the Foundation and one for Rotary, as by then she was our Rotary President. I felt numb with sadness, it was so overwhelming me. Once I had explained everything to Lisa, she just wanted me to stay working with her and the team as long as possible.

With all that had happened, I questioned God, the Universe, Karma, and whoever else I could think of that may have be able to give me enlightenment, an understanding of what my next move would be. I couldn't understand why I had given so much information, knowledge, and passion for something I could have been used to help so many families and now, so cruelly, I was having to return to Australia. It was a Catch 22; to remain in the US I had to be earning in consultancy fees around US$250 K each year. With my last opportunity lost, I knew my time there was ended. Making money was my priority to justify my visa, but it was never in my agenda to make money from any family going through spinal cord injury. I always hoped my skills would lead me to a position of being able earn the money I needed to stay in Carlsbad.

Mostly I questioned why, for a short period in my life, I had finally found a place where I was truly happy, had made amazing friends, and from out of nowhere it was all taken away from me!

I questioned the Universe endlessly. There was so much I couldn't find answers to! I was angry, frustrated and gut wrenchingly sad!

I did make one decision. Once I returned to Australia, I would walk away from everything. Warrior Momz, helping families with SCI; I WAS DONE and I was totally mentally and emotionally broken!

And then something profound happened; it started innocently enough.

One morning I was at the Discovery Center when Lisa was out. She called me, needing me to do a voice over for a radio commercial being produced for the Tip Top Run which was coming up in March.

I didn't want to do it, and said that to Lisa! But you can't say no to Lisa; and before I knew it, the arrangements were made and the appointment scheduled for later the same morning. All I had to do was arrive at the radio station, read the commercial script and leave. It was to be that easy!

I put the address into my GPS and headed to San Diego - the GPS had me heading to La Costa east of San Diego. No matter what I tried I couldn't input the address for San Diego.

Two things I hate in life are being late and getting lost, especially when I am on the freeway system in the USA.

I headed back onto Interstate 5 and rang the Discovery Center, asking them for verbal directions.

Finally, after a frustrating 40 minutes I reached my destination. Very late!

On entering the radio station I was in no mood for messing around. I was frustrated, tired and frankly needed to get this ad over and done with! Having to record the ad was just another frustration to add to my ever growing list!

I read the script, and thought what is this? It made no sense to me. I told the producer it would have to be rewritten. They politely told me I would have to do the rewrite. I looked at them, asking are you serious, and *I* have to do the rewrite? All I could think of was this has to be done, they are not going to do it, so Kay just get on with it.

Finally we finished, and in actual fact I really enjoyed the experience!

While waiting for the audio to be finalized, the producer looked at me and asked me "Kay, why are you here" I smartly answered, "to do this radio commercial!"

Once again she asked, "Why are you here?"

I can't begin to tell you what I was thinking. I just wanted out, but then I realized it wasn't about the commercial, she was asking what had brought me to the USA.

I quickly gave her the three minute Josh story, and as I finished, she had tears in her eyes. I said I was sorry I hadn't meant to upset her. She went on to tell me that she had four brothers and sisters; her mom raised them on her own. One of her brothers had suffered a spinal cord injury 11 1/2 years ago, and such was the severity of it that he died. Her mother had never gotten over it!

Hugging her, I immediately said, "Your brother had to die. I can assure you that your mother would never have been able to look after him and four other children. It would have killed her! Every day she would have nursed your brother; she would never have managed."

I suddenly thought that morning I had put a couple of Josh's books in my car. I said "Hang on a minute I'll be back!" I brought one of the books back for her to give her mom. As I was signing it, I wrote: *with love and hugs Kay Ledson - The Warrior Momz.* Even as I write this now, it makes me really emotional, very teary!

At that moment, I realized my destiny, at least for the next 8 - 9 years. I am building the Warrior Momz network. *I came so close to walking away from it!*

So now I just have to make it work for me, so I can afford to keep up my support network.

Faye arranged a farewell get together, at the Aussie Grill, our old stomping ground. It was a bittersweet night for me, with over 50 friends coming to have a good bye drink. I was numb. I couldn't believe this was happening. I just had to put my emotions on hold and try and be positive. My God, I still don't know how I did it!

Everyone asked me, "What will you do"? All I could say was "I don't know!"

I had put everything into staying in Carlsbad. The only money I would go back to Australia with was what I received for my car.

I loved my life in the USA, and I did not have a B Plan!

I attended my last Rotary meeting, and that was devastating for me!

Saying goodbye to my second family, I was emotionally done!

It was my last Bunko game, and the final good bye to those fabulous Bunko gals. Co incidentally, it was at Lisa's. Wow, what a last night that was; they presented me with a signed picture from them all. It was so hard not to burst into tears!

After everyone left, I stayed chatting to Lisa for what seemed ages.

I enjoyed a final dinner with the Wednesday night dinner crew, Maureen, Kori and Faye.

In my last days in Carlsbad, I took every opportunity to drive the coast road. The view always inspired me, taking my breath away every time I saw it. It was as though I was trying to embed this spectacular vista into my brain, a beautiful memory to help me through the dark days waiting for me back in Australia.

As I boarded the plane to fly back to Australia, I can honestly say, I didn't know how I was going to manage the flight, the coming home. Not that I wasn't going to be pleased to see everyone, it just wasn't the destiny I planned.

I felt so empty, my heart was so sad it ached!

I loved my time in Carlsbad, in my head and heart I will always be part of that wonderful Community. For a window of time in my life I learned to laugh again, be appreciated, be loved, and importantly making friends who will be in my life forever. I will be always grateful for those two very precious years and the generous wonderful Carlsbad community that helped me heal!

Chapter 25. My Heroes

"In life, we try so hard to get things we don't have, but we never sit back to appreciate what we have. Having a spinal cord injury, all I want is to have my life back to where it was! So celebrate what you have; you never know when you could lose it all" -Josh Wood 2012

In my opinion, hero is a word used extremely loosely by today's society. I find it difficult to justify a sportsperson or entertainer, who are well paid for what they do, being called a hero!

Before Josh's accident, I had no idea about Spinal Cord Injury and its cruel effect on the person unlucky enough to suffer it. In addition, its effect on their support network of family and friends is devastating.

In the 15 years we have been living with this injury, I have been inspired by many. I have met genuine heroes. Perhaps you will never hear of them in the main stream media, but against all odds they try every day, battling relentlessly with their bodies, and in spite of most medical opinion, working at the chance to get something of their old lives back. They are totally committed to do whatever it takes, to achieve their goals.

My hope with writing this book is to give a glimpse into the world of someone suffering a spinal cord injury from the view of a loving family member.

Someone once said to me, "The difference with an able bodied person working out in a gym and someone with a SCI working out is that an able bodied person can walk away any time. They can quit their workout and really no one cares, no damage is done. And yet someone with a spinal cord injury works every session to its conclusion; they will never finish early, or never not put in 100%, as in their mind, if they can just keep pushing on to the end of their session, something may trigger their body towards recovery."

I remember that a major achievement for Josh was finally, after 12 years, *jogging* in the last five minutes of his last session at PW Carlsbad 2011. That was something none of us would have dreamed of the day of his accident. Something his doctors in their wildest dreams would never have believed could happen.

There are so many stories, and it is my goal to one day have some of them told in a compilation book *My Heroes*!

I have lived with my son's injury all these years, and yet I really have no idea what he actually goes through. I can't imagine what it would be like to be trapped in your own body. I have sat next to him while he is driving his car, and he is constantly moving trying to get comfortable. It is devastating to me, and yet he takes it in his stride, never complaining.

Personally, I hate having my bed sheets tightly tucked in. The first thing I do before going to bed is loosen them, so I am free to move! My son has no choice but to live in his tightly "tucked in" body no matter what he does he is "trapped" in his own body. I have no comprehension what it is like for my son. I see his pain, but I have no reference for neurogenic pain in my body. I see him struggle to make those legs of his work. I wish I could make it easier for him, but I can't! Sadly, my son lives in a "manual" body, again something I have no reference to.

I move freely without thinking, yet Josh has to make his body react. Everything he does he has to think about, and he has to direct movement, to his legs, arms, etc. Josh says a spinal cord injury "is the loneliest injury" one can suffer, as there is no one injury the same! I truly get this. There are no rules to recovery either. Everyone is different, and everyone has different goals they want to achieve. I try to make Josh's life easier, but in reality all I can do is be there for him and give him love and support; he really has to do everything for himself.

My son is my hero!

Josh is my benchmark for heroism!

Reading Josh's Facebook post on the 18th of May 2014, I realized I had left out a very important chapter in my book. I want to dedicate part of this chapter to Josh. I am going to include a very small selection that. I will call "Woody's Words of Wisdom" consisting of posts and insights he has made over the years.

While reading the following post from Josh I cried for him. I felt sad, and yet he keeps fighting. He is continually mentoring people from all over the world, sometimes with little thanks, and sometimes he is even criticized publicly, yet he never gives up. He never expects anything in return, and I love him more! This is the toughest cruelest injury of all. My son is a humble hero and I totally understand why he posts these posts. Josh's posts are really the good, the bad, and the ugly of the insights of someone suffering a high level SCI.

"My body is tired, angry, in pain, the pains so bad I feel like my legs, back, arms and right hand have been burnt and someone's dragging their nails through my skin, my spasms are so bad that when my wife moves in the bed my body jolts and throws my legs into my chest, just because the bed sheet moved, when I wake up in the middle of the night I need to sit up and attempt to stand and fall towards the wall to catch myself just to stand, if I need to roll over I need to wake up, sit up then turn, I reach for things and my hands won't open, I try to let go of things and my hands won't let go, I can lift weights but I can't peel wrapping apart. The list goes on and it's been like this every single day since June 25th 2000. I've never had a break. I've never even had one second of pain relief in nearly 14 years, day and night. But last night it started getting so bad I could almost have broken down in tears of frustration. But then I thought of these three, my glue that keeps me from falling apart, my mum who has never stopped fighting for me, my family, my mates and all others going through this FUCKED up injury that is more cruel than anyone could ever understand. It's a tough long road but it also makes you stronger than you could ever think you could be. I'm not posting this to sook. I'm posting it to hopefully let people know you're not alone, there are people who understand and the good days outweigh the bad, last night was super tough but I'm awake, I'm alive, I'm loved and I'm going to never stop fighting".

"The harder I work the more pain I am in from waking up my body, just wish I can get some sleep and a break from this shit, life of pain, just one day without pain would be nice. A spinal cord injury is the most fucked up torture ever and there's no cure for the pain, every day my body feels like it's been completely burned and someone is scratching at the burns with a fork, and that still doesn't come close to describing it".

"Today I got to head down to Mountain District Learning Centre and catch up with the year 10's, they were my first school of many that I'll be seeing over the next few weeks as part of my #BeRelentlessGivingBackProgram.

These kids were so awesome, I'm going back next week to hang out again.

I know, I'm excited to head back and from the request of the teachers, and

287

the kids, I'll be bringing Thor and Montana to hang out and play as well. I was given an awesome gift; I got it from the group after my talk ...a hand written poster with messages and thankyous from the kids."

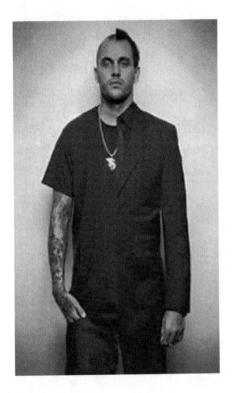

Don't Label Me

Here's the meaning behind this photo: After my accident I was treated differently, because I was now in a wheelchair, even though I had the accident and was paralyzed I was still "JOSH". I wasn't going to be labelled a quadriplegic/disabled or take any shit from narrow minded idiots. I was just "injured". People talked down to me, they slowed their speech, because they didn't think I could understand. I was judged, I was ridiculed when I went out to night clubs! "What's a cripple doing at a night club?"- "Shouldn't you be at home?" People judge others way too easily! Under the hair and suit I'm still Josh, two different looks, exactly the same person! Is my message making sense? Don't judge someone by their looks or what you think you know of them. Until you live in their shoes, don't make assumptions or label them.

This awesome photo was by the amazingly talented and good friend Nick Dale, @nickdalephotography who is also responsible for my cover of *Relentless: Walking against All Odds.*

"Although it's been a tough 13 plus years it hasn't been all bad. The really tough times have made me the person I am today, one of the biggest gifts it's given me is the ability to "MOVE" rooms and change people's lives, to help them find strength and the courage they never thought they had, to find reasons to never give up on themselves and their goals, that the "impossible" is just a word that narrow minded people use.... This picture is at my last talk on Wednesday night....Two things about this picture, first one is that I was only in an emergency hospital 24 hours prior, to tonight, I discharged myself just so I could make this talk and the second is me pointing at a picture of me back on the snowboard 3 years after I was told "I WOULD NEVER GET OUT BED AGAIN, LET ALONE WALK" again....! I love watching the audience's faces when I show them this slide of my goals I had and that I achieved them with support from my family, friends and "off the wall therapy"... Please friends never give up on yourselves... You never know what's around the corner!

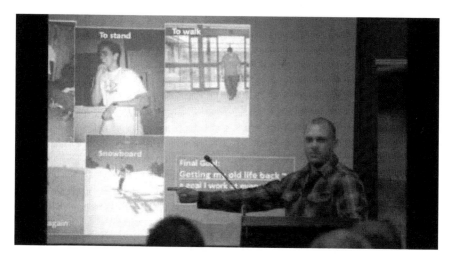

Josh Giving a Talk

Since being catapulted into this crazy world, I have had the privilege of meeting many heroes! Every day I walked through the doors of PW Carlsbad, and I witnessed true heroes. The gym was full of people doing whatever it took them to get their lives back. They chose to disregard their doctors. If you like prove them wrong, many were motivated by the negativity of their medical teams. Against all odds, they chose to take control and recover whatever they could, and were enjoying the journey.

Seeing how hard Josh and so many others work, train, and live their lives has changed my perspective on what's important to me in my own life. I enjoy so much more the "now", take in so much the "immediate" instead of worrying so much about my future!

I want to tell a few short stories, some actually told personally by my heroes. I cannot possibly detail *all* my heroes, as this would fill many books, but I have included a small selection of some of them.

These stories written by my heroes are in their own words, and are unedited.

Michelle Cole

Michelle Cole (Mom), Kolter Beneitone (Son), Florence, Missoula, Montana

My friend Michelle Cole was thrown into this crazy world of spinal cord injury when her son Kolter was in a road accident, leaving him a paraplegic. Although her nursing background told her one thing, in the end she is a mom wanting the best for her son. Since Kolter's accident, she has researched and educated herself in alternative below-injury recovery. She is the go-to person in her community of Missoula these days when someone suffers this cruel, savage injury. Michelle has been an enormous resource for many in our community especially when they need to discuss a "medical" issue. Michelle has taken the courageous step of educating her medical community about the possibilities of below injury recovery. A true Warrior Mom! Michelle has contributed to this section with a few words on her and Kolter's story.

Here are Michelle's words:

March 18th, 2012 on a winter Sunday morning I got the phone call I have feared since I started my ICU trauma nurse career.

290

My son's friend was on the other end of the phone. A group had driven for the weekend out of town to a nearby college town for the St. Patrick's holiday. The boy on the other end stayed calm but I could hear the fear in his voice. He said they were in an accident, they hit a snow storm and Kolter (my son) was thrown from the truck.

I instantly went into nurse mode. He stated everyone else was ok and that Kolter was hurt the worst. I asked the friend to take the phone to Kolter and I tried to ask him where he hurt. His head was bleeding and he was yelling over and over "My back! My back!" I was somewhat relieved to hear his voice knowing he was alive but he was only moving his upper body and could not move his legs. I spoke to the emergency personnel on scene until they transported him to the nearest hospital. My husband and I had to drive an hour and half through one of the worst snow storms; vehicles had slid off the road all along the highway. I received a call from the trauma surgeon just miles before we arrived to the hospital. The news was devastating! My son had broken his back and he now was paralyzed; emergency surgery needed to be performed as soon as possible.

Since that dreadful day our family has been through many ups and downs. I can say the biggest turning point for us was when I met a lady through social networking from Australia that was living in California. Her son also had a SCI and she was living in California working at a facility that specialized in below the level of injury therapy. What I heard from this angel on the other line was HOPE! Kay gave me the support I needed during that lonely time. She was a life line and we have since formed a lifelong sister hood! I can never thank Kay Ledson enough for all she did for me, my son, and my family!

See https://m.facebook.com/daretodefi to keep up to date on Michelle and Kolter.

Reece Wallen

Townsville, Australia

Reece was a young man in the Royal Australian Navy when he suffered a catastrophic spinal cord injury. Initially, I met him and his mum Robyn through Facebook. I had the privilege of meeting Reece personally when he came to Carlsbad in 2013. I was also lucky enough to meet his mum, who has devoted her life to helping him get his life back. I am proud and honored to call Reece and Robyn my friends.

Here is a small snapshot of his story:

In December 2010, life as I knew it changed forever. One day I was a very active 24 year old, riding motor bikes, playing football, fishing and camping, and the next I was a C5/C6 quadriplegic unable to do the things I loved in life. I spent 6 weeks in Intensive Care on a ventilator unable to even breathe for myself or move anything below my neck. All up I spent 6 months in hospital trying to regain any function possible. Doctors told me I'd be using a Power Chair for the rest of my life and never be able to look after myself in any way.

While in hospital, I heard about an intensive training program called "Walk On" which was based off another highly regarded intensive training program in America called "Project Walk".

Since doing Walk On I am now using a manual chair and have gained enough strength to transfer in and out of my chair and a car with minimal assistance. I have also made the trip to America to attend Project Walk where I gained more strength and motivation, and I'm planning on going back again in the near future.

After more than 3 years I'm still getting stronger and making progress towards regaining more independence and possibly to at least being able to stand one day.   https://www.facebook.com/thereecewallenappeal

_____

Erica Predum

Fort Wayne Indiana USA.

Wow, Erica, a true hero and a treasured friend to Josh, Amelia and me. I had been Facebook friends with Erica for a few years when I finally met her at Project Walk. Although she was busy with her therapy, we got to hang out a few times. When Josh launched his book at Project Walk Atlanta, Erica convinced two of her friends to join her on a road trip (something like 10 hours each way) so she could attend Josh's launch and meet him. We were humbled, honored and blessed that she made such an effort to join us, and finally her meeting Josh. Erica, although with only 10% independence raises her two boys, she is the first to step up to support a newly injured person. Erica is generous in her support, and genuinely cares about not just her injured friends, but their families.

I know Erica and I will be friends forever, I bow down to her!

Here are Erica's words:

Seven years ago, lying in a hospital bed, unable to breathe or move, being told I'll never walk again, was the worst moment of my entire life. I was 22, living my life my way, nothing was stopping me from what I wanted to accomplish for myself and all of a sudden, on a typical drive home, my life was changed forever.

My SUV rolled several times on the highway, throwing me out of the vehicle, onto the highway, leaving my 3 year old son, Aidan still inside the vehicle. I suffered 27 injuries, fortunately my son was fine, and he was uninjured!

All of my injuries healed up besides one, my spinal cord injury, I was now labelled a "quadriplegic."

Our lives were turned upside down. I was forced to start over, living a new life in a new body that I had zero control over. I'm still unable to think about the first two years after the accident without overwhelming emotions, those years are just a blur to me, I was in survival mode and wasn't really living life.

My "new life" started coming back together once I met my boyfriend, had a baby (a beautiful boy, Junior) and together we focused on this new life and our family. Eventually, I started to focus on what I needed to do to take care of me and this damn injury for the sake of my health and happiness. It was from that moment on, my life took a turn for the better and it hasn't stopped!

I began setting and accomplishing goals pushing me forward, refusing to let my accident hold me back any longer. During my journey to better my situation, I've met lifelong friends, who I have to thank for showing support, love and guidance whenever I needed it. This is such a difficult injury to deal with, and having friends to lean on, who understand exactly what you're going through, helps me not feel alone or misunderstood. I now focus on pushing my body to get stronger while taking care of my two boys and making sure I enjoy my life as it is, because, nothing is promised and I've seen how bad life can get.

I am just moving forward!

Spencer Fox and Celia Brew

Solana Beach, California

During the time I was in Carlsbad, I had the pleasure of meeting Celia and her son Spencer. Spencer's work ethic at Project Walk was motivating to all those around him; his total belief in his recovery was inspirational. For a young man his attitude towards his recovery was well beyond his years. Spencer was always totally committed to gaining as much out of every recovery session he had.

Celia, his mom, thrown like all of us into this crazy world, was totally dedicated to Spencer's recovery. As a single parent, she managed to balance a demanding position with supporting her son.

Celia was a caring, solid supporter to me during my efforts to remain in the USA. I will be forever grateful to her. Celia and Spencer are respected ambassadors for those suffering from spinal cord injury. It gives me great pleasure to include their story in my book.

Here's Spencer's story, written by his mom Celia. It is honest and real, dealing with some of the many issues facing someone suffering a SCI:

On 2/1/2010, my son Spencer Fox was paralyzed from the neck down in a snowboarding accident.

Four years ago, I found myself in an intensive care unit in Salt Lake City, Utah, with thirteen-year-old Spencer hanging on to life by a gossamer thread, hooked to an overhead canopy of blinking, beeping, life-saving machines.

Heart-stopping alarms sounded with regularity; it was every parent's nightmare.

After two days we were fairly certain he would pull through, but the prognosis was stupefying: Spencer's broken neck resulted in a spinal cord injury. He was completely paralyzed, a quadriplegic. Doctors said he may never breathe on his own, and likely would never recover movement or sensation. "Never" is a very scary word that we could not accept.

Thus began our odyssey, a long journey defined by experiences that give riseto knowledge and understanding. There is no more apt descriptor. It captures the vicissitudes of our heartbreak and triumph. It acknowledges Spencer's fierce resolve to prove doctors wrong and my own determination to lead my son into a bright but unimaginable future. In uncharted territory, along the way we made mistakes. Occasionally we suffered pain, loneliness and grave disappointment; sometimes we trusted the wrong people. More often we were blessed with knowledge, opportunity, and insight. We were forced to experience the world differently and it gave us a chance to define ourselves anew. We found laughter and lifelong friends. We learned that love and compassion are thicker than blood. We endured the death of Spencer's loyal service dog Mojo. And through it all we have been carried by Spencer's valor, his funny, pragmatic attitude, and unceasing work ethic.

Today I look back in awe and exclaim in exaltation, "Here we stand!"

Here is a summary of what luck, hard work, community support, six-rehab- sessions-a-week and four years later looks like for us:

Mobility and Independence

Spencer is driving his own adapted car to school and rehabilitation, no longer dependent on caregivers. He will need some care giving services when he goes to college, but his ability to function independently is remarkable and life changing. Spencer knows no fear, but he is careful to think through the best way to do things so he can do them again the next day and with the least amount of pain.

In December, Spencer walked for an entire day at school. He didn't know if he could, but he wanted to see if it was possible to get by without his wheelchair. At the end of the day he realized he still needs his chair because it was too difficult and painful to walk that much, but what a feat! "How many people said they couldn't believe how tall you are?" In typical Spencer fashion he quipped, "A lot. But I couldn't believe how short some people are."

Spencer went to the desert recently for a weekend with his Uncle John. As I was packing his gear I suddenly remembered his chair. I hadn't considered where it would fit. "Are you taking your wheelchair?" Spencer thought for a minute, "No, I don't think so. I think I can get by without it." And he did. On the same trip, Spencer had the opportunity to try skeet shooting. He fired a shotgun for the first time and hit the first clay disk.

295

Then he missed several, but by the end he was hitting them consistently. The fact that he could stand, balance, lift the shotgun, aim, and pull the trigger, is simply astounding.

Spencer sometimes leaves the house late at night to Jacuzzi with friends, no assistance required. He can pump his own gas. He can surf with a crew of friends. He can walk up and down stairs if need be. He can carry his backpack to the car. He can bend from a standing position to pick something up off the floor. Spencer can do almost anything, though it might take longer.

We honor all of the trainers and therapists who have worked with Spencer at PW and MRK Lab. And we are especially grateful to Matt Audia, who has become much more than Spencer's hand therapist; he is a friend and fan. Matt assures Spencer's hands get stronger all the time, striving always for a functional right hand. Spencer also continues to work on full body strength and balance. He will cope with the paralysis and damage to his central nervous system all of his life, and he will need to manage spasms and pain. Still, his neurological recovery has been off the charts.

I glory in his each and every movement... I take nothing for granted. Nothing!

Academics and Career

Eight weeks after the accident, an occupational therapist at Rady Children's Hospital attached a brace with a pencil to Spencer's left hand so he could write (he used to be right-handed). With great effort Spencer was able to make a huge, childlike "S" on a sheet of paper. I cheered along with everyone else, but inside I felt cold panic and I had to turn away to hide my tears. Before the accident Spencer had been writing papers on comparative economic systems. How would anyone know what Spencer was capable of if he could not communicate with pen, paper or computer?

Once again, the situation called for faith, not fear. Spencer will be graduating from San Dieguito Academy (SDA) high school on June 13 with a robust GPA and excellent scores on his college entrance exams. He completed his college applications to California schools with great science and technology programs. He is interested in becoming an engineer, possibly a chemical or physical engineer. Spencer's college education is critical; his life will always be harder and his costs higher than for most people.

SDA has supported Spencer throughout. We give thanks to his aides, his tireless advocate Mark Easbey, and to a host of great teachers who saw beyond his physical limitations to his limitless potential, with special kudos to Susanne McCloskey, Sheryl Bode, and Stephanie Siers. Likewise, our hats are off to the SDA students involved with last year's Theater for a Cause fundraiser for HelpHOPELive in Spencer's honor, and to Sheryl Bode for promoting our participation in the Surfing Madonna Beach Run. We live in a great community.

Finances

The financial realities of spinal cord injury (SCI) are harsh. The Christopher Reeve Foundation estimates first year ($1,023,000), annual ($109,000) and lifetime ($3,319,533) costs for Spencer's level of SCI. An estimated one in three bankruptcies in this country results from uninsured medical expenses. Most people live one medical crisis away from financial ruin. I could have been one of them. I am a single mom 100% financially responsible for my family. Despite my great job and health insurance, the costs of Spencer's injury were potentially overwhelming. My house was on the market and nearly upside down when Spencer had his accident. I emptied my savings and borrowed to keep and convert my house for wheelchair access to bring Spencer home.

Since then, I have sold everything of value, eliminated expenses, and made two career changes for a higher salary. But I did not get here alone.

We have invested over $250,000 in uninsured medical costs associated with Spencer's recovery; well over half of it was raised by the community through HelpHOPELive.

We are grateful for every dollar. I cannot emphasize enough what a difference every contribution has made. I picture you in my mind as I write thank you notes with misty eyes. I record your generosity and your connection to Spencer's story in my heart.

Truly, Spencer's future would look very different without your support.

At the risk of missing someone, I want to acknowledge some golden-hearted individuals who have made Spencer's cause their own. These people repeatedly donated money, helped with fundraisers, aided at surf events, assisted with the car, kept my family when my work schedule demanded more time than I had, and buoyed our spirits: my sister Lisa and brother-in-law Gary, my twin brother Jake, Debbie Nye, Lori Manroe, Dan and Kaye Hentschke, Jan Uhlman, Steve Cushman, Chris and Katrina Goldsmith, Doan and Mary Beth Hohmeyer, and Jane Morton. I don't know what we would have done without you.

Because of our combined efforts, Spencer is headed towards a good education and an independent life. Spencer, in turn, has started giving back to the community; speaking for adaptive surfing and scholarships for those with physical disabilities; it is a great circle.

The Rest

Spencer is fortunate to have the world's greatest brother, Dane, and sister, Ruby. I have written before about the uninvited change Spencer's accident wrought on the entire family. Recently I remarked to Dane, "Who would have thought Spencer would be where he is today?" and he reminded me, "I did." It's true. Right after the accident Dane maintained that if anyone could recover from this, Spencer could. Dane has unwavering faith in Spencer's ability to do the impossible. And Ruby sees no disability in Spencer. She adores her big brother--they argue about music, TV shows, movies and everything else--but Spencer gently guides her through school, homework and life while Ruby exuberantly shares her artwork and creativity. My kids have become closer and better for all they have been through. I am thankful because it could have turned out so many other ways.

Most important, Spencer has grown into a fine young man. He has great friends who are bright, caring and hilarious. He was the Master of Ceremonies for SDA's Community Day because he loves to entertain. He is in the Spanish Club and he eats every day at the cooking class, though he is not in it. He is wickedly funny and very kind. He has a broad array of interests and can talk on any subject; just ask him. He is very competitive and he thinks board games are a blood sport. He watches a lot of football, has eclectic musical tastes, and plays too many video games (in this mother's opinion). When Spencer finds a book he likes, he reads compulsively to the end. He enjoys being challenged, solving problems and learning about everything under the sun. He is ready to launch.

When Miracles Happen

I am so proud of my family. I shake my head in wonder and marvel at what we accomplished in the past four years. And I have learned something about miracles. I truly believe we have experienced a miracle, though it didn't always feel that way. It often felt more like hard work and struggle, overcoming obstacles, doubt and fear. Fortunately, even when uphill, we tried to move ever forward. And that is what I have learned. *You too, are likely living a miracle, whether it feels like one presently or not.*

In the end, may we all look back on a beautiful, complex tapestry of the life we created and see it as awe-inspiring and miraculous?

May all of our miracles continue!

If you want to help Spencer with his ongoing recovery, please donate through HelpHOPELive. Donations are tax deductible, and donated monies can only be spent for qualified medical expenses, including rehabilitation, caregivers and medical equipment.

Misti Gainan

Missoula, Montana

Sadly, I have not met Misti, but her story continues to inspire me!

Misti and I connected through Facebook and have become great friends. Misti does not have a spinal cord injury. Her paralysis was caused as a result of a brain bleed. Misti, like all of my heroes, is fighting to get her life back. She above all wants to be a great mom for her daughter Ava. I look forward to the day that we meet. She is such an inspiration to me. Misti is very active in supporting our community on Facebook. Along with her photo on Facebook the words read - I CAN AND I WILL - WATCH ME!

During the summer of 2009, I was starting to feel drained. I was a full time college student double majoring, working two and three jobs, and babysitting for a friend. I was pushing myself to do the very best at everything, but something felt wrong. The right side of my body felt numb. I had no balance, horrible daily migraines, and I was tired all the time.

After months of this feeling getting worse, I saw my general physician on September 21 2009. She shined a light in my eyes and told me "You don't have any tumors behind your eyes, but I want you to see a neurologist."

One month later on October 21 I saw a neurologist. He scheduled me to have an MRI of my brain at 9 AM the next morning. I remember looking at the computer screen after my MRI and I saw a big black spot. I didn't know what to think, but I soon found out. My neurologist called and wanted me to get to his office immediately. When I got there they rushed me to his office. His words will always be with me "Misti, in 40 years of practice I have never seen anything like this. Your brain is bleeding." It was called a Spontaneous Caver Noma. My neurologist was in the process of setting up emergency brain surgery with a neurosurgeon who was highly qualified, but unsure how things would go. December 21, 2009 with only a 2% chance of making it through such a risky procedure, I tried it. *I had to fight!*

When I woke up, I was so happy to be alive that it took about a week for it to sink in that I was paralyzed on the right side of my body.

After a month in recovery I had given up on recovering and on life. Then I found out I was 7 1/2 months pregnant.

Twice in one year my life drastically changed, so it was time for me to change! My baby deserved that from me. Since having my beautiful daughter (Ava), I have been attending physical therapy three times a week for three years. I have put literal blood sweat and tears into my recovery and I'm proud to report that I am walking again using a walker! *I am so excited about the next phase of my life*!

Facebook is Misti Gainan and my email is mommamsg@gmail.com

JD Guerrieri & Sherry Pierro

New Jersey

Josh, Amelia and I met JD and Sherry while they were attending PW Carlsbad, and the connection with us all was immediate. JD's accident was particularly tragic! In a few seconds he went from a strong powerful fit young man to being completely dependent on his mother Sherry. Sherry fought for JD's life for months. There was nothing she wouldn't do for him. Together, today they are a formidable team. Even though their focus is on JD's recovery, they always have time to help others. Both Sherry and JD are passionate warriors for the plight of those suffering from spinal cord injury. Recently, Sherry posted an extremely emotional post on Facebook. I asked her if I could include it in my book because it is such a powerful piece written by a very committed loving mother.

JD Take a Stand

Well, where do I begin? Three years ago today, I found my beautiful son JD lying lifeless in the street without any idea as to what happened to him, why he was there, or if he'd ever live to see another day. I watched my baby take his last breath and then watched his heart stop beating....and mine did, too. I know this may sound crazy to a lot of you, but seeing him lying there forced me to do one thing, pray. I knelt down alongside his lifeless body. I placed my left hand over his heart and my right hand over my heart. I bowed my head and began to pray.

I said, "God? God, you have blessed me almost 18 years ago with this beautiful child. And it was 18 years ago exactly that I was faced with a horrible demand from my OBGYN to 'end my pregnancy' due to all of the complications I was facing with this unborn child that, according to the doctors, would never survive. I fought them. I stood up to them because I KNEW that You were with me and that You would see me through it all. And I kept that baby and fought through a delivery that nearly took both our lives and You prevailed because You gave me this beautiful child- a beautiful boy that I have cherished every moment since. I thank you God for all these years You have blessed me with, but 18 years isn't enough. I want to see this child go on and live a good life and bring me more love and joy - watch him grow and fall in love and have a family of his own one day. If you must take him now, I don't think I'll survive the loss because this child has given ME purpose. This child has put love in a place that I never knew existed and I know that You have always been there, because every time I look at this child I see YOU, God. So I ask You again, I BEG You to PLEASE spare this child and please allow him to go on here with me, because if you take him now, if he dies, I will surely die, too. I beg you, Lord, please spare this life, this child, this heart of mine." Just then I heard a voice, I heard a man's voice say CLEARLY "I already saved him."

I jumped up to look around because surely someone else was standing there...and I thought to myself, was I praying OUT LOUD? Did somebody here hear me and answer me back? So I opened my eyes and looked up- I look around and there's not a soul in sight, so I say OUT LOUD, "WHAT did you SAY??!" And I clearly hear the same voice answer, "I SAID that I saved him. I've already SAVED JD. He will be fine you'll see. You will need to stay strong and stay faithful and he will be alright. You'll see. Now GO! GO! GO!" And just like that the voice was gone and I began to hear the sounds of sirens screaming as they approached me, knowing that those sounds were coming for my boy for my baby JD....and it was the most frantic moment of my entire life.

That fateful night was the beginning of a LOT of heartache, a lot of fear, pain, and multiple resuscitations. The coma, the Intensive Care Unit, life support, respirator, ventilator, stitches, clamps, staples, miles of IV lines and a feeding tube for direct nourishment and multiple surgeries to repair a smashed skull, a shattered spine, and collapsed lungs. (And many other things too!)

Then the pneumonias and the staph infections, the sepsis, ALL while in the ICU on life support as I listened to multiple doctors advise me to "shut the machines and let him go"....a mother's worst nightmare to watch helplessly as her beautiful child lay in a coma in a hospital bed surrounded by machines to keep him alive....and all the while I remembered what that voice said, "I already saved JD" over and over again in my head like a bell. Then I have my heart saying, "You know this kid- you KNOW his heart you KNOW how strong he is and how special and different he is. These doctors aren't dealing with Joe Schmoe! This is JD! This is MY super- strong, unbelievable strong willed, physically strong son this is MY BABY they're talking about and HE IS GONNA MAKE IT! HE IS GONNA GET THROUGH THIS and HE IS GONNA PROVE THESE DOCTORS WRONG! JD IS GONNA LEAVE THIS HOSPITAL ALIVE and HIS STORY ISN'T OVER YET!"

NO WAY IS HIS STORY OVER! This is just a HUGE road block in just ONE of the MANY chapters of his book. JD is going to be a name that EVERYONE will know one day because he is going to GET THRU THIS! Through ALL OF THIS! He was a miracle before and he is gonna be a miracle AGAIN!!"

And so it was- he made it one day, then a second, then a third until after a while he opened his eyes and came OUT of that coma! And little by little he fought and he made it another day! Six LONG MONTHS in a hospital bed is a LONG time. And here we are today, three years to the day exactly that our lives changed forever and he is stronger than he was, better than he was, doing more than he was! He isn't out of the woods and you know, maybe he won't ever be, but he IS getting better every day and I BELIEVE he WILL KEEP IMPROVING because he gives 1000% of all he's got to push himself in therapies and keeps himself strong and healthy and POSITIVE!!

I look forward to each and every day that God gives us, like a child that waits with anticipation on Christmas Eve, wondering what Santa has brought them and although this isn't Christmas and we aren't talking about gifts under a tree, we ARE talking about THE GREATEST GIFT OF ALL....LIFE!! We have LIFE and we have God's blessing and His promise and we have the DRIVE and the DETERMINATION to keep pushing forward to keep reaching for the "impossible" because according to the medical world, the odds were against him and it was "impossible" for him to SURVIVE this tragedy three YEARS AGO!!

So today, I would like to say to my beautiful, amazing, inspiring, strong, determined, smart, good-hearted, and wise beyond his years son this: JD you are MY inspiration- you are MY HERO, my world, you are the sun in my cloudy skies and YOU have given ME strength! YOU have given ME love and YOU have given ME LIFE! Life that I can't wait for each and every day- to love you, to BE loved by you, to watch you achieve the IMPOSSIBLE & BEYOND!

Your book has only just BEGUN, baby, and I will be there behind you every moment, every struggle, every joy, and every accomplishment that YOU overcome, experience, and enjoy- you are on the path that God has chosen for you and I AM SO PROUD of YOU!! Proud of WHO YOU ARE- WHAT YOU ARE and WHAT YOU STAND FOR! KEEP ON FIGHTING! KEEP ON PUSHING because YOU WILL BE REWARDED and YOU WILL ACHIEVE ANYTHING YOU PUT YOUR HEAD and HEART INTO!! ANYTHING!! I love you so MUCH and I haven't left your side, not even for a MINUTE in three solid years and I will ALWAYS be here with you FOREVER!! God bless you baby and I KNOW you will get ALL that you want, because you give ALL of yourself to get it!!! Keep up the GREAT work with yourself and all those you help and mentor on this journey!! YOU are a TRUE WARRIOR - a TRUE INSPIRATION and I LOVE YOU MORE THAN WORDS could EVER say!!! Love Always, Mom xoxoxox."

I would like to briefly mention a few more of my heroes.

Bayne "the Magnificent"

(My nickname for him) is a service dog belonging to one of our Warrior

Momz, Tina, another of my heroes. Tina adopted Bayne as a rescue puppy. Tina wanted to personally train a service dog to assist her with her daily living, and she also wanted a trusted companion. Tina has done an amazing job in her training of Bayne. He is truly a magnificent dog and furry friend to Tina and her family. He is a giant of a dog, with strength and intelligence. When I was in Atlanta I had the privilege of meeting Bayne and his "mom" Tina. Tina has meticulously trained him; his demeanor is impressive, and his intelligence is truly amazing. I spent the day with them, which included eating out at a busy southern family restaurant. Once inside and all seated, Bayne curled up under the table and waited quietly while we ate.

Tina and Bayne are examples of the wonderful relationship that can be achieved between a dog and his "mom." I continue to be blown away by the relationship between these two heroes. They were both brought together through a tragedy; a truly wonderful story.

Paul and Jeannie Pickard - PW Atlanta –

Paul and his wife Jeannie were thrown into this crazy world when their son Chris was involved in a motor vehicle accident leaving him a quadriplegic. Paul and Jeannie, along with their son, knew there had to be another option for his recovery. Their research led them to PW. They purchased a license and established PW Atlanta.

I was very impressed with this inspiring facility when I visited it in April 2013. Paul is a motivated leader, committed to helping his clients while supporting his son's recovery. He has a wealth of knowledge on funding and grants that help with some of their client's therapy expenses. Paul is extremely active in the SCI community, attending conferences, learning more, educating others, and always having the time to speak to someone with this injury. The Pickards as a family go the extra step in helping not just the families in our SCI Community but are strongly committed to their church.

I am proud to call Paul and Jeannie "family"

Liza and Amanda Perla - PW Orlando

Liza is a treasured "sister", a bond we have formed through being moms of children who have suffered a spinal cord injury. Liza and I have never met but we have shared so many phone / skype calls and messages we are friends and trusted allies.

Liza and her daughter Amanda founded PW Atlanta after Amanda suffered a devastating spinal cord injury from a motor vehicle accident. Together they run this recovery center of hope and love, while managing Amanda's ongoing recovery. Both Liza and Amanda have hearts of tigers, fighting for recovery for all who enter their facility. Liza is amazing, nothing is too much for her, so often I am asked for help on the East coast USA, Liza is one of my first contact points.

Anyone attending their recovery facility is instantly enveloped in love and an important supportive network. I am constantly inspired by the Face book posts of Amanda and her commitment to walk again.

http://www.projectwalkorlando.org

Chapter 26.   From the Darkness to the Light: 14 Years of Learning

I learned, because of the catastrophic nature of Josh's injury, that I had to "mourn" the loss of my son - the old son, the wild child, the extreme child who loved life and was always so happy and positive. I needed to learn to celebrate the life of my "new" son who looked the same but much, much thinner, still had the same smile, was so positive, but who would obviously have a new life path. So while I did mourn his life "lost," at every moment I celebrated the life we both have fought so hard to rebuild.

For the record he is still my "wild child", my "extreme" child who loves his life and is mostly happy and positive. In truth, he is the same, however in a slightly broken damaged body.

I also had to allow myself to mourn the loss of my old life. It was so dramatically changed after Josh's accident that this became an important issue for me to deal with. I will say up front that this is an ongoing process for me! One thing I have learned is that my "old life" that I thought was so perfect, so full of growth and learning, was lacking in meaning and true purpose; something I embrace every day, and in all honesty, I do not miss it.

To this day I have never cried for Josh, fearing if I did I would never stop!

About three years after the accident, a friend suggested that I should see a physiatrist. The intention was to help me learn to mourn what had happened to Josh. Initially I wasn't sure, but thinking about, it I thought why not, I have nothing to be embarrassed or ashamed of, so I threw myself into my therapy, one hour a week for nearly two years.

These regular sessions became a time for me to gain huge insights, understanding and significant growth. I received so much from letting myself go for that short time every week. After two years of therapy, which of course wasn't just about Josh's accident, it was really about my whole life, I found I had worked out the emotions, the effect of the accident on my life, and I was grateful for the time I spent on me for that one hour a week.

I have no regrets. Josh and I have been on an amazing journey!

Josh now says that the accident was the best thing that had ever happened to him. How much he has learned, how much he has grown as a man, learning what is important to him, and learning to celebrate any progress no matter what or how small, and appreciating life!

Through this time, our own relationship went from strength to strength, although there were times I can honestly say it went to hell and back!

Sometimes the "hell period" continued for weeks, or months, causing us both a great deal of angst. But in the end, our love for each other pulled us through and we would get back on track.

Thank God for the lessons learned!

Positive Selfishness - Self time

In those first months, as a mom, (I never allowed the term "carer or caregiver." NO matter what, I was Josh's mom), you have no time for yourself. You just do whatever you have to do! I pushed myself to a level I never knew I had, in fighting for Josh, his self-esteem, and his life!

I wasn't eating, I probably appeared manic to everyone except Josh, and I was so tired. I learned very quickly that I had to take care of myself. At times it felt selfish, putting myself before Josh and my family, but I knew in those early weeks post-accident that if Josh was to survive I had to keep strong, healthy, fit, and focused. So I needed to somehow find some "me" time.

Those times were cherished by me, even if it was simply having a coffee, reading a newspaper, a walk in a garden, having a massage, or getting my hair cut it. It didn't have to be anything major; simply a time when it was just me doing something for me.

It was invigorating, and truly formed part of my reenergizing without feeling guilty.

When your life changes so dramatically, you feel out of control, confused, frightened, and fearful. You become caught up in this crazy new world, a totally new reality.

You need hugs, the more the better. It's such a tough time emotionally; never under estimate the power of a hug.

You need to see that eventually you will get part of your old life back. It won't be the same, but if you look after yourself, you will embrace it as I do. Frankly, you have no choice in the matter!

I know initially when I realized that I had to take care of me, it did feel selfish. I experienced real guilt, and then one day I was speaking to someone about it, and I said for my survival I had to be "positively selfish." All of a sudden I realized that it was okay for me to take a time out!

These days when I am mentoring families, very early on I emphasize the importance of taking a time out, if you are on your own for yourself or as a family or a couple, the importance of "family /date" nights.

You will be let down *and* there will be always disappointments with this injury; it is so tough.

As a parent, I felt totally let down by the lack of support from Josh's father. Josh and his dad were always so close, they shared so much, but after Josh's accident the relationship changed, especially between his dad and me. Even though we had been divorced many years up until the accident, both his dad and I were totally in tune with Josh's wellbeing!

In those crazy early days just after the accident we didn't seem to agree on anything. This was especially devastating to me, and I know to Josh. For months, even years, his total lack of support for Josh has truly saddened me, and I questioned my 29 year relationship with him. But over the years I have learned to let it go. It's really not my issue, it's his, and I'm sure he suffers the consequences of his actions every day. On a positive note, Josh enjoys his relationship with his dad, and really that's what is important.

Friends and Strangers

Most of my friends were very supportive. People we hardly knew really stepped up to support Josh and to help us, but for me there were two close friends I never saw again. They were friends who had gone through so much with me, but from them there was nothing but silence! Initially it was disappointing, but yet again other positive surprises made up for it. (I only mention this because for those of you suffering through the early days of this injury you will experience disappointments like this, but the sooner you get over it, let it go, and move on, the easier it gets. In the end it's not about you.)

You will get exhausted by people asking you when will "   " get better? When will "   " walk again? You get the picture! Even worse was when Josh was in the wheelchair, with people speaking to me instead of Josh, or speaking loudly and slowly to him. Seriously, sometimes you just wanted to scream "Josh is okay; he can hear just fine, nothing has changed!"

I'm sure you are getting the picture!

You will learn not to be shocked or angered by these sorts of questions. Try using them as an opportunity to educate them on the catastrophic effects of spinal cord injury.

Most people have no idea about the injury; in fairness we had no idea!

What really used to make me really frustrated was the number of people who thought because Josh was in a wheel chair that his work opportunities would be totally limited. I would be asked the following - What sort of work will Josh do now? And then before I could answer, they answered for me offering, "He could always work in a call center!" or "He could work in a job that allowed him to sit in his wheelchair at his desk."

Even his talented medical team dismissed his work opportunities. The following is a direct quote from one of his surgeons from Josh's medical report dated 06/25/2001: "As a result of his injury, his choice of work in medium to long term will be restricted. No manual work, no standing, or bending or twisting. Employment will be restricted to sedentary work that will accept a wheel chair. In a similar fashion hobbies and sporting pursuits will be significantly restricted. As a result of his devastating injury he will never be able to undertake manual work. He will be restricted for the rest of his life in relation to walking and standing."

I always thought, "Are you serious?" To this question my reply was always the same -, especially in the early days, "Josh has a full time job - getting a little better each day!"

Today Josh mentors injured athletes, is building a career as a Corporate Motivational Speaker, influencing young Australians to believe in themselves through his school program.

SCI Community

I love this community. Josh, Amelia and I have made countless lifelong friends, but sometimes you are shocked by a comment or reaction to a situation. I have had a mother say to me "I got lucky" when Josh walked. I was disappointed. She never took the time to understand what Josh actually needs to do to walk, what he deals with every step he takes, and that in reality his life would be possibly easier in a wheel chair. Some people are quick to make unqualified judgements!

My feeling with this injury is that we are such a small community, and we need to stick together. I am the first to admit that I don't really understand the injury, and sometimes because of this I "put my foot in my mouth" but it is never intentional, and I totally understand that not everyone will walk that has this injury. What I do know is that below injury recovery is possible!

At times I felt I had to apologize for Josh walking! Obviously I never did, but people need to understand that everyone is different and no one spinal cord injury is the same. I personally have no idea who will walk and who won't. As I often say "Walking for someone suffering a spinal cord injury is totally between the person suffering it and their God."

Naively, I expected Josh to walk with the never ending work and therapy we did with him. I knew he was an athlete, used to training, and so my expectation, with all the therapists and healers we had over the years, was that he would walk! I truly never really understood the injury until much later in his recovery.

Josh and I have stated on several occasions we have never researched spinal cord injury. Still today I rarely look at a site unless someone has referred me to it!

Josh is very generous with his time when asked to help someone with an SCI, although I am devastated for Josh at times. There was a young man who Josh mentored at his request for many months after his injury. All Josh ever did with this young man was advise him on what had worked for him. Josh made himself available whenever he called, to get him through the tough times. I know Josh spent hours mentoring him, as I did his family.

After 12 months, he wasn't walking. He criticized Josh publically on social media twice, basically saying he did everything Josh told him to do and nothing happened. He still wasn't walking! Well, all I can say is Josh is not a healer, he is no clairvoyant, all he ever does is *volunteer* his time to help those battling with this injury, as I do!

What that young man failed to understand was through following Josh's advice/mentoring, he was a lot more fit. He was setting his body up for recovery by keeping fit. With his spinal cord still swollen the importance of fitness cannot be overstated...especially getting him into an injury mentality rather than one of disabled! There is NO quick fix to recovery from spinal cord injury.

Ignoring the odd criticisms (there haven't been many, but they do hurt), we have had worked with hundreds of families who genuinely are grateful for our support of them, in offering them a "light of hope" when all hope has been taken away by the medical profession. We are the first to say, though - to gain recovery from this injury is hard, hard work; a total commitment, being prepared to work harder than you've ever worked in your life. There is no easy recovery option with this injury. It is repetition, repetition, repetition... finding out what is working and keeping on doing it!

Sadly, insurance companies in most parts of the world do not cover below injury recovery programs, which puts enormous financial pressure on families to be continually fund raising. Josh and I try and promote facilities that offer scholarship programs but sadly they are few and far between. It is devastating to us to advise families thrown into this crazy world of SCI to start fund raising when they have so much else to deal with.

Faith

I was raised a Christian, and as a child I attended Sunday school. But as I grew older religion really did not play a part in my life other than through my own beliefs. The more I travelled the more religions I experienced. Over the years, if asked, I would say I definitely believe in a higher power. My beliefs ran across Christianity, Hinduism, and Buddhism. Josh's accident certainly challenged my belief system and we were not let down!

As I write this book, I have never been more challenged financially and personally in my life. A strong believer in karma, my belief system has been seriously challenged these past four years (2010 – 2014), but I am mindful of the times when in desperation we have been supported spiritually. The messages I received in the early hours after Josh's accident definitely came from a higher power!

I was rewarded with names when I needed them. I was clearly told Josh would walk within 2 1/2 years. Within nine hours after the accident I was guided to look out of the square in Josh's recovery journey. The people I needed to help me were there already in my life, and many had worked through other injuries Josh had had, so I trusted them. My father, Josh's grandfather, who had passed away when Josh was three years old, supported Josh in spirit in those dark and challenging early days after his accident. There were times he appeared to Josh, always smiling, during the intense healing sessions with Isobel.

In those early days when Paula meditated, more often than not she received messages in relation to Josh's ongoing healing. Sometimes she couldn't explain what she had been told; she needed to draw the instructions.

Josh's two furry kids were definitely gifts from the Universe. They have wisdom far beyond any dog we have ever had, and they both totally understand Josh's injury. Both doggies came into our lives when we needed help and love, and I can't add the amount of times in Josh's "dark times" that they gave him to will to keep going.

I know Josh's friends who have passed over are with him always. They have his back; they protect him, and they motivate and inspire him. He is in contact with them through his personal spirituality, memories, and the great love he had for them.

Amelia came into Josh's life at a time when both of them were on paths of self-destruction. Together they have forged a team of love, strength and total commitment to each other, which is inspiring to all who know them. Their relationship has helped heal my broken heart, and I have total confidence in them both continuing to grow and learn together.

Expectations

By this I mean expectations of recovery. It was not me that made Josh walk, he did it himself. He knew I totally believed he would walk. I never doubted it, moving through his recovery journey, and seeing how hard it was to make those uncooperative legs move, I asked him more than once if he thought he would be better off in a wheel chair. He always just glared at me and said "I can't believe you said that. I hate the wheel chair."

This is the toughest injury of all. I can honestly say, and many who walk will agree with me: Sometimes it is tougher to walk, due to the level of cord damage, to fight a body at every waking that doesn't want to cooperate!

If Josh wanted to walk again, then I wanted Josh to walk for himself, not for me!

Sometimes families and friends try so hard to make it easy for their injured loved one, encouraging them to keep improving, wanting them to succeed more and more. But I have found that everyone who is injured has different expectations of what they want to achieve in recovery. Many are happy in the wheelchair, and build successful inspiring lives around it, and there are some who will continue to do whatever it takes to constantly improve.

There is no right or wrong here. Like the injury, everyone is different, and therefore everyone's attitude to recovery is personal and individual.

Unconditional Love

There have been so many times when Josh has said to me, "Get on with your life, I am okay." I simply say when you are a parent you will understand the unconditional love you have for a child. This injury is particularly difficult for parents and their loved ones. I can't simply walk away!

As a mother I look at Josh struggling with unbelievable and unrelenting neurogenic pain all over this body. Witnessing his constant fight with an uncooperative body devastates me! Knowing there is nothing I can do to help him, it frustrates and saddens me! At times I feel that I have failed him. I know that's not the case, but it is very hard, nevertheless!

I watch Josh give so generously to those who have asked for his help through his knowledge of the injury. I have watched him break his heart over friends lost through accidents and this cruel devastating injury.

I have watched him struggle to make this broken body of his work, when it just won't play the game.

I burst with pride when I hear him speak publically about his journey, his power, his growth, his never ending commitment to get that little bit better every day; he rarely complains.

I have experienced seeing the fear in his eyes when his body starts to shut down. His terror, his inability to control his body, and yet he bounces back. He has a positive attitude, no matter how hard his life becomes.

My son is a humble man, but above all else Josh is still my wild child, the extreme child who loves life, is always smiling, and no matter what life has thrown at him, there has always been something that gave him the strength and courage to keep pushing ahead! Through his injury we have certainly experienced the most thrilling, wildest, scariest "Roller Coaster Ride of Life."

There is so much I have probably left out of this chapter. There have been so many experiences we have learned from over the years it becomes blurred.

ABOVE ALL ELSE, WE HAVE SURVIVED!

Chapter 27. Leaving No Stone Unturned - Josh's Journey of Recovery

I realize there are huge areas missing in our story of recovery. My focus with this book, especially in the first chapters, was really to concentrate on the early days and weeks of Josh's injury. I wanted those reading my book to gain an insight of the pre accident Josh, so they gained an understanding of the history we had shared that helped him and me work out his recovery options.

With this chapter I will endeavor to put a time line to Josh's journey, to give those reading an idea of the things we tried to assist him gain his recovery.

From the outset, I want those reading this book to understand that everyone who worked on Josh in those early days was known to us. They were trusted friends; as Josh became stronger we extended our team through referrals. I make no recommendations regarding what we did. I will simply tell you what worked for Josh and remind you that every spinal cord injury is different.

In those frightening dark early days, our primary goal was to keep the energy flowing through his broken body. Since Josh was completely paralyzed he couldn't do this, so we had to figure out a way to do it for him! We knew we had to commence immediately, yet we were in an environment (the hospital) that made this seemingly impossible. Yet we did it, by thinking out of the box.

We set up a custom of closing the curtains around Josh's bed every time anyone visited him, day or night. By me gaining an understanding of the ward's staffing in the evening, we worked out a system that would allow for our trusted "healing team" posing as visitors to perform their magic without being interrupted safely within the "cocoon of the curtains" I sat on guard watching the nurses station through a small crack...we were never challenged!

To achieve the recovery Josh has made, and continues to make after nearly 16 years, Josh needed to adopt the mindset of a gold medal winning Olympian. Training his mind through visualization and his body through physical training was his only focus.

From those early days, he has always trained with the belief that he was injured, not disabled.

Over the years he has developed his visualization skills to a super level; from those early days, when he was totally paralyzed, he would lay in bed for hours trying to connect his broken body back to his brain. Through his memory he visualized the process of various movements, including weight bearing movement to achieve an action, i.e., jumping a motor bike over a hump; what he needed to do with his weight and movement, actions he had to do while he was preparing to jump, and hitting the ground after the jump. He visualized the movement of gliding his snowboard through the snow, and how he shifted his weight and moved his legs and arms. His memory of all these activities, and more, became the basis of him reconnecting the pathways of his body.

An example he uses when he speaks is to "Imagine you are in a darkened room, and the only light is your brain. You see a flicker of light somewhere in the room, and the challenge with my injury was to teach my brain to connect those flickers back into it. I used this visualization exercise to connect the flickers of light in my body back into my brain." Slowly the connections began to join together.

From the end of the first week in the hospital, he maintained this regime for several hours every day, until he really commenced the reconnection of those remote areas of his body to his mind. This intense daily process went on for 3-4 months.

Day 1 – We commenced massaging his fingertips, fingers, hands, toe tips, toes and feet, combining the massage with essential healing oils. Sandalwood was our preferred oil due to its ancient healing processes.

For Josh to regain his hands and finger function - as he became stronger we encouraged Josh to visualize the area we were massaging, again trying to get him reconnecting with his extremities.

I have learned an important part of rehab for a quadriplegic is the intensive massaging of their extremities – this being their toes, feet, hands and fingers.

The more we massaged his extremities, the harder Josh worked to commence reconnecting his brain to the endless massaging. These exercises were critical to maintaining the connections. Looking back, I believe these exercises, although Josh couldn't feel anything, were crucial in ensuring the movement memory of his nervous system was maintained.

Wendy brought in a stress ball to the hospital a few weeks after the accident. In those early days Josh couldn't even hold the ball. It would sit on his lifeless palm. Many a time I would return to his room to find Josh staring at the ball sitting on his palm. I would ask "What are you trying to do?"

"I am visualizing getting my hand to try and close around the ball."

Over a period of weeks he managed to clasp the ball, and over a longer period he could hold it applying pressure. Josh used the same methodology to learn to clean his teeth and use cutlery, eventually enabling him to feed himself.

Today, Josh's hands for a quad of his level are very functional. Mostly he can achieve all tasks, including threading a needle, something his mother can no longer easily do!

Day 1 - until today. Regular checks with our personal doctor Graeme Baro. He has been Josh's personal doctor for over 18 years.

Day 1 - until today. Chiropractic care – Dr. Simon Floreani visited Josh (at my pleading) the first days after the accident, and commenced adjustments (not near injury) the weekend following the accident (once we had possession of Josh's MRI's). Simon had been Josh's chiropractor for two years prior to his accident. We had total trust in Simon. He was our friend, and everything he did was with our permission and at our request.

In hospital and rehab, Simon would work on Josh for between 1 - 1 1/2 hours each session, once a week. His primary goal was to ensure the Josh's energy was flowing through his body.

Since his release from rehab in November 2000, Josh has continued to see Simon for regular adjustments, to this day.

Week 2 - until 2008. Paula (physic healer) would work on Josh with a mixture of crystal healing and massage for up to 90 minutes weekly. Paula commenced her work on Josh within two weeks of his accident, both in the hospital and later in the rehab for several hours each week. Josh continued to have healings with Paula as he thought he needed them or when she called him to come to her home for a healing session. Josh has had no healings from Paula since 2009, due to her ill health. We will be forever grateful for her visionary work and inputs regarding Josh's recovery. She never stopped believing in Josh's ability to continue to recover and gain more movement.

Week 2 – 2002. Chakra realignment and in depth healing massage. While in hospital and rehab, Isabel would work on Josh for 1 - 2 hours weekly. Once Josh was discharged, it was whenever he needed to see her. He hasn't worked with Isabel since 2010. Isabel has a special and unique talent. When healing Josh she always sought messages and guidance from "spirits and guides" in her healings with him. Again, we have been blessed with special, gifted healers.

Week 4 until approximately Week 20. Weekly reflexology with Jackie (through our chiropractor Simon). Jackie would come to the hospital or rehab, usually on Saturday evenings, working her magic on Josh for about two hours each session. We always enjoyed a laugh when she was working on Josh, sharing Chinese takeaway and a glass of wine out of cardboard cups.

Week 7 - until 2008/9. Once Josh could have weekend leave from the hospital / rehab, an acupuncturist Bing, who was trained in Acupuncture and Traditional Chinese Medicine in Shanghai, China, worked her magic with her unique understanding of acupuncture combined with massage. She would work on Josh weekly for between 90 - 120 minutes. At the time, Bing could speak little English, but she and Josh found ways to communicate. She was amazing - truly understanding Josh's injury. Thanks to Bing, Josh achieved amazing results.

2014 - Josh has recently returned to seeing Bing, hopefully on a regular basis.

2000 - First month. Josh is trained in transcendental meditation. This enabled him to wean himself of his pain killers. Josh embraced the TM very early on in his recovery and still uses this technique today.

2000 - First month. Paula trained Josh in visualization techniques. Not an easy skill to master, especially with all the issues Josh was dealing with at that time, he truly embraced visualization as a core healing technique. I would say he has mastered this skill to an extreme level with what he has achieved.

Visualization is a CORE technique. Josh continues to utilize in his healing journey up to today.

2000. While still in the hospital, Josh received a "body energy flow" analysis by a team of TM healers from India. Paula had arranged their visit. They came to the rehab unit, and I don't know what the nurses were thinking when these three people came into visit Josh, fully dressed in their traditional Indian saris. I cannot explain their techniques; it was really about checking Josh's pulses, heartbeat, and blood flow. After about an hour, through an interpreter, they made some recommendations regarding Josh's immediate diet. Josh embraced their recommendations for about two weeks, admitting to feeling much better, but he is a carnivore, and as much he followed their diet, he truly missed meat and he resumed his old diet.

2000 - Getting His Driver's License back - While Josh was in rehab, we asked about getting his driver's license assessed. Once he was injured, Josh's driver's license was no longer valid, and he had to go through an onerous process to drive again. We were told it would take months. We asked why, and the rehab team gave us a list of tasks Josh had to be able to complete in order to gain his license back.

"Can we have the list?" The rehab team, in their usual "positive" (not) way said "It will take months!"

"Well, just give us the list."

Finally we were given this magic list of tasks Josh had to master!

Josh loved driving, so he threw all his energy into preparing himself, and he set a goal of two weeks. He asked me to bring his car in and leave it in the rehab parking lot. During the day he would roll his chair out to the carpark, transfer from his wheelchair into the car, and sit and listen to his music. This was an important part of his rehab, helping him in "feeling normal" by completing a normal task on his own.

Within two weeks Josh had mastered the list of tasks, and his car was taken to have the necessary engineering work done on it. To drive his current car, the only modifications that were needed were for the accelerator pedal to be moved to the left hand side, so he could accelerate with his left foot. He didn't need a modified steering wheel because his hands had improved so much with his therapy, and he could manage steering normally.

So the drama started again with his rehab team, who never had a sense of urgency regarding the scheduling of his license assessment – Yet again we asked "When can Josh get his test?"

"It will take weeks." "Why," we asked.

"Because it does!"

Finally I said, "Look, Josh has done everything you have asked, just organize it!"

Not long after, Josh took his test. He passed with flying colors, and he was able to get around on his own again. Awesome!

On his release from rehab, Josh would spend hours at home practicing his transfers in and out of the car. His goal was to not see his wheel chair, so to achieve this goal he practiced wheeling his chair to the trunk of his car, and standing holding the trunk lid, he would collapse his chair, get it into the trunk, and then holding on to his car "crab" around to the driver's seat and get into the car. Once he was confident he could manage the process, he would take himself to the gym, or to any therapy he was doing on his own. In the beginning it took a great deal of effort, but the more he persevered the more proficient and stronger he became. It's really the much used phase: repetition, repetition, repetition.

No matter how much we offered to help him, he resisted, saying over and over again, "I want to do this myself, if you help me I'll never get it, and I will never get my independence back."

2000, approximately 3 -4 months after his accident, Josh had two sessions of hypnotherapy. These sessions cleared up any doubt about the accident being anything but an accident. He had done nothing wrong, and seemingly made no mistakes.

During the first session he went back to when he was lying on the roadway. Immediately after his crash, he saw himself fighting for his life, trying desperately to stay alive. During the session, Josh reached out and picked something up from the road and forced it into his neck.

His second session was very powerful. In the hypnotic trance he journeyed back into the operating theater to the night his medical team was rebuilding his shattered vertebra. He could "see" the doctors working on him.

As I have mentioned earlier, Josh has, from the morning after his surgery, felt that his right leg was "empty" and not functioning properly in his body.

He "saw" the doctor, who was removing the bone from his right hip. The doctor was saying this kid is f#4@ed.

This further confirmed in Josh's mind that something had been missed

322

when the procedure was completed on his right leg. It would take him nearly 12 years to find the answer.

The sessions proved enlightening. This was another part of his understanding of the accident, certainly contributing toward Josh's acceptance of his accident. The important part of the hypnotherapy was that Josh took responsibility for the accident, and began to move on with his life.

2000 - 2004 On his release from rehab, Josh wanted to get into training. Not knowing any better, he returned to his old gym, initially with Dutchy.

We asked around the gym, and a personal trainer called Ben Robinson was introduced to us. Ben was a gifted committed professional, knowing little about spinal cord injury, but he did what we had already successfully used. Ben embraced logic.

He knew Josh had balancing problems, so that was a focus as well as his core strength. Josh trained at a normal gym, always transferring out of his wheel chair to work out. Josh and Ben worked together twice a week for four years. Our gym also had a pool, so Josh would wheel his chair to the edge, transfer to the poolside, and get into the pool and swim, using the opposite methodology to get out and back into his chair. Josh never wanted me at the gym. This was his space, his time.

May 2001 Josh travelled alone to the USA for specialist chi therapy. He spent six weeks undergoing this therapy. We were breaking all the rules with this therapy, but it worked ... and really helped Josh learn the importance of him holding his chi energy.

2002 – Josh was experiencing constant nagging pain in his right little finger.

The pain was never-ending and it really began to get to Josh. Paula, never giving up on finding someone to help Josh, was told about a French healer who had skills passed down generations from his family. He had a talent for moving exposed nerves back into their sleeves. He believed the problem with Josh's finger came from an exposed nerve in Josh's neck.

We arrived at his home in an outer Melbourne suburb. Immediately he said in broken English, the halo Josh had worn had caused a burn scar on both sides of his inner soul on either side of Josh's lower neck. We explained Josh never wore a halo, in fact the very area of the scaring, was where the "big angel" worked on him through Isobel in those early weeks after the accident. The healer immediately dropped to his knees and started praying. After a while he composed himself and started working on Josh's neck. This was just another one of our unusual experiences we encountered through Josh's recovery.

Bali - Josh's first trip back to Bali was in 2004, when several of us decided to take a break for two weeks. There were about eight in our group. For company, Josh brought his friend Lee with him. Lee was recovering from Lou Gehrig's disease, so they were both very challenged in their walking ability. It didn't stop them partying and totally having a ball while there, though!

We all stayed at the Bali Mandira, right on Legian Beach. The Mandira had two pools, one on the ground level and one at the top of a very steep staircase. Well, you can guess which pool Josh and Lee chose. Several of the guests, including all of us, were in terror of one of the boys falling, especially after they had spent the afternoon drinking Bintangs, but fortunately neither did, both of them worked out the safest way to master the stairs.

During our stay in Bali sister Asri brought in two Muslim healers that specialized in deep raw ginger massage. They would come to the hotel twice a week and work on both Josh and Lee for two hours each time. Both boys found the deep ginger massage really helpful, even if only for the short time they were in Bali.

We travelled to Bali several times over the following years, and Asri always found new healers for Josh to work with. The Balinese have no understanding of spinal cord injuries, so they work from the messages they get from the body; they have no boundaries, so to the uninitiated you need to be very careful. But we have a long experience with Balinese healers so we are confident they understand.

Afron was one of the more talented healers to work with Josh in Bali in January, 2012. From a spiritual level he just "got" the injury. It was fascinating watching him work with Josh, using Josh's MRI's to track the neural pathways. He would work on Josh for sometimes over two hours charging us less than $12.00. Afron was the one who told us that Josh's hip flexor muscle was not re attached after the operation in 2000.

We don't recommend anyone with spinal cord injuries racing off to Bali for treatment. We were very fortunate to have a Bali family that finds these amazing people for us. Also, Josh has so much experience

working with alternative healers, he can easily recognize who is helping him or not.

In 2008/2009 Josh and Bronte ate a diet of "pulse foods" for 40 days and 40 nights. An American healer spoke to them about the healing properties of this super nourishing food. So Bronte and Josh decided to commit to the program for the 40 days and 40 nights. Now both these guys are meat eaters and enjoy drinking alcohol, so this was a huge commitment. The only fluid they could drink during this fasting period was water.

I decided I would join them to lose some weight. Well, folks, I lasted a week, and after that I was done! Josh and Bronte lasted the distance, and at the end they both felt fantastic, but felt it was too drastic a diet for them to maintain. To this day I don't know how they did it!

2011 - 2012 in total 5 1/2 months at PW in Carlsbad, CA.

2012 for 4 months Doug (Chiropractor) and Uschi Schneider (Cranial Sacral Therapist) Encinitas, CA. Josh and Amelia had weekly sessions with Uschi and Doug – covered in a previous chapter.

_____

Over the years Josh has worked with many talented healers, with all manner of therapies, massage, and healing techniques, some for many months, sometimes years and others for short periods, or one-offs.

Josh has worked with Shamans, and healers from all walks of life. He has gone through an extremely traumatic rebirthing, worked with naturopaths, physiotherapists, cranial sacral therapists, the PW trainers, and personal trainers. He has maintained a gym program of cardio and weights consistently throughout his life, even before his accident.

He usually is on some kind of additive program, and Amelia, his wife, keeps him eating healthful foods as much as she possibly can, although it's a difficult argument when we try to get him to give up his much loved McDonalds.

Something that continually frustrates me is when someone says to me "Josh is lucky!" To achieve what Josh has achieved is through total determination, using massive will power to be able to deal with never ending pain. To never give up. When someone says to me Josh is lucky I simply say read his book, and then tell me he is lucky!

What I can say is since the morning after his accident, Josh has set himself huge goals, breaking each goal down into small achievable goals, understanding that to achieve each goal, he has to achieve the smaller goals sequentially. For example, to walk, he had to transfer from his bed, he had to master the wheelchair, he had to learn to stand, etc. The final and yet the most important goal was to get his old life back, something his doctors said was impossible.

Being lucky has nothing to do with it. My son has the strongest mind of anyone I have ever met. I have seen him near exhaustion from working out, and yet he never stops a session early. He sets goals and achieves them! *He is not lucky, he just never gives up!*

Over the years, I have come to realize that by thinking out of the box from Day 1 with his recovery, using and integrating all the things we have tried, Josh has been able to retrain his neuro pathways.

It is hard to believe that his 5% functioning cord at C6 and C7 is responsible for all his body movement. To me, and obviously I am no expert, it seems that all the intensive stimulation in those early days commenced the process of rebuilding or re-purposing his neuro pathways. There seems to be no other explanation.

For the record, in January 2014 I sent a personal letter to two of Josh's main specialist doctors from his medical team in 2000, offering to work with them in a research program. We acknowledged that they didn't misdiagnose Josh, but we are still awaiting their response. The silence is deafening!

For your information I have included the letter, with names and contact information removed for potential legal purposes (my apologies for the gaps):

████████████

PRIVATE & CONFIDENTIAL

Re: Josh Wood

Dear _____:

It's been many years since we first met. In fact it's been over 13 years since Josh was admitted to the XXX ICU, on the 25th June 2000.

In our opinion the timing is right for the Austin Hospital to take the lead by researching - Josh's recovery from a medical perspective.

Josh and I realize there will be no significant change in the treatment of those with spinal cord injuries until the medical profession starts to adopt a "recovery belief."

Sitting down with Josh, and taking the time to understand what we he did would present an enormous opportunity for the Hospital and its Spinal Unit.

Over the 13 1/2 years of Josh's injury we have learnt:

That the XXX's medical team's original prognosis of Josh was correct - he was admitted complete, and in the words of the admitting doctor that night *"Josh's spinal cord is so badly crushed it is likely he will never get out of bed. If he does he will be in a motorized wheel chair using mouth controls"*.

We also have in Josh's medical records that were passed to us that the belief in any recovery was about 3%.

We had the XXX's prognosis verbally verified/confirmed (2000) through our U.S. based friends who took his MRI's to XXX in Los Angeles, where they met with an orthopedic surgeon.

So there were never any thoughts in our minds that Josh had been misdiagnosed medically.

Fortunately for Josh, I knew his capacity for recovery and with the greatest respect to you all, we ignored the teams prognosis and commenced "Below Injury Recovery" stimulation and rehabilitation, while he was still in the acute spinal unit.

To this day neither Josh nor I have ever researched spinal cord injury. (We never wanted any roadblocks in his recovery goals.)

We also know Josh received the very best surgical treatment during his surgery to reconstruct his vertebra and remove pressure from the spinal cord at the XXX.

Our only area of concern was his right hip flexor muscle area, something Josh felt from the morning after the operation wasn't right. You probably

327

don't remember, but Josh was adamant that something was wrong, but when you checked the notes everything appeared "text book" and there was no film of the procedure. We raised concerns again after Josh went through hypnotherapy a few months after his accident, and yet again we were assured all was correct. We recently discovered (2012) that his right hip flexor muscle was sown back/placed back incorrectly. The amazing thing about all this is, even though Josh was totally paralyzed at that stage, the morning after surgery he knew there was something wrong. He kept saying to me "my right hip area feels empty".

Anyway, this is not what this letter is about. Just thought it was worth mentioning as Josh knew from Day 4 that there was a problem, even though he was without any sensation.

I believe you know by now that I smuggled Josh's chiropractor, Simon Floreani, amongst many other alternative healers, into the Critical Spinal Unit the day after he was moved there from ICU. Simon and the others, worked on Josh behind closed curtains for several months while he was in the XXX facilities.

Simon now has a 15 1/2 year history on Josh; he was Josh's chiropractor, for two years before his accident, treating Josh for a L5 injury he sustained in Switzerland. You both must agree this is a very valuable history of Josh's recovery, through alternative methods. I know Simon would be willing to share his notes.

We can advise you both that Josh continues to recover after all these years and has recently discarded his walking stick. He struggles without it, but he is determined to keep improving. Another thing Josh recently discovered was: he was riding a "spin" bike at the Gym, his wife texted him. He answered, but realized once he focused on the text, he forgot to keep moving his legs and they stopped. He is now focusing on training his mind to "multi skill"/"task".

In his second stint at Project Walk in California, his trainers actually got him jumping consecutively down a rope ladder placed in the floor. This was the first time he was able to co-ordinate his "feral" right leg in a continued jumping exercise.

Josh has just released his book *Relentless - Walking Against All Odds*. In it he discusses his recovery. It is a brutal tale of never giving up. You really get an in depth view into his thinking.

_____, I remember well that morning in the training area at the XXX in 2001, when you invited Josh to talk to the team. Josh was put through the wringer with the consensus being even though he walks now, he won't for much longer.

_____, you stood up saying "no one has ever walked from an injury such as Josh's, we need to learn from him". We are still waiting for this opportunity.

We have been told many stories from people that have asked the doctors and nurses from the XXX about Josh, and they are usually told "he wasn't that badly injured" or "he preaches false hope." These comments sadden us deeply.

Especially when we know the original prognosis was correct.

This is not about Josh, this is about both you and your team taking the time to learn from him, and maybe the XXX SCI team may learn something about the power of the human mind to recover, along with the integration of alternative therapies / modalities with mainstream western medicine.

Josh has never been asked to mentor patients from the XXX. In fact we know _____ you don't welcome him there. This is bigger than Josh or either of you. Living in the USA as I do now, I see recovery of sensation / movement on a regular basis. It's not easy, and it requires training and commitment, but it is happening! Unfortunately, the medical profession is playing catch-up in this area.

This letter is to ask you both to take the time to speak to Josh, learn from him, accept what he has done and research him medically. Josh's is a positive story; neither he nor I ever gave up.

The XXX already has precedent in looking at alternative treatment of cancer through its XXX facility. Why can't you replicate this through a research program for below-injury recovery from SCI?

The University of Montana's New Direction's Wellness Center under the guidance of Susan Ostertag, PT, DPT, NCS, Clinical Assistant Professor, Director, UM Physical Therapy Clinic, University of Montana School of Physical Therapy and Rehabilitative Sciences, is part of a neurological network that is researching the possibilities of below-injury recovery. The work/ research being done through this facility is exciting and all medically documented. I presented Josh's recovery to students there, and it was well received.

Gentlemen, I am returning to Melbourne briefly in mid-February for three weeks. Josh and I would welcome the opportunity to meet with you both.

The best way to contact me is by email: _____ or Josh can be phoned on _____. A message can be left on my sister's mobile phone _____.

Looking forward to hearing from you.

Sincerely,

Kay Ledson

Chapter 28. Only a Mum!

I have written at length about my time in California, those two wonderful years where I suddenly realized that for the first time in a long time, I had time for myself, just me. I also felt Carlsbad had become my "safe Kay cave," a place where I wasn't anybody's anything, not a mum, not a sister, not a daughter, really just someone who had friends, a life, and became someone who had learned to laugh again.

Recently I looked in the mirror and was shocked! I had started taking notice of me for the first time in a long time. I realized I had aged; there were too many wrinkles on my face, and my eyes seemed to have disappeared. Umm, when did all this happen? - I really need a facelift hahahaha - a new goal. Obviously I had looked in the mirror many times over those years, but I guess I never really noticed; there was always something more important. I realized I hadn't thought about myself or my appearance in a long time.

Then I started thinking about the past nearly 15 years - everything - the highs, the lows, the experiences, amazing and some so very sad, the people we have met, the "lifelong" friends I no longer have, my new friends, my career, my business and financial security that were totally destroyed through no fault of my own; totally beyond my control.

Continuing to reflect, I felt so grateful for our amazing family, especially my sisters. I thought of the tragedy and sadness of losing my much loved Mum - Dottie Dearest – and all the other experiences and life events that had occurred. I also thought about when I turn 64. I suddenly realized that although 14 years had passed since my 50th birthday, in my mind I hadn't aged at all in years. The year I turned 50 was my big year with so many plans, so much to look forward to, so much yet to achieve. It obviously took a totally different turn on June 25th 2000, but here's the thing: I am still 50 years in my head. In my 50th year I came very close to losing my only child - I know at times Josh feels guilty for what happened, and how his accident changed all of our lives. But he should never feel guilty. We all had choices, and my choice was to give Josh his life back; and more importantly his independence, or as much of it that we could get back.

Sure, my life took a turn that no one could have ever envisaged, but what a time of growth, of learning, and understanding the strength and power of the human spirit I have learned.

I have had the privilege of sharing an amazing journey of discovery and healing with my son and now with Amelia, his wife. It's a journey that hopefully very few will experience (due to the devastation of the accident.)

As a mum, I have watched Josh fight for his life, fight for his independence, and fight to survive. I have experienced my son growing as a man to a level I would never have dreamed. I have been with him when he is mentoring someone suffering a spinal cord injury. He exudes confidence, and yet is humble. He always goes to lengths to explain that long term recovery is the hardest of roads, but a fight worth having; the rewards are worth it.

I watched him marry his soul mate Amelia, in a beautiful wedding ceremony surrounded by our doggies, our family, and friends - who enjoyed every minute of the day. There is never a day that passes that I wish his accident had never happened, but there is only one reason I wish this: It's really the constant unrelenting pain Josh is always in. There is nothing I can do to help him with this, and the pain Josh goes through gets even worse as he recovers more function...it seems so cruel...it is the nature of this vicious injury... but it doesn't stop him; he just keeps going.

As I enter my 65th year I have no regrets with where our lives have taken us. I am so in awe of my son's strength, commitment and compassion, his great love for Amelia, and their great love for each other, and his presence.

Really when it all comes down to it, I am not jaded by age, because really in my heart and soul I am still 50, albeit with a few more wrinkles and lines.

I hope you have been helped by and enjoyed my story. I know the book isn't a literary masterpiece! I simply told my story from my heart and soul, to help others on a similar journey, and to give light and hope.

For the record, I never cried for my son's injury, although there have been many "happy" tears along the way. It's a little easier; not so hard these days!

The end...well, not really the end; you could say a new beginning..

Chapter 29.   Emerging From the Darkness, One Hour at a Time

I dedicate these chapters to Wendy. Without her I would not have existed financially. She has provided me with a roof over my head, helped me buy a car, and made sure I had enough money to live on. She never judged me, but I know she was extremely worried about me. My sisters - Susan, you have given me unconditional love and support, and Asri who gave me love and support, and made me laugh so many times.

Jamie, Lisa, Kori and Maureen, thank you for your love, friendship and support through this difficult time! And yes, Lisa, I have pulled on my "big girl panties." I am so lucky to have my sisters and sistas!

After completing Chapter 28 "Only a Mum," I really thought my book was finished; only recently I admitted to myself, over the months since my return from the USA, that I personally had suffered some of the darkest times of my life. For months, I was totally overwhelmed by a feeling of hopelessness, a dread that had really enveloped me since the fateful lunch in Carlsbad when I realized my dream to stay in the USA was over.

In hindsight, that lunch was certainly the catalyst, but in reality it was the final straw in my journey that started the night of the phone call in June 2000. This really was the culmination of my story, my journey. The accident was certainly the event that changed my life, but where I find myself today is simply the result of me not dealing with the emotional side of that event. It was not in any way Josh's fault; it was simply my attitude in not emotionally dealing with the trauma and the grief that has caused me to be where I now find myself.

I knew my current journey would never be finished, unless I dealt with this issue completing the writing of my book.

The darkness was so subtle. Every day, once I returned to Australia, I felt a little worse. I was totally detaching from everyone and everything. I was still managing to make it through each day, and most people wouldn't have noticed; I hid it really well. The nights were the worst. I would wake up shaking, feeling so desperate, so totally out of control, angry, disappointed, really wondering when things were ever going to improve, for Josh, Amelia and me.

As I mentioned in an earlier chapter, the last six weeks in the USA were a time of disbelief, disappointment, and overwhelming sadness, knowing in my heart and soul that my dream of living in Carlsbad was over. I was happy to see everyone before leaving, but I struggled to get through every day. Lisa had been great allowing me to stay working at the lagoon for as long as I wanted. It was busy, so for those few hours each day I felt normal.

Arriving back in Australia in mid-February, I knew I had to somehow get through the next three weeks before we left for Bali. I decided it had to be one hour at a time, and honestly that's how I managed.

I didn't set goals. I didn't think about anything too much. I just focused on getting through each hour. I spent a lot of time in my room sitting on my bed writing my book, only leaving if we had something organized; dinner, sightseeing, or a planned event.

Getting around was hard not having a car, and knowing for the first time since getting my license I didn't have a car of my own was devastating to me. I had always loathed public transport, yet it was the only way to get around, so I had to get used to it.

Wendy went out of her way to make things easier for me, making her car available when she didn't need it.

In early March, Wendy, Susan and I travelled to Bali to stay with our sister Asri in Jimbaran Bay. They were staying two weeks and I was going to be there for a month.

I needed to work on my book, and would take advantage of the extra time away to do this. I also wanted to look at some potential business and work opportunities up there. There was a part of me that thought I would rather live in Bali than Australia, but I had to be able to make a living there. Otherwise there was no way I could stay there.

I was in denial about living in Australia, and in my mind it wasn't an option. I was looking for any opportunity *not* to live there.

During our trip I would celebrate my 64th birthday. I was looking forward to this, as my birthday is always the beginning of my new year. I needed to be in a better head space to enter my 65th year.

Bali has always been my safe haven. I love the simple uncomplicated life. I always manage to lose myself in the humdrum of Kuta and Legian.

For me, walking 12 - 15 kilometers every day was so healing. I didn't have to think about anything except just placing one foot in front of the other - simple!

I was struggling with my relationship with Josh. I wanted to see him get on with his life with Amelia, and yet they had so little money. So many who had promised him work, speaking or mentoring, had let him down; seeing him struggle to pay the most basic of things like rent, broke my heart even more.

In the past I always had the money to help him, and although he wanted to support himself the situation we all found ourselves in was causing me constant stress and frustration. I struggled with it so much.

I couldn't believe how much things had changed. In 2008 I had the money to retire comfortably in 2010, yet here I was in 2014 with little savings, living off my sister's generosity, and unable to help my son and his wife in any way.

This situation further added to the darkness and frustration, which continued to dog my every waking moment.

My way of coping was detachment; just going further and further into myself.

Finally we arrived in Bali. The weather was fantastic, and I immediately felt I would be all right. I just needed time to recover, dust myself off, pick myself up and move on!

We enjoyed a fun two weeks together. We kept our lives very simple, swimming most days, having healing sessions with a local "medicine man", eating out at local restaurants (costing next to nothing), helping out with a little Rotary business, and reading. I actually read three books. (Finally, I was beginning to feel less dark, seeming to be coping a little better.)

My birthday arrived, and to celebrate this special day we were going to a new resort hotel, the Mulia, located on the magnificent Geger Beach, near Nusa Dua to enjoy a sumptuous birthday brunch.

I have loved Geger Beach, for many years. It's a beautiful beach to relax on, and the waters are safe without the surf of other Bali beaches. It was somewhere I truly loved. Sadly it was now changed forever with this huge resort development. I was assured that the locals who harvested seaweed from the waters for cosmetics were all provided for, with some still maintaining their "industry."

The hotel was luxurious, and we enjoyed cocktails in the bar before moving into the enormous restaurant for brunch. Wow, there was so much to choose from, with international food kitchens set up throughout the restaurant. I reflected momentarily on my first trip to Bali in 1981, when I was pregnant with Josh. Bali had changed from a romantic undeveloped island, to now being the home of magnificent hotels, and luxury shopping malls. Yet, thankfully, there were still parts of the island that had never changed since my first visit there in 1981; who would have thought?

I felt so spoilt! My sisters gave me exactly what I needed, love and support, never questioning me, just accepting. I was slowly working through my sadness.

We had such a lovely day. We took lots of photos. I really felt I would be all right, I would survive, and I could confidently enter my 65th year.

All too quickly it was time for Wendy and Susan to return to Australia. I had two weeks left to commence researching the property market for ex pats. I had been asked to look at the various legal structures for property purchase in Bali, so it was time for me to get into the work mode.

Another group had asked me to look for accommodation sites for a health fitness retreat, making suggestions for "Balinese experiences" to be included in the program.

For the first time in weeks, I was busy and loving it. I attended some expatriate Rotary meetings to commence the building of my expat network. On all my past visits to Bali over the years, I had always hung out with Balinese friends, rarely interacting with the ever growing expatriate community, so I was enjoying meeting all these amazing, interesting people.

My last two weeks quickly evaporated. Towards the end of my trip the Balinese Ceremony "Nyepi - the Bali Day of SILENCE", was approaching.

Nyepi is a day of silence, and it involves fasting from 6 AM to 6 PM, only allowing contemplation and meditation; keeping one's mind quiet. The airport is closed, there are no cars on the roads, all shops are closed, and people have to stay in their homes and guests must stay within their hotels. The streets are totally empty, the beach is deserted, and everything is closed up...there is only silence!

I made a decision to become a Balinese for 48 hours. I would totally immerse myself in the culture and the community!

The commencement of Nyepi starts the previous 24 hours, with everything going into slow down. The day before fasting, Asri and I went to Jimbaran Beach for cleansing, and we dived into the ocean. We had to cleanse our eyes, ears, and head with ocean water allowing it to roll down our bodies. Then we had to swill our mouths with seawater. Anyone who has experienced Bali knows that cleansing my mouth was truly an act of faith, when you see what flows into the ocean.

I was enjoying floating in the salty water once we were finished.

Asri said, "My mum says it's cleansing to pee while you are in the water, a great cleanse." I answered in shock, knowing I had been swilling my mouth with the sea water, "Did you pee in the water?" Asri laughing said "Yes." Shocked I said "Well, I just swilled my mouth out in the water YUK." Still laughing Asri said "Sis, it's a big ocean."

We left the water and enjoyed breakfast at a beach Warung.

Later in the day, we visited Asri's local temple for praying and a blessing with holy water from the priest. I dressed in traditional Balinese attire for this ceremony. I think there is nothing more bizarre than seeing me in all the "local" gear, it never seems to look right on the big "bulai" (Balinese for white person...used affectionately, of course).

Returning to the house, we grabbed drums, and saucepan lids walking through both of Asri's houses into every room making as much noise as we could to scare away the evil spirits. It was so much fun.

We had dinner, and then we went into the streets of a nearby village to enjoy the evening celebrations. The locals got dressed up in hideous costumes and prepare scary, grotesque floats to parade through the streets to scare away the evil spirits.

Asri and I would have walked for miles following the parade looking for vantage points to view the spectacle. In all the times I had been in Bali I had never experienced anything like this. I was really getting into the spirit of the celebrations and really enjoying this unique festival. There were families, individuals, and people from all walks of life laughing, happy, making as much noise as possible, and scaring away those evil spirits. It was an amazing experience, with everyone joining together determined to frighten the evil spirits away.

While I was in Bali I felt connected, unlike the feelings I had experienced in Australia of detachment and disconnection, combined with that dreaded feeling of being out of control, akin to being in the ocean in a storm on a small yacht being battered in every direction, having no control.

Arriving back at the house, we went to bed early, as we had a 5 AM wake up call, to eat breakfast, have a huge drink of water, (as we couldn't drink anything, either) before our fasting started at 6 AM.

Finishing breakfast, Asri suggested going back to bed for a few hours.

Climbing the stairs to my room, I thought no way would I sleep; I was awake, I had just eaten, and yet I went into a deep sleep.

I thought to myself, geez, maybe this Nyepi Day of Meditation, Reflection, and Quiet really works!

I woke up at around 8 AM. I threw my bathing suit on, and grabbed a sarong, deciding to spend my day by the pool, in the Bale.

With my book in hand, not being able to do any work at all, I was wondering how I would get through my day. This, in my mind, was going to be a very long day.

How wrong was I!

My day was totally for meditation, contemplation, praying to the gods, resting, and with Asri opting to stay inside her home, I was on my own!

It was so quiet. No planes, no cars, no people, just so peaceful. It reminded me of the times experiencing the Australian outback, and in the Gobi desert (China). No sounds, only of nature, the birds and the wind, and even the Bali dogs were silenced.

To my surprise, the day flew by. I swam, I was quiet, I slept, I read, I reflected on my life, the past four years since the dramas and tragedies of 2010, how it had taken a 360 degree turn in 2000, my journey with Josh, the friends I no longer had, the new amazing friends who had come into my life, the career I was so proud of gone in a morning, my time in

Carlsbad, the healing that occurred for me there, and how grateful I was for this; in my heart I knew if I hadn't gone there I would be no longer on this earth plane.

And then it was 6 PM, time to eat.

Without being able to use lights until midnight, it was dark inside the house and outside. Asri and I sat talking for what seemed hours, but in the end the darkness enveloped us totally. We couldn't see each other, so we decided to go to our rooms and sleep. And I slept like I hadn't in so long. I was refreshed and calm, feeling great; something I hadn't experienced in a long time.

I loved the experience of Nyepi Day, and will be back to Bali to do it again. I felt enlightened!

And then it was time to return to Australia. In my heart I knew I wasn't ready, and I needed more time in Bali to research opportunities. I was researching two developments and venues for retreats. There was more work to do there, yet it was time to leave. In my heart and mind I knew I needed to make a decision about where I would live, and here I was returning to Australia.

I arrived home, to uncertainty for not just me, but for Josh and Amelia. Once again Josh had been let down over some promised work, he had little money, and I could no longer help him. What a disaster it was!

It was so stressful for us. I could not believe I was in this position. I kept thinking what do I have to learn from this?

I knew going to the USA had cost me everything financially, but there was no way I would ever regret it, but there was no denying, I had paid a huge financial price for my health and healing.

I found myself constantly pleading with the Universe, for answers; why was this happening? Why after all we have done to help families, giving light and hope, why was this happening to us, what more do we have to do? What more lessons do we have to learn?

Soon after returning to Australia, I called Josh. He said he had a migraine and was going to bed to sleep it off! Within an hour, Amelia called me saying she had called an ambulance and Josh was being taken to Emergency as his body had started to shut down.

Not having a car, Wendy drove me to the hospital – I was in so much fear for Josh; all I could think of was what else has to go wrong?

Josh and I were scheduled to speak at a client seminar for a financial planner in Melbourne the next evening. It had been in place for several weeks, and both Josh and I really wanted to do it.

In my heart I knew if it was only a severe migraine, once he was given the right medication he would be fine. The problem with anyone having a spinal cord injury finding the drug that will work is not always easy.

The other issue far more concerning was trying to get the medical team to understand they are essentially dealing with a complete quadriplegic. This is always an issue with Josh. They see his mobility but can't get it into their heads that he has so little cord function. At times with drugs being administered it's akin to playing Russian Roulette with his life.

We always attend the same ER. Over the years the team there has accumulated a reasonable history on Josh, so I am reasonably confident in their capacity to treat him. After our warnings of taking extreme care with the drugs the medical team were preparing to administer, they decided to try a low dose to see the effects. The doctor we were working with was sensational. Josh was drifting in and out of consciousness, so every time he increased the dosage, he brought Josh around asking him what was going on with his body. In all the years we have dealt with emergency issues, we have never worked with an emergency room doctor who really was listening to Josh and us.

It took several hours. The doctor tried 5 -6 different drugs, and finally Josh started to respond. We were in awe of the doctor. It was the most positive experience we had ever had at a hospital in all the years since Josh's injury.

Adding to the stress and tension, the financial planner, out of concern for Josh, wanted to reschedule the evening. Josh was determined to speak. It was important to him. I had an obligation to her, but I was confident in Josh. He understands his body so well that if he felt he would be all right, that was good enough for me. The decision was to proceed with the event the following evening; Josh was relieved!

Finally around 8 PM, Josh was discharged, preferring to sleep in his own bed rather than spend the night in the hospital.

I caught the train back to Carnegie from the hospital. It was late, it was dark, it was cold, I was feeling totally devastated, and I was neither happy nor comfortable. Here I am sitting on the train, in truth thinking, what else has to go wrong before things get better?

I found myself back in the land of numbness and detachment. Actually, all day while at the hospital I realized I had been going through the motions of dealing with doctors, supporting Amelia, praying that Josh would be fine, and yet I was totally detached internally! I really think it has become my mechanism for dealing with the horror of seeing your child going through this vicious injury!

As usual, outwardly I was strong, confident, but inwardly I was feeling totally done in!

I was totally fed up with this cruel unrelenting injury. It has the capacity to keep on giving challenges and obstacles, just when everything should be all right! Oh my god, how I hate it and what it does to our loved ones suffering it. Amelia was exhausted. She had been amazing, supporting Josh all through this, and never once did I doubt her great love and commitment to Josh and their future. It must have been so frightening and stressful for her.

On arriving home, I called Josh and Amelia. They had stopped on the way for food, and Josh was heading straight to bed. He planned to sleep as long as possible so he would be "on point" for his talk the following evening.

The night of the "Son and Mum" talk was on us. Josh looked tired and washed out, but other than that he was in fine form. He seemed a little more subdued than usual, but powerful nevertheless and hitting home to everyone there concerning the vulnerability for those suffering this injury. I felt totally "done in" from the emotions and events of the day before. After I finished speaking, Wendy said "I came across as being really angry." I felt sorry, if that was the case. I felt personally that I spoke with passion and commitment. Well, it was no good beating up on myself.

A few weeks later I listened to the recording of our talk, and I still think I was more passionate than angry! Anyway, if my message reached one family regarding the importance of insuring their children, then I was successful.

The feedback on the evening was very positive. We were hoping to be booked for some more talks. Together we are a powerful force, yet nothing eventuated!

341

To keep busy, I continued to work on my book. I was determined to finish it! I had rewritten it four times and was now I was onto the 5th draft.

I was more unsettled than ever, unsure of where I wanted to live, what I was going to do! I was seriously considering walking away from the whole spinal cord injury recovery network, allowing me to completely focus on helping Josh and getting some work. *But there was always that nagging thought of knowing personally what families go through and the difference it could make if I could just help one family!*

Internally, I felt that horrible feeling of loss and hopelessness. I had left Bali, in a state of limbo! For my own wellbeing and sanity, I HAD TO MAKE A DECISION!

One Sunday morning, after a sleepless, stressful night, I booked a flight to Bali using my frequent flyer points. I was going for a month. With the small amount of savings I had left, I booked a month's accommodation in low cost hotels in Legian, Seminyak and Kuta, all within in 300 meters of the beaches.

One month's accommodation for $1,200. Oh, how my life had changed! I used to spend $200 plus a night in Bali, and now my budget was $40. I felt happy and relieved that I had made a decision!

My living expenses for the month would be $2,000 ($66 per day). Umm, this could be a challenge as I needed to pay for all my food, transport and anything else I needed.

I was determined it had to work, as I felt I had no other option than return to Bali this time totally alone!

I still had a month to kill in Australia before I left.

Again, I felt the devastation of failure. I was struggling emotionally, and crying a lot. I was feeling totally done in. I was let down once again by someone I thought of as a true, supportive friend, as far as work was concerned. He was deleted from my life!

Josh and Amelia's financial position was becoming more desperate every day, and I was beside myself with worry. I tried to be positive; it was the nights in bed that I hated.

I wasn't sleeping. Lying in bed I would shake and cry, constantly questioning the Universe nonstop. It was like everything had finally caught up with me. The effects of the last 14 years since Josh's accident, the frantic crazy pace of the stressful yet lucrative business I had run since 1997, the sadness's of 2010, Josh losing his four friends, nearly losing him, when he plummeted out of control, the stress of that crazy time, the loss of my dear mum, the loss, and total destruction of the company I so proudly built, and how an industry I helped build turned its back on me.

Night after night this "devastatingly sad action movie played out" over and over again!

Somehow I managed to make it to the day I was to fly out to Bali; through all this, my sisters were there for me. I know they were really worried, but they were in no position to help me other than to love me.

A bright light through this time was my regular contact with my Carlsbad buddies through face time. They made me laugh. After speaking to them though, I cried, mourning the loss of my life there.

At last the day had arrived for my return to Bali!

Once on the plane, I experienced a great sense of relief. I was on my own, I would only see people if I wanted to, and I was in control for the next month!

My simple plan while in Bali was:

- ✓ Finish my book, find an editor in Bali through the expat community, and check out the potential of self-publishing my book through an Indonesian Printing House.

- ✓ Attend "expat" Rotary Clubs there, and hang out with non-Balinese, something I had never done before. I wanted to visit several residential developments while there, really learning the ins and outs of purchasing property on the island. It was easy for me to buy property in Bali if I wanted to, as I had my Bali sister, but for expats with no trusted connections making property purchases it was totally different. I had to be absolutely confident in the process before presenting properties to potential buyers back in Australia. I needed to come to terms with the complicated legal issues of ownership by non-residents.

- ✓ *Sort my headspace out once and for all and walk.* Something that I always found healing for me, especially in Bali.

343

✓ Make a decision as to where I will live and stick to it - no regrets!

True to form our Australian low cost airline arrived nearly an hour late, but I managed to get through visa and passport control in record time.

With the arrival delay, I calculated I would be in the hotel by midnight. I wasn't prepared for the extended wait for luggage to come off the plane.

It was 12:45 AM by the time I climbed into the taxi for the long trip to my hotel.

To say I was nervous was an understatement. Bali is like a second home to me, but I have rules: never be out after midnight and never travel through Kuta late at night. Yet here I was in a taxi moving through the crazy streets heading to my hotel.

I chatted to the driver. He was a nice guy, working hard to support his family. I promised him a good tip for getting me to my hotel safely.

Arriving at the hotel at around 1:15 AM, I was pleasantly surprised with my hotel choice. I had been allocated a room in the rear section, on the ground floor. Initially I was nervous about this, but the staff assured me the security was very good. I would be there for two weeks.

My room was surprisingly spacious. The king bed was comfortable, and the bathroom was okay. What a bonus; I was only paying $32 per night.

I was determined to get myself emotionally sorted out and mentally focused over the coming month. I had to if I was going to move on with my life. These next 30 days would go a long way towards determining my future. I was absolutely certain of this.

My feeling of relief was invigorating. I was finally on my own, with only me to answer to! (It wasn't that I didn't appreciate my family or friends, it was just that I needed the space of solitude.)

The following morning I was up at 6 AM commencing my planned regime of walking 12 plus kilometers every day.

Walking in Bali is a very healing experience for me. After the devastation of 2010 it was my daily walks in Bali that provided me with clarity. It's a time for me that's totally about me, doing something I didn't have to think about!

Very quickly I morphed into my routine, getting up at daybreak, walking about 10 kilometers along the beach and back through the streets, eating a healthful breakfast, and back to the hotel for 2-3 hours to work on my book.

Afternoons I would walk, sometimes catching up with Asri for lunch or dinner. Mostly keeping to myself, I was enjoying the anonymity, the silence!

If I could have, I would have chosen to live this life forever!

My second weekend, Asri, Angeli (Asri's granddaughter) and I went up into the mountains about two hours northwest of Legian. It was so very beautiful, peaceful, and silent except for the noises of the jungle. The view of the sunset over the ocean through the mountains was magnificent. We sat drinking gin and tonics enjoying the brilliant red and orange sky.

That night we slept in a typical Balinese hut in the middle of a jungle resort. It was so quiet, very rural, and stunningly beautiful.

For the first time in ages, I was feeling like I was living in the now. There was so much in the past that represented too much sadness; my future was still unknown, yet for the now it was bearable!

I started to feel the heartbreak of leaving my "home" in Carlsbad a little more bearable!

Emotionally, I still felt numb. My present focus was getting through each day, trying to feel a little better.

In my life there had been so many tough times, and I had always pulled myself out of them. This time was different. I felt tired of constantly fighting to stay positive, and tired of trying to project a happy persona. It was all too hard for me these days; I needed to face the reality of where I was personally, emotionally and deal with it...no more pretense!

I attended three different Rotary Clubs while I was there. Asri's, where I knew most of the members in Kuta, and a "local" Rotary where I met some of the members of a predominantly expats club, just north of Seminyak.

They invited me to attend one of their weekly meetings.

The meeting was held in a magnificent old Balinese mansion, which had been turned into a high end hotel. Positioned on the ocean, it was magnificent. *(Telling Asri about it later, she said the "locals" thought the house was haunted.)*

The members were friendly and so committed to helping the Balinese community, which is something I felt really strongly about. It was a fun night. I managed to meet many of the members; they were so welcoming. The membership was like a mini United Nations, with members from Australia, England, Indonesia and Europe.

I was invited to their "Changeover Dinner" the following week. I thought why not, what have I got to lose?

I was continuing to research real estate opportunities there. As well as inspecting properties, I met with various legal experts, finding out that there were many different legal structures, making me increasingly nervous.

In the end, I decided it was all too hard and crossed real estate off my potential income earning opportunities in Bali.

Through Rotary, I was told about a woman who was a highly regarded editor living in Bali. She also advised on publishing options. I was given her name by three different people, so I knew I had to meet her before I left.

Through telephone conversations and email we finally set up a meeting for an evening about 10 days before I was due to return to Melbourne.

As well as my daily walks and writing my book, I enjoyed lying on the beach, swimming in the surf, or having a massage. All about me!

Every night I would choose a different restaurant for my dinner. My many years of "solo" work travel had gotten me used to dining alone, so I was comfortable eating by myself enjoying a few cocktails all the time while watching the brilliant ocean sunsets. Oh, how I wished I could live this life forever! Some nights I would chat with other diners, but for the most I indulged in people watching and the views.

I set myself longer and longer walks. I was averaging between 12 and 18 kilometers a day. My longest daily walk was 21 kilometers.

Strangely, I wasn't losing any weight, and yet I felt I was getting fitter.

My simple Bali life was without stress or worries. I had left all my problems in Australia, and didn't even think about them!

I "face timed" the Carlsbad gals, always feeling better after hearing all their news. For a few minutes, I was able to be reconnected to my old life.

After two weeks I moved to Seminyak. While the hotel was well located, I didn't like it, and wished I had stayed three weeks in Legian. The one bright spot was the fantastic spa, where I enjoyed several relaxing massages. I maintained my walking program, still walking each day to my favorite breakfast spot.

I finally met with Sarita, who would hopefully agree to be my editor. We met at her home. It was so peaceful, in a tranquil area on the island. We chatted for hours. After the disappointment over the editing of Josh's book, I was extremely nervous, and yet I felt a deep trust of Sarita; as mothers we connected.

Sarita was very honest with me, saying that she had several projects to finish before she could even look at my book.

I sent her through some information, agreeing we would meet for lunch the following week.

I left feeling relieved. I had found someone that I was confident would ensure my book would be professionally edited.

My book was finally finished, and I moved to a hotel opposite the beach in Kuta.

It's ironic that so many travelers to Bali these days would never stay in Kuta, preferring the more luxurious remote resorts, but for all the years I have visited Bali there is something I love about Kuta that is special to me! Mind you I don't frequent the Aussie bars and local night clubs; it's more the beach and some of the restaurants that I really love.

Yet again I was pleasantly surprised with my choice of hotel. My room was large on the first floor, the bathroom was roomy, I had a fridge, and a balcony overlooking the pool. I was paying A$43 per night, and Kuta Beach was directly across the road - perfect!

With only eight days remaining before returning to Melbourne, I felt at least for the next six years I needed to accept my home would be in Melbourne. This realization settled me down. I knew I would return to the USA for holidays, but my dreams of living there for the time being were over! While I was sad, I was also very relieved!

Following my strict routine in Bali, I knew that as soon as I returned to Melbourne I had to set up a routine that allowed me to continue to heal and accept that my life was there for the immediate future.

My new Rotary colleagues were encouraging me to attend a Wellness Seminar the day before I was to leave. Frankly, it was the last thing I wanted to do, but something made me say YES!

Umm, what was I thinking, spending my 2nd last day cooped up in a hotel, a 1 1/2 hour taxi ride from my hotel.

It was approaching the 14th Anniversary of Josh's accident, a day always cloaked with sadness for me, and yet it was certainly a time to celebrate our journey. Emotionally, it's a day tinged with sadness for what the accident has done to him physically, although having so much joy and pride in seeing the man he has become!

Two days earlier, Josh returned to the hospital he had been admitted to all those years ago to visit a young man who had recently suffered a spinal cord injury, and his family. Josh had given them a copy of *Relentless* to hopefully offer inspiration to them.

After Josh left, the young man was on his own. A nurse, seeing the book said "Don't take any notice of this book. Josh Wood preaches false hope."

Josh was devastated on hearing this later. He thought, I am going to show them once and for all anything is possible.

Discussing this with Amelia, they made a decision to walk from the Rehab Centre where he had ultimately walked out from to the hospital he was admitted to 14 years earlier.

This was a journey of seven kilometers, mostly up hill, and he needed to cross two very busy, dangerous roads in the process.

He advised me of his plans. While I totally supported him, I was extremely nervous as he had damaged his knee and would need to rely on crutches, adding further to the difficulty of the walk. Since his accident, Josh hadn't walked more than a kilometer at any one time, so a seven kilometer walk was a huge task for him. I was totally aware of his determination, so I was confident he would make the distance. My concerns were what he might do to himself in the process.

I was glad I wouldn't be there with him, since this was another step in my journey of me letting go, and I totally trusted that Amelia would keep a watchful eye on him. I decided to walk the same distance along the beach, leaving the same time as Josh. We posted Josh's "Relentless Move to Change" walk on Facebook.

It was a beautiful, calm morning walking along the beach. Finishing the seven kilometers I raced back to my hotel. Facebook was in meltdown; Amelia was posting their journey, and Josh was going really well!

I was updating the Warrior Momz, our little support group. They were all commenting, and sending their encouragement. It was so exciting!

Josh completed the walk in just over two hours and 40 minutes, a truly sensational effort. There was no fanfare, just a small group of supporters, but through this walk a new initiative emerged "RELENTLESS Move for Change." Watch this space for more details to come from this!

My last days in Bali were filled with walking, walking, and more walking. With *Warrior Mom* finally finished, I had removed a huge weight from my shoulders. I felt there would be more books but for now I was done!

I spent time with Asri and Angeli, relaxing, eating, and preparing for my return to Melbourne!

Attending the Wellness Seminar was one of the best things I had done in many months. I connected with many amazing people there.

Two men that I met have potentially opened up two exciting opportunities for Josh, one for further healing and one for speaking. I was so glad I had made the effort to go!

Chapter 30. When Death is the Alternative, You Draw a Line in the Sand or You Die!

Arriving home in early July, I felt a sense that everything would be okay. I was positive, and although not back to normal, I knew I was on the right path.

Wendy offered to help me buy a car. My credit rating was solid, but not having a deposit was a problem. Wendy offered to lend me the deposit, so we went in search of a car. To obtain finance it had to be a new, so we looked at what was available.

Deciding the Korean cars represented excellent value, I finally decided on a KIA Cerato. I financed it over five years, so my life would at least be focused in Melbourne for this time. Yet again, I felt a sense of relief. I had made a decision! Again my realization in Bali to commit to Australia for at least 5 – 6 years was reinforced.

My living costs in Australia were about $2500 a month so I had about one month's living expenses left from my meager savings.

Josh was trying hard to get speaking and mentoring work, and yet nothing was happening for him.

I rang my contacts, but there was nothing. In fact many never contacted me back, which I found extremely disappointing. I knew there was nothing left for me in the investment side of financial services. I was really at a loss of what I would do.

I applied for some casual positions, and was interviewed for one.

I liked the idea of contracting to the company, but it was all commission based and in the area I would be focusing on, I had no contacts.

After committing to extensive research on the company, I accepted the role. I spent a month developing contact lists and gaining understanding of the position. I knew this would be a great opportunity in the long term, but in the short term it wouldn't bring me in the money I needed.

Josh and I had spoken to Simon about creating a recovery program for people with spinal cord injury through his wellness center in Middle Park.

Josh would work with Simon and the clients in establishing individual recovery programs based on the work we had done with Josh in those crazy early days that we believed had set him up for his ongoing recovery.

I was excited for Josh! Once launched, Josh would earn regular mentoring fees, and in the long term as the business grew I could receive fees for marketing and assisting with programs.

All very positive, but no immediate income for me! I was continuing with my Warrior Momz radio program, but that was costing me valuable money as well as taking time to put together the programs.

Every day was a fight to stay positive. I went to bed early but wasn't sleeping again. The nightmares of failure, of disappointment, of fear started again! I knew I had the power to reverse this attitude of mine, but for some reason I couldn't make the physical or mental effort to do it. This alone was very frustrating to me!

After all my healthy eating, walking, and swimming in Bali, I lost interest in everything active once I returned home.

It was easier to have a short walk in the morning, eat whatever was in the fridge, and enjoy a glass or two of wine every night. Mentally, I was not in a good place!

I kept on reflecting on my old life. I had always achieved so much career-wise, but to achieve the success I had pushed myself to extraordinary levels. I was relentless in my work ethic. Nothing was ever too much or too hard, and yet now I found myself knowing what I had to do, but lacking the energy or the willpower to make it happen!

I realized that I never stopped to think about my journey with Josh and his recovery, and for nearly 14 years I had never let up, or taken time out to smell the roses. I was always fully focused on earning the money needed to fund his recovery, maintain his self-esteem, and support our lifestyle.

I had no other priorities. Every year I would take two or three trips overseas to recharge my batteries, and then it was straight back into the frantic pace again! Even when my mother was dying (June 2010), as much as I tried to be there for her and my family, due to my work load at that time of year, I had to divide my priorities between my family and my marketing team. This caused me great anguish, sadness and stress, but I had no alternative!

Up until September 2010, the work I did was extremely stressful, demanding, and time consuming! My earning potential was what many dreamed to earn, but in return, I traded everything to maintain it!

It all ended in a huge economic disaster, thanks to the global financial crisis! In the space of a morning, I went from travelling forward in life at 100 mph, to crashing and burning, seeing everything I had created destroyed in the space of two hours.

Since that crazy September morning, over the next four years everything I had accumulated financially had been eroded away, until I found myself where I was today living off my sister's generosity, and not being able to help my son.

I was also becoming increasingly devastated and disappointed for Josh. He was always available to help someone in need, but when he needed help there was no one there for him.

Since returning to Australia, I had some old "friends" contact me, wanting my help and insights, but not wanting to pay me. This was frustrating. In the space of a few hours meeting I would give them so much, but when it came to them helping me with work, oh, that was another story.

Rock bottom for me was when I had to borrow another $2000 from Wendy to pay my bills for the next month!

Over the next two weeks, twice I had gone to bed asking the Universe to end my pain and let me die in my sleep; put me out of my misery! Even then I worried, "If I died, how would Wendy be paid back? What would happen to Josh?" I never considered taking my own life. I would never do this. I rationalized if I woke up in the morning things would be all right, I was meant to be here.

Then a series of small things happened, making me realize that I was the only one that could change things, and the only way I could change my present situation and my future was to take charge of my life and not rely on anyone to help me. I had to do it myself!

Some random incidents came together to set me back on the road to recovery. I knew from the start it wasn't going to be easy, but I was confident that by talking small steps, taking it an hour at a time, I would be finally heading in the right direction.

I had been following Scott Lopez on Facebook. Ironically he was an ex-Marine Corp fighter pilot.

He invited me to join his new page *Ascension Success Formula*. I started reading the posts, and so many things were resonating with me, inspiring me. I reached out to him, and he sent me a webinar to listen to. He was very supportive, messaging me and offering help.

I began to realize that if I was to be successful again, I had to use the skills I had learned from my old life to totally rebuild a new life!

I had to be tough; ditch the sadness, the anger, the disappointments, and importantly the "hangers on" from the past that were happy to utilize my skills but not prepared to pay for them. They had caused me so much grief and sadness.

I needed to keep the positive friends with me, but totally eliminate, *delete,* the negative influences. *There would be no going back!*

My new definition of success would be managing a work/life balance, and earning enough money to ensure financially I would be all right, being happy internally and externally. I would never resume the "tiger lady" I had needed to become in my previous career. Frankly, it held no interest to me anymore!

Even though I had the two business opportunities, it would be some months before I could count on a regular income. I needed money now!

I had to do something; I needed to get a job! In the end ego and pride don't pay bills!

I registered on casual and part time employment sites.

Remember, I had been working in senior executive positions in financial services from 25 years of age. I was multi-skilled. I could train, run teams, build teams, understand banking and finance, financial planning, sales and marketing, but what could I do that was simple, stress free and could bring me in a regular wage?

I could sell! So I applied for retail sales positions. That weekend I applied for five positions. I knew I was over qualified, but I needed a job.

I submitted the applications on line with covering letters, CV, and a link to my LinkedIn profile.

Within an hour of submitting the applications, I was called for a retail position, selling high end beds and bedding. The interview was scheduled for Sunday at 3 PM. Wendy was positive, wishing me luck. I was desperate, I needed this position.

I was interviewed by the franchise owner who was about 28 years old. Every finger had gold rings on them. He had a gold necklace and gold bracelet. I felt sick but I had to be positive. The interview went well until he asked me where I saw myself in six years. I would be 70. Without hesitation, I said "Walking the Camino De Santiago in Spain". He looked at me and asked how long this would take. I answered 4 1/2 months, and he nearly fell off his chair. I knew then I would not get this position.

The next day I was contacted by a recruitment group, and the following week I attended a very professional interview. I was appointed to a part time sales position in a major department store.

Yay, I had a job, I will earn money! Slowly the sadness was untangling itself.

Writing these last chapters have been part of my journey of recovery, growth and preparing myself for the next phase of my life.

I know it will be awesome, because I am not afraid to be different. I am not afraid to back myself, and I am not afraid of the future!

My story is not over; it is really just beginning!

Reflections, January 2015

As everyone sets their 2015 goals, I have spent a lot of my spare moments these past few days, reflecting on 2014.

I realized that 2014, was my "final wall" and that for the past 14 1/2 years I had been running a marathon - a marathon consisting of triumph and tragedy, celebration and darkness, of wonder and disbelief, and of tremendous learning and understanding!

A marathon I never planned, never trained for, and at times, never saw myself finishing!

Anyone who has run a marathon knows it's those last few miles that are the hardest and most challenging! You have to dig so deep to finish!

After hitting the "final wall" from January to September 2014, I am now confident I have finally finished this "amazing life" race.

There were no accolades at the finish. I'm not even sure of the exact moment I crossed the line.

Even now, I have a feeling of quiet relief, yet I feel numb, somewhat detached from the triumph of the journey.

It will take me some months to truly reflect on this great race.

What I do know is - I survived that final wall. It had challenged me in a way I never thought possible!

My "marathon" support team of my sisters: Wendy, Susie, and Asri, who have never failed me. As sisters they have gone over and above in their support of me, especially Wendy, who without hesitation was instrumental in getting me over this final painful wall.

There has been small group of "sistas" who have consistently encouraged me, picked me up even in those darkest early days; they never left my side!

The marathon has been a time of making new friends, and along the way learning to delete those in my life who tried to trip me up!

The catalyst for commencing this marathon was Josh's accident! He feels bad that his accident changed my life so dramatically.

I can honestly say, other than seeing the pain he goes through every waking minute, I would never change anything.

Although through much of this marathon, my running buddy was Josh, we always managed to run our own races!

I am so proud of my son, his journey, his growth, his commitment to his recovery, his commitment to the future, and dealing with all he goes through! Today, I am resting, regrouping, and getting ready to commence my next life marathon, knowing that this race has been prepared for. I have spent nearly 15 years training for it.

"NEXT: MOVE ON"!

Chapter 31. Media

This chapter is a reproduction of articles I have written over the last few years.

Depression and SCI

After the recent tragic death of Robin Williams, I was prompted to write this post for the Warrior Momz network about depression and suicide. I would like to make some observations from my / our experience with spinal cord injury - I want to say I am not an expert; I am just a Mum/ Mom, who has lived with this injury.

Josh and I have been in this crazy world of SCI for over 14 years. Over this time I have spoken to many families that are dealing with this injury, as well as trying to understand what my son Josh was going through.

A spinal cord injury in my opinion is the toughest injury of all, especially a quadriplegic injury, where is most cases, at least for a period, everything is lost to that person suffering the injury.

It is really important to give someone suffering the injury so much love, respect, and support, while at the same time encouraging them to try and gain recovery, even then as a loved one you have no idea what those suffering the injury are going through.

My goal for Josh was to help him gain his independence back, and keep him fit and focused. OMG, I can't tell you how hard this was especially after Year Three.

Josh discusses it in his book "the darkness", the being "trapped in his own body", the constant never ending nerve pain he suffers 24/7 from C5/T1.

He has said for many years that a spinal cord injury is the loneliest injury of all. There is no one injury the same; every injury and every recovery is different.

Josh never had a mentor, someone that understood what he was going through. He was on his own for all those years, and then after Bronte had his accident, for the first time in over seven years Josh had a "soul mate," someone that understood to a certain extent what each was going through. They were there for each other, and then we so tragically lost Bronte, and that was devastating to us ... beyond words.

There were things I found out about Josh while we were writing his book that I had no idea about. The drugs, the total devastation he went thru after losing is grandmother (my mother), and his four mates in the 12 month period (2010,) his questioning of himself, and what was the point of living a "good life." Where had it got him?

During this period he went on a path of self-destruction. I had no idea what to do; all I could say was I love you, we will work through this.

Relentless, for anyone reading it, is a roller coaster of emotions, dark and euphoric...for many years Josh resisted writing his book, but once he made the decision to do it, he knew he had to make it honest and true.

In the end, the only things that pulled Josh from the abyss was the understanding that he had to live for those boys that had died. His grandmother had faith in him always continuing to recover, and the love of his dogs, and then he met Amelia.

Realization for me during that period was that I could have lost him!

I am rambling, but depression is a real issue with SCI. That's why I established Warrior Momz and that's why we are active in the community...supporting each other!

A hero of mine, an Australian who had an SCI at the same level as Josh, wrote a book that was given to me a few days after Josh's accident. I never met him, but this book became my bible. He had been in the same hospital and same rehab as Josh and I related to him and to his passion in dealing with his injury. So many times when things were confusing and scary to me in those early days I referred to his book. After that, I read everything he wrote. He was a leader in the community here in Australia. I loved his passion, and then one day he committed suicide. I was devastated, angry, and scared. My thoughts were that if this young man can commit suicide, what hope is there? This was a tough time for me personally, and yet I knew I had to be positive for Josh so we worked through it.

These days, my family and friends who love and care about me tell me to walk away from what I do. Focus on me, especially after what happened in the USA. But I can't; I know that devastation, that fear of watching your child "caught up in the horrors of this injury," and in some cases being helpless to help them...with all that has happened, if I can help one family it's worth it.

What I know is, as loved ones we have to recognize the darkness of this injury and do everything possible to bring light and hope to our loved ones...to help them through it.

Reflections from the Warrior Mom

Josh 14 years on - reflections from the Warrior Momz

Josh and I always refer to 25th June 2000, as Josh's Twice Born Birthday. I was thinking about this while in Bali and realized it is also my rebirth birthday and I need to celebrate it. On that day my life changed forever too, and with all I had done to save my son's life, all I really had in my corner was my track record as a mother.

Josh's "rebirth" 14 years ago has caused me to reflect on my part of his recovery.

At 2.30 AM on the 26th of June 2000, nothing in my life had prepared me for Josh's accident - nothing in life can prepare you for such a catastrophic event. I guess writing my book and assisting Josh with his has caused me to go through a period of deep reflection.

What I can say is that Josh and I have become an invincible team. In those crazy early days we backed each other, and we trusted each other! Now we have three more team members in Amelia, Montana, and Thor, along with my sisters and a group of friends who have been there for every step, through all these years, along with the new friends.

Up to June 25th, 2000, I truly thought I was invincible from a career perspective, yet at 2.30 AM on the 26th June, I realized my goals and my successes were all "BS". Nothing else mattered or counted, but how I was going to save my son? For days I watched my son fight to live. I also experienced his medical team put him in a position where he nearly lost his battle a further two times. This from the hands of those who should have helped him...

In those crazy days, I prayed like never before. I actually did deals with the devil to save my son, promising he could have me in the place of my son. I think this is why I find myself in the position I am today!

In those early days, I have never felt so scared, so inadequate, and so vulnerable! Only a parent going through the same experience could relate to me!

In those crazy first weeks, nothing was important, nothing was relevant. My only focus was to save my son!

My past successes, the money I had earned, and the amazing teams I had built all paled in to insignificance!

My track record as a mother was all I could offer Josh in the fight of his life... I was:

- ✓ Not perfect

- ✓ Worried too much, over-stressed myself, and pushed myself to hard in everything I did

- ✓ For me, if you weren't going "full out" you were failing!

- ✓ Yelled and screamed too much, but I -

- ✓ Had never made a promise I had 't kept

- ✓ Understood nothing great happens without hard work

- ✓ Loved my son, and was prepared to do whatever it took

- ✓ Had an amazing network of healers

- ✓ Was willing to do whatever it took for my son to get his life back. I had no choice if I wanted my son to live

Through all this, I have learned:

Success is how you behave as a person, not how much money you make. Ego is irrelevant when you are facing your Maker.

No matter what, make your judgements and decisions with the attitude and belief of *NO REGRETS*!

Recovery Below-Injury for Spinal Cord Injuries is Possible!

Jan 27, 2015

Over the past nearly 15 years, since we were thrown into the world of acute spinal cord injury, I have learned so much about the power of the human mind to contribute to healing. I understand that there is no injury alike, and every injury, sadly, is different. Like the injury, there is not one Recovery Program/ System which offers all that is required to achieve ongoing below-injury recovery.

What works for some is ineffective with others! Through our experience with Josh, I have learned the power of having the injured body in alignment. To me this is the most basic of recovery needs!

To understand my attitude towards recovery, you need to understand why I confidently say "below injury recovery is not one system, one program, it is simply a total belief in the philosophy of recovery", and being prepared to continually seek both traditional, and in some cases, out-of-left-field recovery modalities to achieve the recovery goals.

Josh and I have been criticized because the common view is that we are only interested in the recovery outcome of walking. This is a belief about us that is far from the truth.

We understand one's goals could be to feed yourself, to sit up, to use a standing frame, and move from a power chair to a manual chair.

Our belief is doing what you have to do to achieve your own personal goals, whatever they may be.

In our experience, any goal achieved over the initial medical prognosis is fantastic!

It's interesting that in our experience, athletes understand the philosophy of recovery, because they are used to training, and doing whatever it takes to overcome their injuries.

Briefly, Our Journey of Recovery -

On the 25th of June 2000, my son Josh's life and all those who loved and cared for him, were changed forever. Josh crashed on an alpine road, while attempting a snowboard jump. He barely survived the impact; sadly he was left a complete quadriplegic from C5 - T1.

The night of the accident, his medical team made their diagnosis, and that was it. We knew they would operate to rebuild his shattered vertebrae, removing the bone fragments from his cord, but in their minds that was where it ended, not started. From the medical team's view, Josh had, if he lived, less than 3% chance of any recovery. His spinal cord was so badly crushed that in their view he was destined to spend the rest of his life in bed, or at best using a motorized wheelchair operated by mouth controls.

My son Josh, in their professional "learned" eyes, was now one of the "Silent Epidemic" of predominantly young males who were now "complete quadriplegics/paraplegics".

(The average age of spinal cord injury in Australia is 14 – 28 years, with over 85% of those injured being male.)

In those early hours, I realized that if Josh was to live, I had to find a way to help him recover. The medical system was all about us accepting the "new normal" (Josh would be bedridden for the rest of his life). If this was the case, I knew Josh would die. He was the kid who was so active, loved being outside, always living life on the edge!

I can't describe adequately the fear I felt in those early hours. There would be no medical life line for us, no hope was given by any member of his team, there would be no miracle, and somehow we had to figure out a recovery program!

With a career in financial services, I was hardly in a position to become an expert in below-injury recovery of a spinal cord injury, and yet somehow I would have to be! I made my mind up that I would NOT research the Internet!

Fortunately, Josh agreed, and we decided we didn't want to understand spinal cord injury. We didn't want anything stopping our belief in his recovery.

The morning after the accident we commenced massaging his toe and finger tips for hours every day. Josh couldn't feel us doing this, but he was annoyed by it. We simply told him that when you can move your toes and fingers then we'll stop.

Josh instructed the nurses to take away any medication that wasn't lifesaving. Josh's chiropractor Simon was smuggled in to the acute ward. Simon's only goal was to ensure the energy was flowing through Josh's body, and that his body was aligned.

As part of his recovery program, Josh was taught visualization and meditation. At this stage Josh was totally paralyzed. He wasn't able to move, and all we had was his brain and strong mind to work with. We were fortunate that I had a close friend Paula who was a psychic healer.

Utilizing her meditation skills and knowledge of the healing properties of crystals, she would come into the hospital 1-2 hours a week and weave her magic. Also part of our initial team was her daughter in law Isabel, who worked for hours in those early weeks realigning Josh's chakras, ensuring his chi energy was flowing through his body unrestricted.

During this period, it was all about the mind, the language, keeping the focus! Within a few weeks Josh felt internally more centered. He was dealing with this horrendous injury, and yet even though he couldn't feel anything, internally he was beginning to feel less stress. While in hospital, every Saturday night a friend Jackie would use reflexology on Josh's feet, which while stimulating the area of his foot enabled her to work on his organ function.

As his condition stabilized and we could get him out of hospital, we had a Chinese-trained acupuncturist named Bing work on stimulating Josh's broken body. Once he was home, Josh returned to his old gym in his wheelchair. Always training out of it, he worked with a personal trainer (who had no knowledge of spinal cord injury, but had a degree in sports science) twice a week for nearly four years. During this period Josh did not drink alcohol and ate a balanced nutritious diet.

In the May after his accident Josh went to the USA and worked with a well- respected Chi master for six weeks.

Over the years, we have left no stone unturned. In 2011 we learned about a recovery facility in Southern California; Josh had to attend!

Once there, initially he was very unsure, as he had never trained in a facility with other spinal cord injured people. It didn't take him long to settle in. He trained with an experienced team of professionals, Eric, Josh, Jason, Kimber, and Genn, to name a few, who just understood the body movement and rhythm, and really CARED about their clients. In some respect they formalized what we had worked out ourselves. Sadly, none of Josh's trainers are there any more, which is the reason why we have decided to follow Josh's old team, and recommend their new facilities.

While at the facility on his second visit, because of his constant desire to look for more recovery options, he was introduced by a friend to Uschi, a physiotherapist and kinesiologist from Encinitas, who in Josh's eyes was the second best person, next to Paula, who had ever worked on him.

With all that Josh has tried and learned over the years, the modalities he uses daily and weekly to this day are: meditation, visualization, chiropractic, acupuncture, gym work, yoga, and diet.

Finally, there are no magic answers with spinal cord injury recovery. It is hard work, needing an unbeatable attitude...always with the belief that with the right people in your team anything is possible.

One thing that Josh and I are extremely careful of is recommending a recovery facility to someone.

Our basic criterion is that the client has to be treated like a valued family member, first and foremost. Understanding that bone density and health issues have precedence over everything, we don't care how good the program is, without the "care factor" there is no way we will recommend any facility no matter what their reputation is!

It goes without saying that facilities have to be profitable, but fundamentally they are dealing with families that are desperate to help their loved ones, the care factor has to be the dominant attribute, not the money that client brings to the facility.

For the record, Josh's spinal cord has never recovered. It is actually worse due to scar tissue. Medically, he has 5% cord function at C6 and C7.

The cost to me personally over all these years has been in excess of $1.6 million. I don't regret one cent of what I have spent. Josh has turned the word impossible into I'Mpossible!

The Son and the Mum

Josh Wood - the Son

On the 25th June 2000 at 3.30 pm, at 18 1/2 years, Josh's life was changed in a heartbeat.

In a split second, Josh went from a potential professional snowboarder to basically being a head and a brain. Josh was attempting a snowboard jump across an asphalt road, something went terribly wrong, and he landed upside down on his neck.

Once stabilized on the mountain road, Josh was medivaced by helicopter to a hospital in Melbourne, where he was diagnosed as a complete quadriplegic at C5, C6, C7, and T1. His spinal cord was crushed. Josh was left with a non-functioning body, and his prognosis was extremely grim.

The view of his various medical specialists and medical team was that Josh had less than 3% chance of *any* recovery. His future, according to them, would be spending the rest of his life in bed. From the night he was admitted, Josh was pigeon holed as an 18 1/2 year old male complete quadriplegic.

All his medical team was interested in was making Josh and all who supported him accept their belief he would never get out of bed. Josh and his mum quickly realized that his medical team would mend Josh, not heal him. It was going to be up to the two of them to find a way for him to get his life back. Fortunately, Josh and Kay had shared an apprenticeship utilizing alternative recovery therapists to heal his various injuries over the years, so naively; they adopted an "injured" mentality rather than one of being "disabled."

It was very tough in those early days, as everyone connected with Josh and his family had all been thrown into this crazy terrifying world that no one can ever prepare you for. Kay knew that to save her son she had to commence his recovery immediately, so she set up a routine. Every time Josh had a visitor, the curtains would be closed around Josh's bed, allowing an alternative therapy team, which Kay had commenced to build from day one, to work their magic on Josh. Josh had a chiropractor, who Kay introduced to his medical team as his snowboard coach. Kay smuggled in massage therapists, who aligned his chakras, ensuring his chi energy was flowing. She also brought in a reflexologist every Saturday evening for about eight weeks. All this therapy would have been wasted, if Josh had not adopted a RELENTLESS attitude to his recovery!

Within the first week, Josh set a series of goals, and each goal needed to be achieved to get to the next one. His ultimate goal was "to walk down the road with his mates without them having to wait for him." He has recently, after 14 years, achieved this goal! *He never gave up!*

Family and friends commenced massaging Josh's toe and finger tips the day after his accident for hours; Josh was taught meditation and visualization within the first 10 days.

Josh set a goal to walk out of rehab before his 19th birthday, which was nearly five months from when he was admitted. He achieved his goal, walking out of rehab 4 1/2 months after he was admitted. Within two years he no longer used his wheel chair. He used elbow crutches for another two years, relying on a walking stick up until 2012, when he finally "ditched his stick" and walked unaided, even though he still has less than 5% functioning spinal cord at C6 and C7.

All through his recovery journey, Josh has mentored and inspired people from all over the world. Although he has little money, he never charges anyone. Basically, Josh is available 24/7 to help someone with this injury. When Josh has the opportunity, he loves to do motivational speaking and mentoring.

His story is really about the power of the brain and the human body to recover under extremely dire circumstances, and not sweating the small stuff that can put you off achieving your goals. Understanding the big goals can't be achieved unless you get the tiny steps right.

He speaks about the effect his accident had on all those who loved him and his regret of this.

He tells of his two friends lost to this cruel injury through poorly prescribed prescription drugs, and how he, himself, wanted to commit suicide when told four days after his accident of his prognosis. His message is unilateral, appealing to diverse groups, from school children, to the corporate world. All who hear him have been moved by his story.

Josh has recently told his story through his book *Relentless - Walking against All Odds*. It's a real, gutsy, honest story of his journey to recovery over nearly 13 years. The reviews he has received have been truly humbling. Josh loves speaking at schools, and positively influencing Australia's future leaders.

Here are some student comments from a recent Year 12 Retreat Josh spoke at in Victoria: "Josh showed me how dedication and a strong will can get you to where you want to be in life" "honest and inspirational," "he emotionally connected with our age group" "very touching and inspirational" "It definitely made me grateful for what I have" "he was a strong role model" "amazing story, changed my life". Josh spoke to a grade six class last year, and one of the comments that brings tears to people's eyes every time they hear it is "a magical person came into my life and showed me that anything was possible."

Kay Ledson - the Mum

It's 2.30 am 26th June 2000, and the specialist calmly advised Kay that her son Josh was now a complete quadriplegic. He said Josh would spend the rest of his life in bed and, if lucky, be able to use a motorized wheelchair. Devastated, Kay looked the doctor in the eye and said "my son will walk again because he is so strong and has a powerful mind."

The doctor replied "Ms. Ledson, that's the problem - mothers like you. If you do not accept that your son will never walk again, then I feel sorry for your son."

In total disbelief Kay retorted, "You don't know me, and you don't know my son, and he will walk again."

Josh walked out of rehabilitation 4 1/2 months later, with the only support being his elbow crutches.

In a heartbeat, Kay was thrust into a world she had never experienced; a world of abject fear, negativity, and acceptance of the "inevitable". Everything inside her knew her son would walk, but there was no support for her from those who should have helped her: her son's doctors and medical team!

Ill equipped for dealing with this tragedy, she quickly realized that the doctors would weave their magic and mend her son's broken, shattered vertebra but they wouldn't heal him. That would be totally up to her! *Her son's life now depended of her, to find a way to help him recover. If she didn't, he would die!*

Even though she had spent her entire working life in financial services, and with all her experience and knowledge, she was still totally unprepared, as most of us would be, for the emotional, legal, and financial ramifications of Josh's accident. Although she was more than adequately insured, with the range of protection a single mother would have, she had not considered insuring her son.

Over the past 14 years, Kay has spent in excess of $1.6 million on maintaining her son's recovery and life style.

These days, Kay mentors families throughout the world, helping them to deal with this devastating injury. In April 2012, Kay established Warrior Momz, a positive support network for families dealing with spinal cord injury.

Through her blog radio program, she has interviewed leaders in spinal cord injury research and the families that are working on ways to rehabilitate their loved ones who suffer this injury.

Kay's story to financial planners, their clients, and the insurance industry, offers a rare vision and understanding into the unexpected devastating situations facing parents and loved ones when such a tragedy occurs. Along the way she gives unique insights into the strategies she used to help her son rebuild his life.

She frankly discusses the financial implications of Josh's accident on herself and her family, giving a personal insight into the financial planning issues confronting families when faced with such a devastating event. She describes how insurance can go a long way to protect families from this potential financial disaster!

Kay has recently completed her book *Warrior Mom*. In her book she devotes a chapter to the financial implications of a catastrophic event such as Josh's on a family's financial security.

Don't Leave the "Kid" to the "Kids" - Financial Planning for your Disabled Child

Jul 6, 2014

Many years ago I had a conversation with an MLA regarding a very distressing meeting he had with one of his constituents. He was approached by a mother asking him to help her arrange the humane "putting to sleep" of her severely disabled daughter.

The story was devastating and extremely sad, leaving the MLA in a desperate situation. The mother was suffering a deadly cancer, with little time to live. Her daughter, an only child, knew no other companion than her beloved mum. There were no relatives, no money, and the mum was desperate!

I never did find out the outcome of this tragic event, but it took me in a direction within financial planning where I realized that if this mum had sought financial planning advice when her daughter was born, or as she was growing up, the situation the mother found herself in now would have been possibly avoided, or at the very least provided more options.

Unfortunately, financial planning is probably the last thing parents with a disabled child think about; this is an extremely sensitive area, presenting a huge challenge/opportunity to financial planners.

After this experience, I spent two years researching families, the legal profession, and charities regarding financial planning strategies for parents with disabled children who require long term care. Sadly, I found that the solution for many families was their able bodied children, with the parents assuming they would look after their disabled sibling! Although many were prepared for this eventuality, many were devastated and angry that their parents assumed they would gratefully take on the carer role of their disabled sibling!

A comment made to me by a sibling was "most people think their parents will leave them real estate or investments when they die. My parents are leaving me my sister; this is so unfair." Sadly, comments such as this are repeated over and over again.

Financial planning for children with long term disabilities is an emotional and yet necessary issue.

These days, with more sophisticated structures available, there are real alternatives that can be utilized.

Life insurance can form a solid foundation to ensure that the financial stability for those precious children is, to a large extent, guaranteed.

Financial planners, once knowing about a disabled child, need to have the conversation with the parents early in the process. This is crucial!

You have no idea how much I thought about all my research, all my knowledge as I sat watching my son hovering between life and death in those crazy early days after his accident. Here I was. I knew the statistics, I had developed the strategies, I had insured myself to ensure my son's security, but I had never taken out insurance on Josh. With his injury, it is now nearly impossible for him to obtain life insurance and the normally expected insurance a young family needs as Josh and his wife Amelia contemplate starting a family.

Accidents to our children are so tough on parents. Learning to let go once they are recovering is the hardest! Learning to trust other people with your children is unbelievably hard, and the feeling of fear never leaves you! It's so tough being a parent in these circumstances!!! Accident anniversaries are the hardest of all. You are grateful, and yet you are sad!

A Dedication to the Families Dealing with the Horror of Spinal Cord Injury

When reading my book, some may wonder why I have gone into detail regarding some aspects of my life these past 14 plus years. Well, it's simple to explain. On the 25th of June 2000 at 3.30 PM, my life changed forever. All my short, medium, and long term goals evaporated in a heartbeat, and my life totally changed, as did Josh's. Since then I have not set any long term goals. My focus has been to get through one day at a time, and to keep my son fit and focused.

My journey, triumphs, celebrations, and fears to get to this moment in time are all a result of one phone call. If Josh hadn't decided to make the jump, I would have quietly gotten on with my life.

This book has been written for the families, to show that no matter how hard it gets, if you just keep moving forward, albeit at times at a snail pace, there is light.

My journey has not been easy, but as I reflect through the writing of this book I would not change anything.

In the end, I still have my son!

Chapter 32. Three Lives

Joshua John Wood – born Frankston, Victoria, Australia - Friday November 13th 1981 – 25ᵗʰ June 2000, 3:30 PM

Twice Born - Joshua John Wood reborn asphalt road, Mount Buller Ski Resort 25ᵗʰ June 2000 at 3:30 PM

<u>AJ</u> Malcolm Andrew **Wood** born Werribee Birthing Clinic, Victoria, Australia 22ᵗʰ January 2016 7:21 AM

November 13, 1981

Josh was born on a hot November day. He was an extremely sick baby; the placenta had died and he had existed in my womb gaining only basic nourishment to survive. From the moment he was born you knew he was an old soul and from the moment of his birth he was a fighter. Spending two weeks in the special care nursery, he slowly gained strength and weight.

For 18 ½ years Josh lived life to the fullest. He was extremely popular, and had many friends. He was the party man, bringing an eclectic group of friends together to have fun and hang out. He struggled through school managing to finally graduate in 1998. He loved travel, partying, but he worked hard; just prior to his accident he worked three jobs.

The weekend of his accident, he had finally found work on the Mountain, which would have ensured his stay for the season on Mt. Buller. He was to sign a lease on an apartment in the Village on the Monday. That weekend his old coach had spoken to him about a potential professional sponsorship opportunity in the USA. It was all coming together…

He was on the verge of achieving his dreams and goals of professional snowboarding…and then he decided to build a jump across an asphalt road in the Village.

June 25, 2000

As Josh propelled himself through the air something went wrong, seeing him turn upside heading head first into the asphalt, at the point of impact Josh managed a "commando" style roll – his neck and shoulder taking the impact of the crash. He heard his neck break, but he stayed conscious telling the boys who raced to his side not to touch him. Slowly they packed snow around his neck! There was a moment as he lay twisted on the road, that he had a decision to make: "TO LIVE OR TO DIE!"

It was a defining moment. He felt his body shutting down, and he wanted to say to Daniel "look after Kze." Something stopped him. It was at that moment he decided to live, and from that moment onwards he has never given up his fight for life, importantly living his life!

Anyone who suffers a spinal cord injury understands they now have two birthdays, their actual birthdate and the 2nd, which is the instant they suffered their spinal cord injury.

Accident dates are always remembered as a time of gratefulness, and tinged with sadness for what was lost.

After all these years, I am now convinced that the accident was Josh's destiny, as sad as it is, for all the pain he endures and fighting with a body that will never let him rest. Yet he has survived – he is wise, insightful, has great knowledge about his injury. He has inspired so many to believe that anything is possible. Together he and Amelia have created a circle of life! Josh never uses the word miracle about himself, in fact he hates anyone discussing his recovery using the word miracle. Yet from day one when they found out Amelia was pregnant, he has used the word miracle!

To the world he will be AJ, but to all of us that have ridden this crazy rollercoaster of spinal cord injury, we all agree he is our little MIRACLE!

AJ

The men in my life!

Sitting next to my son as he fought to stay alive after suffering a devastating snowboarding injury June 2000, his doctor's best prognosis was "if he lived Josh would get around in a motorized wheel chair using mouth controls." According to his doctors, Josh's life as we knew it was over. I can't say the last 16 years have been easy; there have been times our belief in his ongoing recovery has been tested to breaking point. But doggedly Josh and his dedicated team persisted. Our own strong relationship has been tested to stresses and limits that at times seemed irreversible, but our love always won through.

On January 22nd at 7 21 am, our 16 years have been rewarded with the safe arrival of AJ Wood, a miracle created from the true and absolute love of Josh and Amelia.

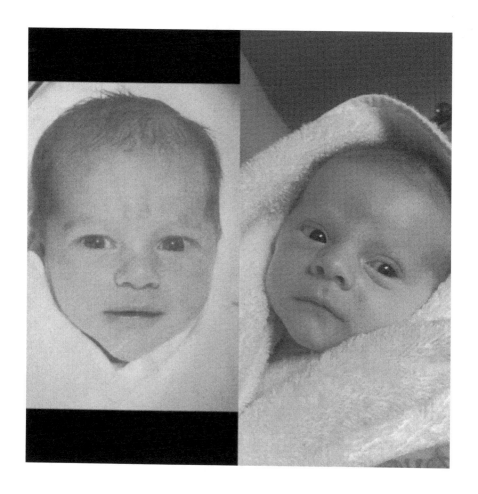

My Dad and Me (Josh at One Week and A.J. at Three Days)

Our little man is another old soul like his dad! AJ is a chilled out little baby, charming all who have met him. The nursing staff has been amazed at his calmness throughout all their testing regime on him. He is relaxed, and all his tests have been perfect. He has stolen our hearts! He has even been for "checks" with our much loved chiro Simon, who has also given him a huge heads up as a healthy "well adjusted" baby.

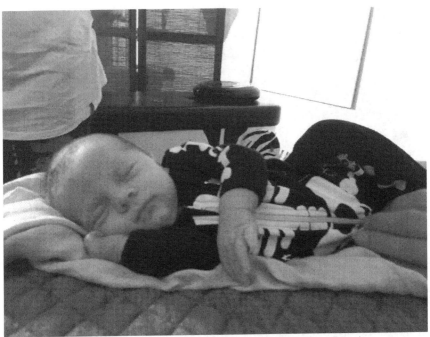

Visiting Uncle Simon, My Chiropractor (Age Five Days)

The book is finally finished. It's ironic that *Warrior Mom* would never have been written if Josh hadn't had his accident. The book was started with Josh hanging onto life, and it is fitting that it should end with the introduction of a new life, the birth of Josh and Amelia's son. Since AJ's birth the world seems brighter. There is a feeling of hope, and the belief that finally after all the sadness, we all have so much to look forward to!

I wrote Warrior Mom for all those families who have had their hope torn away from them by doctors who still don't understand the power of the mind, and the determination of the human body to recover....

Thank You and Acknowledgments

My sisters, Wendy, Susan and Asri, I could never have made it without you!

Daniel, Luke (Dingo), Jeff, and the boys who were there at the jump, you saved my son. You didn't panic, and you kept him calm. After all these years, you are still there for Josh - THANK YOU.

How lucky we were in those early dark days of June 2000 to have our core team of Paula, Simon, and Isobel. Combined, your love, commitment, and extraordinary skills were instrumental in Josh's recovery.

Dana and John Goyak, your support in the USA was critical to Josh's early recovery. We will be forever grateful to you both.

To all the many others who helped in the healing of Josh: Jackie (reflexology), Bing (massage and acupuncture), Ben (personal trainer), the T'mers (meditation and diet), Dr. Graham Baro (our family doctor), the Vitality Chiropractic team, Uschi and Doug (USA), your skills and love are beyond description.

Josh's talented, committed PW trainers and former Director of Research and Development Eric Harness, we love and respect you all. Project Walk Atlanta, you and your team are like family to us, allowing us to launch Josh's book within your Atlanta facility; such a humbling experience. And thank you Project Walk Orlando team for your love and support and ongoing commitment.

And thank you to the scores of therapists and healers we have met on our journey, some for a short time, some for a long time, yet collectively your skills and support formed a crucial part of Josh's recovery and for Josh getting his life back as much was humanly possible.

Josh's healing journey will continue for the rest of his life.

To Josh's wife Amelia, who loves him unconditionally, and is always there for him; you are truly soul mates. Thank you from the bottom of my heart.

Amelia, you gave Josh the belief that he had a future in creating his own family with you. In those dark days of 2012, your love grew stronger.

Josh and Amelia's love and support for each other is truly a match made in heaven!

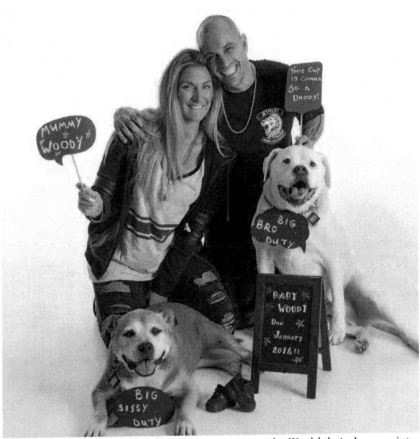

Amelia, Josh, and the Furry Kids Announcing to the World their Journey into Parenthood May 2015

It would be remiss of me to not individually thank two people who were my rocks and always had my back through this journey of recovery: Paula (Paula's name has been changed to protect her identity) and Simon Floreani, our fabulously talented chiropractor.

Through her daily meditations, Paula was given information that became crucial in helping us understand Josh's injury. Her daily meditations and messages from the Universe really set up the path to the alternative healing road we travelled. Paula was and still is a good friend, but sadly her health has been poor, and we have protected her identity through our love and respect for her. Paula never gave up on Josh; even with her failing health she was still actively interested in Josh's recovery. Thank you my friend; we could never have done this without you!

Simon, you are family! Simon, my goodness, what a journey we have all had together! You were my rock in those scary early days and you continue to be all these many years later. You have gone over and above with your responsibilities as our chiropractor. You have guided and supported us all these years. We are grateful; we love you and your family.

For teaching me to laugh again, and helping me to heal, I thank my Carlsbad Buddies, especially the members of Carlsbad Hi-Noon Rotary, the Carlsbad Chamber of Commerce, and Lisa Cannon Rodman, friend and boss; you went over and above to support and help me to stay in Carlsbad. I am forever grateful to you!

Yvonne Brant Murchison Finocchiaro, who was a supportive friend and mentor, my Cobber Digger Mate, Jamie Hartnett "friends forever", Kori Cash Dolkas and Maureen Simons your unconditional love and friendship will always be treasured - you ladies taught me to belly laugh again; I'm so grateful to you both, the Bunko Gals, you all rock! Patty Johnson (my painting buddy and friend) and the Agua Hedionda DC team, I love you all!

Special thanks to my first California friends Shirley and Bill Harmon. You have loved and supported me unconditionally. My thanks to my Sonoma sista, Lesli Luchsinger John, her husband Curtis, and mom Doris. The Sonoma crew, Laurie K, Donna, I love you all, thank you!

My Warrior Momz "sistas"; a sisterhood created through tragedy, and united together through the love of our children and loved ones: Michelle Delgado Cole, Jeannie Pickard, Liza Perla, Sandi Campbell Barbknecht, Tammy Ceja Potts, Tammy Lydic- Reddick, Erica Predum, Tina Mc Crory, Celia Brewer, Sherry Pierro, Georgina Pizzey, Renny Abbica, and Misti Gainan. To all the momz I haven't mentioned, I love you all. Thank you for your support; we are slowly making a difference.

Thank you to everyone who has been there for us on Josh's amazing journey of recovery. New friends and old, family members who have shown patience and encouragement, you all have played huge part in our journey.

It has taken a village, or I should say a small city, to help Josh to get to where he is today. Thank you one and all!

To my father Peter: As a dad you were never there for your four children, but I can honestly say you were a loving grandfather to Josh in life and after your death over 30 years ago. You have been constantly there for him, supporting his recovery journey in Josh's darkest hours. You were with him, and for that I will always be grateful.

My final thankyou is to the Master / Mistress of the UNIVERSE, the highest power of all. I know beyond doubt YOU exist.

I am not a religious person, but I am extremely spiritual. I do believe there is a higher power that guides us, and in some cases, our lives are truly destined.

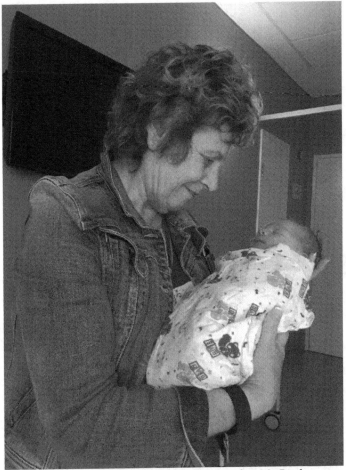

Grandma Kze Holding Me Minutes after My Birth

I know I was destined to be Josh's mother and Josh to be my son. I know there were incidences which haven't been mentioned in either of our books because they were too private - those occurrences were proof of a much higher power at work and who was actively involved in Josh's recovery.

In those crazy early days, Paula was the catalyst for these messages being heard, the catalyst to pass these onto ourselves and Josh's team of healers. I know Josh's accident was his destiny, and as I watch him grow into this amazing man, I know he is destined to change lives. Both of our furry kids were gifts from the Universe; even our Church apartment was part of the plan.

Amelia, who came into Josh's life when both their lives were on disastrous courses; truly a gift from the Universe.

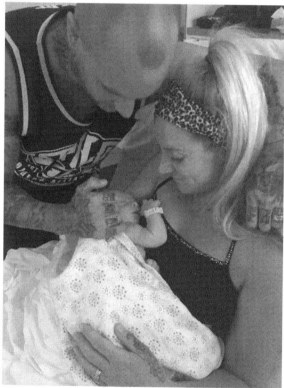

Meeting my Mom and Dad

Me, having the earning potential I had in those crazy years, and losing everything just when things should have been better, was all part of my destined journey. When Josh was born I was told several times I had birthed an old soul. I truly believe this was the case, and I am honored that I was chosen.

The photo below is a fitting way to finish this book. It is the Son and the Mum walking alone on a dark Melbourne Road, competing in the Melbourne Wings for Life World Run 2015. The picture was captured by my sister Susan – it is so special and is a beautiful way to end the story of our journey of love, healing, discovery and faith.

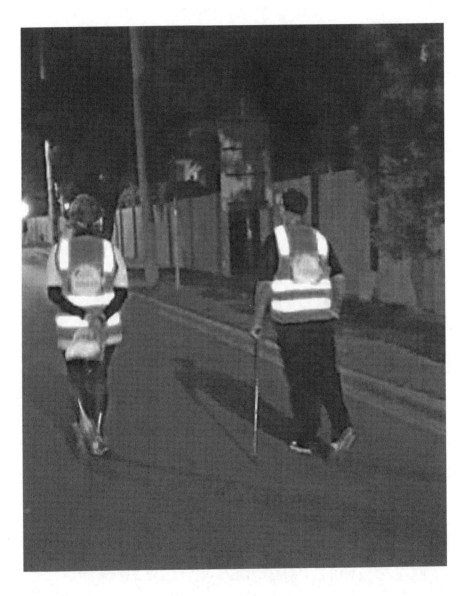

Mum and Son on a Hike

30891042R00213